W9-DEW-130

Better Food for Kids

Second Edition

Better Food for Kids

Second Edition

Your Essential Guide to Nutrition for All Children from Age 2 to 10

Joanne Saab, RD, and Daina Kalnins, MSc, RD

Better Food for Kids, 2nd Edition
Text copyright © 2010 The Hospital for Sick Children
Cover photography copyright © 2010 Masterfile
Food photography and illustrations copyright © 2010 Robert Rose Inc.
Cover and text design copyright © 2010 Robert Rose Inc.

No part of this publication may be reproduced, stored in a retrieval system or transmitted, in any form or by any means, without the prior written consent of the publisher or a license from the Canadian Copyright Licensing Agency (Access Copyright). For an Access Copyright license, visit www.accesscopyright.ca or call toll-free: 1-800-893-5777.

For complete cataloguing information, see page 341.

Disclaimer
This book is a general guide only and should never be a substitute for the skill, knowledge and experience of a qualified medical professional dealing with the facts, circumstances and symptoms of a particular case.

The nutritional, medical and health information presented in this book is based on the research, training and professional experience of the authors, and is true and complete to the best of their knowledge. However, this book is intended only as an informative guide for those wishing to know more about health, nutrition and medicine; it is not intended to replace or countermand the advice given by the reader's personal physician. Because each person and situation is unique, the author and the publisher urge the reader to check with a qualified health-care professional before using any procedure where there is a question as to its appropriateness. A physician should be consulted before beginning any exercise program. The author and the publisher are not responsible for any adverse effects or consequences resulting from the use of the information in this book. It is the responsibility of the reader to consult a physician or other qualified health-care professional regarding his or her personal care.

The recipes in this book have been carefully tested by our kitchen and our tasters. To the best of our knowledge, they are safe and nutritious for ordinary use and users. For those people with food or other allergies, or who have special food requirements or health issues, please read the suggested contents of each recipe carefully and determine whether or not they may create a problem for you. All recipes are used at the risk of the consumer.

We cannot be responsible for any hazards, loss or damage that may occur as a result of any recipe use.

For those with special needs, allergies, requirements or health problems, in the event of any doubt, please contact your medical adviser prior to the use of any recipe.

Health text editor: Bob Hilderley, Senior Editor
Recipe editor: Sue Sumeraj
Proofreader: Sheila Wawanash
Indexer: Gillian Watts
Design and Production: Kevin Cockburn/PageWave Graphics Inc.
Illustrations: Kveta

Food Photography
Photographer: Colin Erricson
Associate Photographer: Matt Johannsson
Food Styling: Kathryn Robertson
Prop Styling: Charlene Erricson

Children Photography
(In order of appearance): 1. © Masterfile. 2. © Masterfile. 3. © Masterfile. 4. © iStockphoto.com/ James Tutor. 5. © Masterfile. 6. © Veer 7. © Masterfile. 8. © Masterfile.

We acknowledge the financial support of the Government of Canada through the Book Publishing Industry Development Program (BPIDP) for our publishing activities.

Published by Robert Rose Inc.
120 Eglinton Avenue East, Suite 800, Toronto, Ontario, Canada M4P 1E2
Tel: (416) 322-6552 Fax: (416) 322-6936

Printed and bound in Canada

1 2 3 4 5 6 7 8 9 SP 18 17 16 15 14 13 12 11 10

Contents

Acknowledgments

Were it not for all the encouragement and support of many friends, family members and colleagues, *Better Food for Kids* would have been a much more difficult project to undertake. We were inspired, too, by the enthusiastic response to our previous book, *Better Baby Food*, which showed us the great demand that exists for more information on children and nutrition — and for more tasty and nutritious recipes! Our thanks to the many people who contributed so much to this book.

To the friends and colleagues who assisted us with reviewing and revising the information provided, heartfelt thanks to Dr. Deborah O'Connor, Dr. Paul Pencharz, Dr. Milton Gold, Dr. Sanjay Mahant, Leanne Falkner, Gloria Green, Jess Haines, Diana Mager, Sarah Farmer and Kellie Welch. For all the hard work and attention to detail in preparing the recipe analysis and calculations, thanks to Linda Chow, Gurvinder Sehra and Jessica Posthuma. And for their encouraging words and advice, we thank Randi Kirshenbaum, Wendy Lands, Terri Hawkes-Sackman, Jeff Sackman, Patrice Banton and Abbe Goldman Klores.

For the people who shared their recipes, and who tested ours, a special thank you to Leya Aronson, Joan Brennan, Christine Dunlop, Lucy Dardarian, Denise Hawman, Joyce Hawman, Inta Huns, Ilze Kalnins, Karen Kurilla, Jacqueline McKenzie, Lori Moreau, Erika Munro, Gisele Poulin, Maria Roso Rosa, Chantal Saab, Connie Saab, Jhana Shimizu and Jaye Shintani. Daina would also like to thank testers Matis, Natali and Blair for their honesty, and for those incredible facial expressions (MR)!

And to all those friends and colleagues at the Hospital for Sick Children, whom space does not allow us to name individually, our thanks for your professional support and encouragement.

To our publisher, Robert Rose Inc., thank you for your support of this project.

For the editorial, design and production work that made this book a reality, thanks to the team at PageWave Graphics Inc.

Thank you to the following colleagues who offered their expertise in reviewing material for this second edition of *Better Food for Kids*: Mary Barron, Susan Dello, Linda Gillis, Gloria Green, Joann Herridge, Inez Martincevic, Valerie Renn, Rivanna Stuhler, Laura Vresk and Kellie Welch. Special thanks to Debbie O'Connor for all your ongoing support. We'd also like to thank Len Piche and Kimberly Zammit for the nutritional analysis. Special thanks to Sue Sumeraj and Bob Hilderley for editing.

With sincere thanks to Eva Almario, Rindy Bradshaw, Elizabeth Munro, Christine Micules and Maureen Buchbinder for their contributions to recipe suggestions.

With sadness, we also think of and remember our dear friend Linda Chow, who was such an important part of the preparation of this series of books. Linda completed the recipe analyses for the original edition of *Better Food for Kids* as well as for *Better Baby Food*, *Better Food for Pregnancy* and *Better Breastfeeding*. Linda left this world far too soon (2009). Linda will always be thought of when we open these book pages.

From Daina

To Joanne, once again, thank you so much for making this project a great experience. I hold such a great deal of respect for your knowledge, commitment and drive. I am so very grateful for your friendship.

To Blair and my children, Natali and Matis. Natali and Matt, thanks for always (well, usually) trying new foods presented to you, and for doing at least the lick test for unfamiliar foods or for my new recipes. So proud of both of you. Blair, how lucky I am to have your support for all I do. Milu Jus.

From Joanne

To Daina, thank you for being such a great partner. I value your work ethic and your ability to work under pressure! It is always a treat when we write together. I am so happy to call you my friend.

To David, Katelyn and Avery. For always testing and eating all the recipes we tried out and for all your encouragement. Thank you for always supporting whatever I do. I love you all so much.

Introduction

The most important influence on our health is the choice we make about the foods we eat and drink. For our children, a healthy approach to eating will give them lifelong health benefits — many of which we have known for a long time and many of which we are still learning about. Unfortunately, this knowledge is not universal. Recent surveys indicate that a significant number of adults do not meet their nutritional needs as recommended by food guides, and that they may not be aware of the health benefits of specific foods. If adults do not lead by example, and if they do not have this knowledge, then how can they educate their children on good nutrition? Other surveys indicate that children age 4 to 8 years do not consume enough fruits and vegetables. About 20% of the calories they consumed were from foods that are considered of poor nutritional value. While these surveys do not portray a healthy picture, it is still possible to make changes by increasing awareness of healthy eating. It is our hope that *Better Food for Kids* will increase this awareness and be of benefit to you and your children.

The information in this book has been gathered through careful research, using established and current studies that have been reported in leading professional journals. We also bring to the book our skills as registered dietitians as well as considerable knowledge we have gained by teaching programs for children, parents and health-care providers.

In this second edition of *Better Food for Kids*, we provide nutritional information that every parent and caregiver needs to know so they can provide a healthy diet for their child. Children also need to be educated on the health benefits of choosing nutrient-rich foods. For this second edition of *Better Food for Kids*, we suggest ways to encourage your children to participate in choosing and preparing food. Following the advice of families and reviewers, we have added a chapter for 6- to 10-year-olds, where we present more lunch options and discuss how to provide meals and snacks while participating in sports activities and living our busy lifestyles. In the nutrition sections, we have added more information on the role of specific nutrients in maintaining health. We have also expanded on the allergy and obesity sections. Stories about our own trials and successes in encouraging our children to eat well show how good nutrition habits can be developed. We have selected some of our favorite recipes in the different chapters, tested by families — and our kids have provided theirs as well!

Nutrition Advice in Brief

Here, in no particular order, we offer our top 10 recommendations for parents of young children. Each provides references for additional information within the book.

1. Whenever possible, serve your child homemade rather than prepared or convenience foods. Commercially prepared foods can add excess calories (including many derived from fat) and salt to the diet. They can also displace fresh foods such as vegetables and fruits.

2. Limit your child's intake of juice. For quenching thirst, water should be the main beverage of choice.

3. Encourage consumption of fresh fruits and vegetables by having a constant supply readily available.

4. Eat meals with your children whenever possible. This time spent together as a family has many benefits, including the opportunity to demonstrate to your children your commitment to healthy eating practices which, in turn, will influence theirs.

5. Make sure you are knowledgeable about food and nutrition, and its overall effect on health and well-being.

6. Share your knowledge of nutrition with your children. Use games or arts and crafts to teach kids about all the good things in the food they eat.

7. Make sure that iron-rich foods are part of your child's diet. Iron deficiency can have serious consequences on the health of young children.

8. Don't rely on vitamin supplements as a substitute for a healthy, balanced diet.

9. Enjoy an active lifestyle together as a family. Exercise, along with healthy foods, can help decrease the incidence of obesity in children — and adults!

10. Variety is the spice of life — and essential to healthy and enjoyable eating. Experiment with new foods and try new recipes (starting with those in this book!).

About the Recipes

The recipes in *Better Food for Kids* are actually not just for kids, but are intended to be enjoyed by the entire family. We have made every effort to ensure that most of the recipes are quick and easy to prepare. We provide simple breakfast ideas that are well balanced. Lunches include soups that can be made ahead, as well as a number of alternatives to traditional sandwiches. Dinners range from simple pastas to special evening meals that may require a little more time to prepare. Snacks and desserts include everything from healthy yogurt dips to more indulgent chocolate treats.

Many people might believe that our recipes — since they come from three registered dietitians — must necessarily be focused on serious, "healthy" foods, with little attention paid to foods that are fun to eat. But the opposite is actually true. Dietitians believe that healthy eating depends on enjoying a variety of foods, with a balanced diet that includes all four food groups, as well as moderate amounts of sugar and salt. Children should not be placed on restrictive "diets," and we have tried to reflect this message in *Better Foods for Kids*.

Nutritional Information

In keeping with the public demand for information about the nutrients in food, we have supplied with each recipe a detailed analysis that specifies the number of calories, as well as the amounts of protein, carbohydrate, fat, fiber, calcium, iron and sodium per serving. All nutritional analysis data is calculated on metric measurements of ingredients in each recipe. The larger number of servings was used where there is a range.

The nutrient database used for recipe analysis was the ESHA Food Processor SQL, version 10.5 (contains entire Canadian Nutrient File 2007b), Salem, OR. The nutrient analyses were based on:

- the smaller amount where there is a range;
- the first ingredient listed where there is a choice;
- the exclusion of "optional" ingredients; and
- the exclusion of ingredients with non-specified or "to taste" amounts.

CHAPTER 1

Feeding
Your 2- to 4-Year-Old

As your child passes the age of 2 years, the experience of eating becomes more rewarding — and challenging. Feeding skills continue to improve, which makes mealtimes less messy (although not exactly mess-free). As children become more independent, they are less willing to accept the purely passive role in feeding that they had as infants. They are both more curious and more demanding about the food they eat. For parents, this provides an important opportunity to guide and educate their children in making healthy choices that will last them a lifetime.

Young minds want to know

Between the ages of 2 and 4 years, children absorb new information at an astonishing rate, and this is particularly true when it comes to food. A parent or caregiver should therefore be prepared with at least some basic information on food-related topics, such as where food comes from and why it is important for our well-being, so that a child can begin to understand the importance of good nutrition.

Here it helps to provide information in a way that relates food to other aspects of a child's experience. For example, you might tell your child that eating is important because food contains energy, which is essential for play and learning. This may not always transform a finicky eater into a child with a healthy appetite, but it will encourage him or her to start thinking about food in a wider context. And as you are probably aware, children do not forget!

Consistency is the key

A consistent approach to feeding is usually best for children between the ages of 2 and 4 years. A variety of foods provided in three meals and two or three (or more) snacks every day will supply the energy and nutrients your child needs to meet the demands of continued growth and weight gain. A diet of balanced meals and snacks will also ensure that your child has the energy for learning, playing and interacting with their peers.

Feeding milestones for children between 2 and 4 years

AGE	MOTOR SKILLS	SOCIAL/PERSONAL SKILLS
2 to 3 years	Holds cup in hand Puts spoon straight into mouth Spills a lot Chews more thoroughly than at 18 to 24 months, but choking still a concern	Has definite likes and dislikes Insists on doing things "by myself" Ritualistic Dawdles Has food jags Demands food in certain shapes, whole foods Likes to help in kitchen
3 to 4 years	Holds handle on cup Pours from small pitcher Uses fork Chews most food	Improved appetite and interest in food Favorite foods requested Likes shapes, colors, ABCs Able to choose between two alternative foods Influenced by TV commercials Likes to imitate food preparer

Note: This information is provided so parents and caregivers will understand what tasks most children should expect to have mastered by a certain age. It is important to remember that children grow and learn new skills at different rates.

ADAPTED FROM: Canadian Paediatric Society, *Little Well Beings*, 1994.

Expanding food horizons

While young children become more curious about food as they get older, they still require encouragement to try new and unfamiliar foods. Toddlers will generally reject a new food when given for the first time. But with a little patience and persistence, they can often be tempted to try it. Here the key is to provide a variety of different foods, prepared in a variety of ways, on a consistent basis.

It is important that the child be given the choice of whether or not to eat a particular food. Research indicates that children's food habits are influenced by many factors, including availability of a variety of foods, and by the behavior of their parents at mealtimes.

Balancing acts

Energy and nutrient needs vary in children because of several factors, including age, gender, body size, growth rate, appetite and activity — all have an effect on food intake. Parents often wonder if their children are getting

Family food diary
In praise of rapini

How can you get your kid's to eat "yucky" new vegetables? Recently, there has been considerable media attention on cookbooks for kids that recommend disguising vegetables by puréeing them and mixing them into favorite foods. While in principle this sounds like good advice, it doesn't encourage our kids to eat vegetables and enjoy them.

Research indicates that it can take kids between 15 and 30 exposures to a specific food before they are willing to try it. At our house, I try to prepare a variety of vegetables beyond the usual same carrots and corn. David and I particularly enjoy rapini and asparagus. While my daughters are still not fond of rapini (frankly, it took me a while to enjoy it), we still put it on the dinner table and the girls are encouraged (but not forced) to try it. While they now eat lots of different vegetables, including squash, sweet potatoes, and, yes, even asparagus, I'm still holding out for the rapini. One day soon... *(Joanne)*

Tips for introducing unfamiliar foods

"Try it … you'll like it," we tell our children. Here are some tips for encouraging your children to give it a try — and for increasing the variety of foods in their diet.

1. Engage children in preparing new foods, for example, slicing a new fruit or vegetable, mixing tofu with marinade or sauce, or mixing and pouring a batter.
2. Teach your children how to set the table.
3. Show enthusiasm for new foods and sample them together. Be a good role model.
4. Keep serving sizes appropriate for children, especially with a new food. A small slice or one teaspoon (5 mL) is enough to sample. Even a simple lick can help create a taste for unfamiliar foods.
5. Encourage your child to try new or unfamiliar foods in the presence of other children their age.
6. Don't force children to keep trying a new food the first time they taste it. Instead, try it again at another meal. It may take several tries.

a balance of the right amount of nutrients through their diet or, in some cases, worry that they are getting too many calories.

In most cases, such concerns are unfounded. If you provide your child with a variety of different foods — including breads or cereals, fruits and vegetables, and milk and milk products, as well as protein foods such as meats, chicken, fish, legumes or lentils — then chances are he or she will get all the energy and nutrition required. See pages 19 and 39 for examples of balanced menus.

Dealing with dairy foods

For 2- to 4-year-olds, milk and milk products (such as cheese and yogurt) provide an adequate source of calories (energy) for growth and, in most cases, are the main source of vitamin D and calcium, both of which are essential for the normal development of bones and teeth. (See pages 76 to 81 for more information on these nutrients.)

That being said, however, it is important to recognize that consuming too much milk — for example, amounts greater than 24 oz (750 mL) per day — can lead to a deficiency of other nutrients. When milk intake is high, a child may have a diminished appetite for other foods. This is particularly true for younger children who are still on the bottle, which, research suggests, tends to encourage excessive consumption of milk. Because this may replace other important foods, and can lead to iron deficiency (which can affect appetite and behavior), children over the age of 2 should be given milk in a sippy cup or regular cup instead of a bottle.

Although milk and milk products do contain some iron, these amounts are inadequate for a growing child's needs.

How much milk fat?

Whole milk contains the highest amount of fat and calories compared to lower-fat varieties, such as 2%, 1% and skim milk, and it is this type (whole milk) to which infants are usually introduced when they make the transition from breast milk or formula to cow's milk. After the age of 2 years, however, children do not necessarily require whole milk, and can be offered the lower-fat varieties. The exception is if a child is not gaining weight adequately, in which case whole milk is still recommended.

First milk

Whole milk is recommended as the first milk to serve after breastfeeding or formula-feeding at 1 year of age, but a recent study suggests that lower-fat milk may be safely offered at 1 year of age in those families with a history of obesity or heart disease. Check with your family physician to see if this is the right choice for your child.

Good sources of iron include meats, chicken, tofu, beans and legumes if eaten with a source of vitamin C. (See page 73 for more information on iron.)

Nutritious dairy foods also include cheese and yogurt. Slices or strips of Cheddar or cottage cheese with sliced fruit are good for snacks. You can also choose from many flavors and varieties of commercially prepared yogurt, although many of these contain a substantial amount of added sugar. A better choice may be to buy plain yogurt and mix in your own fruit. Alternatively, you can buy a sweetened variety and dilute the sugar content with plain yogurt. Fruit smoothies made with yogurt are also great ways to provide calcium for growing bodies.

Your child's daily bread

Foods with carbohydrate content, such as whole-grain breads and cereals, fruits and vegetables, grains and legumes, are also rich sources of many minerals and vitamins, as well as fiber. Although low-carbohydrate diets have been popular in the effort to lose weight, dietitians and other health-care providers recommend including a variety of healthy carbohydrates in the diet of adults and children. Carbohydrates are a great source of energy and are relied upon by athletes as fuel to sustain their energy for short or long periods.

Whole-grain breads and cereals provide important minerals and vitamins, including iron and B vitamins, as well as carbohydrates for energy and fiber to help keep bowel movements normal. Since children tend to enjoy these foods, it is usually not difficult to get them to eat breads and cereals. Yet about one-quarter of children age 4 to 8 do not get the recommended amount of grain products daily, according to the 2004 Canadian Community Health Survey. Good examples of breads and cereals include whole-grain bread, rolls or bagels, as well as whole-wheat pasta, brown rice and quinoa. Whole-grain or whole wheat varieties have more nutrients and fiber compared to plain white varieties.

Calcium deficiency

The 2004 Canadian Community Health Survey found that one-third of children age 4 to 9 and about two-thirds of children older than 10 do not receive the recommended amount of milk or milk products daily. This means that these children are at risk for being calcium deficient if they are not eating other good sources of calcium.

tip
Children really do learn by example. Continue to try new foods and flavors yourself, and you may find your children following your lead.

Vegetables matter

Vegetables are an important part of a young child's diet, providing a rich source of different vitamins and minerals, as well as fiber, which helps maintain a normal bowel routine. The fiber in vegetables, along with an adequate intake of fluid, can help to prevent constipation (see page 60 for more information).

However, in one study looking at the dietary intakes of preschool children, researchers found that children ate less than 25% of the recommended number of daily servings of vegetables. In fact, 40% to 50% of the children studied ate less than 2 servings daily of fruits and vegetables. These children did not meet their daily needs of vitamin A, vitamin C or fiber. The Canadian Community Health Survey (2004) also found that 70% of children between the age of 4 and 8 years (and about 50% of adults) did not get an adequate number of servings of fruits and vegetables daily. Five servings of fruits and vegetables per day is recommended for children.

So how do you encourage children to eat more vegetables? Do not say, "Better eat your vegetables or there's no dessert," or "You may not like them, but they're good for you." Presented this way, vegetables may not be very appealing to children — or adults, for that matter. To make them more appealing, prepare vegetables in a variety of ways that can be enjoyed by your child as well as the whole family. For example, try adding a little low-sodium soy sauce to cooked spinach. Green beans or carrots can be perked up with a dip of ranch-style salad dressing. Corn on the cob is usually popular; by the age of 3 years, many children can eat whole corn on the cob.

The recipes in this book also include a number of tempting vegetable dishes, such as Zucchini Sticks (page 200) and Swedish Potatoes (page 286). We think you'll discover (as we have) that it is possible to get young children excited about vegetables.

Are vitamin supplements the answer?

If we know that children are not eating enough fruits and vegetables, shouldn't they just receive a vitamin pill to supplement their intake? Well, the answer is no. Not only do fruits and vegetables provide vitamins and minerals, they also provide phytochemicals that help our immune system and much needed fiber. Consider also that if children are not eating fruits and vegetables, what are they eating? Often the answer is snacks that provide little in the way of nutritional value, but are high in calories, salt and fat. Increasing fruit and vegetable intake should be a family affair, as we know that adults are also not eating the advised amount of these foods.

Apples and oranges?

Let's compare the nutritional value of a fresh medium-size orange to a cup (250 mL) of orange juice.

NUTRIENT	1 medium orange	1 cup (250 mL) orange juice
CALORIES	69 kcal	112 kcal
FIBER	3.1 g	0 g
VITAMIN C	82.7 mg	97 mg
CARBOHYDRATE	15 g	27 g

Note: You can see that orange juice has more calories and less fiber than a fresh orange. While the juice does have slightly more vitamin C, a child needs only 15 to 45 mg per day, so a fresh orange meets daily needs. Contrary to what many people may believe, even if juice with pulp is chosen, there is minimal fiber, only about 0.5 g per 1 cup (250 mL).

Cool, clean water

Make water the thirst-quenching beverage of choice in your family and ensure adequate milk intake as a second beverage. In a recent study of the drinking habits of 1- to 5-year-old children, 1 in 5 did not drink any water daily, while 1 in 4 drank at least one sugar-sweetened beverage every day. Drinking more water helps to keep children at a healthy weight. A recent study of 2nd and 3rd grade students in Germany found that after installing water fountains and encouraging children to drink water, kids actually did drink more water, and were much less likely to become overweight, compared to the children who were not encouraged to drink water. It could be that children who have the habit of drinking water stay hydrated and may eat less, as they will no longer mistake feelings of thirst for feelings of hunger. Especially for overweight children, water should be encouraged before snacks or meals to ensure that their thirst is satisfied, and then they can more easily recognize if they are really hungry. This is good practice for adults as well!

The whole fruit

Many parents believe that fruit juice is an adequate substitute for whole fruit. But this is not the case. Whole fruits provide fiber, which juices do not, and are lower in sugar. For this reason, make a point of including seasonal fresh fruit in your child's diet. Experiment with different fruits, introducing your child (and perhaps yourself) to new and interesting varieties. Keep a supply of cut-up fruit on hand for snacking at any time.

What about canned fruit? While not as flavorful as fresh, canned fruit is an acceptable alternative. Just make sure that it is packed in fruit juice or water — not heavy syrup.

Fruit juice abuse?

There are few things more popular with parents and young children than fruit juice. Parents like the fact that it contains important vitamins and minerals (such as vitamin C), and they appreciate the convenience of juice boxes and straws, which are easy to pack for lunch boxes or traveling. Kids like juice simply because it's sweet and tastes great. Still, it's always possible to have too much of a good thing — and fruit juice is a perfect example of this.

In a study of preschoolers, fruit juice was found to account for more than 50% of all fruit servings consumed. This means the children were not getting the fiber that comes from whole fruit. Children only get about half of the fiber that they need daily. In addition, the high intake of juice was almost certainly displacing other foods that could provide a balance of various nutrients.

While the occasional juice served with a meal is perfectly acceptable, constant sipping of juice is not. This habit results not only in unbalanced nutrition, but can contribute to higher rates of tooth decay. (See page 27 for more information.)

So what's the alternative? Encourage your children to choose water as their beverage of choice. It's refreshing, and essential to good health. And ensure adequate intake of milk as a second beverage option.

Choking hazards

Between the ages of 2 and 6, children become much more adept at the art of self-feeding. They are better able to chew and swallow a wider range of foods with different textures, so the risk of choking would seem to be less than when they were younger. However, the highest risk of choking is reported to be between 2 and 4 years of age. Food items are the most common cause of choking (60%), while candies are associated with 19% of choking episodes, according to one study conducted in a hospital emergency department.

Still learning

As toddlers continue to learn new feeding skills, it is important to remember that they are still learning and are at high risk of choking from foods — or other small non-food items that may be around the house. Small children are more susceptible to choking than older children and adults because their airways are smaller and foods can more easily block them.

Juice pretenders

Often sold side by side on supermarket shelves, fruit juices and fruit drinks may appear to be the same. But they're not. Fruit juices contain 100% juice, while fruit drinks typically contain a much smaller proportion of juice, which is supplemented by water, as well as excessive sugar and other ingredients. Although some fruit drinks and even water are fortified with vitamins, they are still less desirable than real juice, and are generally not recommended for young children.

Hard to swallow

Foods you shouldn't give to children under 4 years of age:

- popcorn
- cough drops
- sunflower seeds
- whole carrots
- hard and gel candies
- whole raisins
- fish with bones
- chewing gum
- peanuts/nuts
- snacks with toothpicks/skewers
- hot dogs (unless cut in quarters lengthwise)
- grapes and grape tomatoes (unless cut into quarters)
- chewing gum
- uncooked peas
- fruit with pits, such as cherries and plums (unless pits are removed)

Know your CPR

Sign up for a first-aid course. Try to arrange a class with other families and caregivers, including grandparents and older siblings. Ask your babysitters if they have been trained in first aid, and if not, include them in courses you are taking.

It is especially important that children are seated and that they are supervised while eating. This can prevent the sudden inhalation of a food piece that is not yet chewed. (It's also easier to keep an eye on them if they are seated in one place.)

While we have listed many of the higher-risk foods to avoid, parents and caregivers must also use common sense to determine which items are safe.

Tips for preventing choking

How can you minimize a child's risk of choking? Here are some important tips.

1. Avoid giving foods considered unsafe to children who are less than 4 years of age (see sidebar, page 17). Or modify unsafe foods — by slicing hotdogs lengthwise, for example, or by grating carrots, quartering grapes and chopping sticky foods such as dates.

2. Give children foods and beverages only if they are sitting upright. Do not provide liquid in a bottle while they are lying down; they may choke on the fluid.

3. Children should not be force-fed.

4. For young children who do not yet have their incisors or primary molars, be sure to cut food into small pieces.

5. A child should always be sitting while eating. Do not let toddlers walk (and especially run) around while eating.

6. Always watch your toddler while eating. The risk of choking can be minimized if parents and caregivers are aware of their toddlers' chewing and swallowing abilities, and are able to react quickly at the first signs of choking.

7. Choose toys that are appropriate for your child's age. Keep him or her away from older children's toys, which may be unsafe.

8. Most importantly, be prepared to help children in the event that they do choke. Learn how to perform the Heimlich maneuver — and other first-aid techniques. If you don't know how to provide this assistance, contact your local community center or the Red Cross to organize a training session.

9. If serving nut butters, be sure to spread thinly, as thick butters can cause a child to choke.

Kid cuisine

Sample menu for a 2- to 4-year-old

BREAKFAST		
½ cup	Weekend Breakfast Quiche (see recipe, page 151)	125 mL
½	orange, sectioned and seeded	½
½ cup	whole milk	125 mL
SNACK		
½	banana	½
½	apple	½
¼ cup	granola cereal	50 mL
½ cup	water	125 mL
LUNCH		
½ cup	Tasty Tofu (see recipe, page 202)	125 mL
½ cup	brown rice, steamed	125 mL
½ cup	green beans (with 1 tsp/5 mL butter)	125 mL
1 tbsp	ranch-style dressing	15 mL
½ cup	whole milk	125 mL
½ cup	water	125 mL
SNACK		
4	low-sodium whole-grain crackers or pita chips	4
1 oz	Cheddar cheese	25 g
¼	apple	¼
½ cup	whole milk	125 mL
½ cup	water	125 mL
DINNER		
½ serving	Macaroni and Beef with Cheese (see recipe, page 215)	½ serving
½ cup	grated carrots	125 mL
½ cup	whole milk	125 mL
1 piece	Chocolate Chip and Banana Cake (see recipe, page 334)	1 piece
about ½ cup	water	125 mL

Note: Provides approximately 1500 calories and 60 g protein, and meets 100% of calcium and iron needs.

Packing some protein

Meats, fish, eggs, chicken, beans, lentils, nuts and seeds and tofu provide energy, protein and iron for a growing child.

Meatier meals

Parents sometimes find it difficult to get their children to eat meats because they are usually not as soft or appealing as foods from the other food groups. Parents sometimes fear that protein or iron needs are not being met. If meats or poultry are not enjoyed or are refused by toddlers, there are some excellent protein options:

- Softer meat choices (e.g., meatballs)
- Tender chicken thighs instead of drier chicken breast
- Thinly sliced roast beef
- Baked or grilled fish
- Baked beans
- Semi-firm tofu
- Scrambled or soft-cooked eggs
- Canned tuna or salmon

tip

Fresh fruits and vegetables, cut up and presented at the play table, will help replace less nutritious, higher-salt and higher-fat processed foods.

Snack on this

Snacks are an important part of daily eating, especially for growing bodies. About 25% to 30% of total daily calories should come from snacks. Unfortunately, snack choices for children tend to be high in fat and sodium, and low in vitamins and fiber. By replacing processed food snacks with fruits and vegetables, salt and fat intake decrease, while fiber and vitamins increase.

Snacks can be offered at least 1 hour before meals; otherwise, food intake at meals may be reduced. However, every child is different, and especially if children are active, snacks may be offered closer to mealtime.

Great snack ideas for children — and adults!

1. Fresh cut fruits: slices of apples, strawberries halved, orange sections, mango slices, kiwi slices and berries
2. Fresh cut vegetables: shredded carrots (kids *love* this), cucumber slices, celery cut in bits, broccoli flower pieces, tomato slices
3. Pita bread served with hummus or avocado (guacamole) dip or thinly spread nut butters
4. Shelled edamame (soybeans)
5. Cheese: shredded (kids *love* this), cubed or sliced, with low-sodium whole-grain crackers
6. Pita crisps: homemade or low-salt commercial variety
7. Plain or vanilla yogurt with berries
8. Homemade muffin with milk
9. Homemade cookies or biscuits with milk

Family food diary
A family that snacks together...

My kids' favorite snacks include a variety of vegetables, fruits and other energy- and nutrient-rich foods. Here are some examples of what you may see on our kitchen table after school, or what they may be snacking on while traveling to a hockey or soccer game:

- Cherry tomatoes, olives and feta cheese on a plate
- Celery, cucumbers, carrots with ranch dip
- Pita bread with hummus or guacamole
- Plate of mango, kiwi, strawberries
- Bowls of grapes, blueberries or raspberries
- Smoothies made with frozen berries, a ripe banana and yogurt and milk
- Crackers with goat cheese
- Chocolate chip cookies (homemade) and milk
- Pistachios or cashews
- Shrimp with sauce
- Small bowl of quinoa
- ½ panini sandwich
- Shelled edamame
- Fresh bread dipped in extra virgin olive oil, along with feta cheese cubes

(*Daina*)

I'll eat it my way

Because young children tend to be curious about the foods around them, they generally look forward to eating. At the same time, however, their growing independence often manifests itself in clearly expressed likes and dislikes about food. Some of these may appear to be quite arbitrary — for example, your child may insist on having a piece of bread sliced diagonally instead of straight through the middle, or on eating the same food for lunch every day for a few weeks.

Such preferences may often be difficult to understand. But it is important for parents to recognize that children are simply exploring their ability to make decisions in situations that they are able to control — specifically, at meal and snack times. Encourage this independence, and respect that your children have their likes and dislikes of food (as you do). This is not to say that you should not set limits, of course, but you should allow children some degree of latitude in requesting certain foods at meals, and understand that their appetite may not always be consistent from one day to the next.

When dealing with your child's likes and dislikes, remember that opinions formed at this age are changeable and subject to influence. Foods that are rejected outright today may be requested tomorrow. The brown rice that is spurned at your dinner table may suddenly become palatable when served at a friend's house. As you did with your children when they were infants, try not to let your own dislikes of food serve as a negative influence. Children love to imitate their parents or caregivers, so act accordingly.

Keep mealtime as calm and pleasant as possible, no matter how tiring or hectic your day has been. Children read cues and will not respond positively to your attempts to influence them unless they feel that at least some of their decisions are being respected. Social interactions and changes in appetite will influence the choices of food your child makes.

Taking part

As they become more independent, young children like to feel that they are actively participating in family life, and this includes food preparation, selection and tasting. Foods that your child has helped to prepare or select at the store are much more interesting — and consequently more likely to be eaten with enthusiasm.

Tips for boosting energy

While childhood obesity is on everyone's radar these days, there are children who are struggling with not gaining enough weight. They are sometimes described as picky eaters, or as observed by their parents, seem to have smaller appetites than other children their age. If their weight is lower than expected for their height, or if they have not gained sufficient weight in a certain time as determined by the family doctor or pediatrician, higher-energy foods may be needed in order to promote weight gain. Here are some ways that you can boost your child's energy intake.

1. Offer whole milk instead of 2% or 1% milk.
2. Offer higher-fat cheese and yogurt.
3. If the child is older than 4 years of age, offer nuts or nut butters thinly spread on sliced bread or on crackers as snacks.
4. Add gravies or sauces to meat, chicken, vegetables.
5. Add extra oil, butter, margarine to meats, pastas, vegetables.
6. Add avocado slices to sandwiches or to salads.

Feeding frustrations

Does your child take forever to finish a meal? Does he or she seem abnormally fussy or difficult about eating? Well, you're not alone. In fact, behavioral research into children's eating habits reveals that over 30% of parents of toddlers describe some feeding-related problem, including slow eating, poor appetite, unhappiness during mealtimes, rigid food preferences or other negative behavior. The important thing for parents to realize is that, in most instances, these behaviors are relatively short-lived. It is only in a minority of cases, where children have been slow feeders for a number of years, that a more detailed assessment of their feeding skills may have to be evaluated.

Consider, for example, the sample menu shown on page 25. While the amount of food may seem quite minimal (at least, compared to the menu given on page 19), it still provides more than 70% of the child's nutritional requirements (except for iron). The occasional

Picky eaters

So what do you do until children grow out of their "picky eater" stage? Like most parents, you may be concerned that the child is not getting enough to eat. But you probably don't need to worry. As long as your child is growing normally, chances are that he or she is receiving an adequate supply of energy and nutrients.

Eating out

Finding the right kind of care for your child can be a stressful time. When a child starts going to daycare (or some other facility outside the home) and, eventually, to school, the important role of feeding the child is no longer exclusively that of the parent. Instead, it becomes shared with outside providers, who will also have an influence on your child's attitudes toward food and nutrition. How can you ensure that your child eats healthy meals away from home? Check out our tips on page 26.

"picky" day will generally not affect your child's nutritional status. Children are very good at self-regulating their overall energy intake — at least, when we allow them to do so, and give them the freedom to indicate when they are hungry or full.

Stocking up

While lack of time is often cited by parents and caregivers as one reason for not cooking meals and buying prepared meals instead, parents should plan to have some basic food items on hand to prepare a meal and snacks. Stock cupboards, refrigerators and freezers with some of these recommended food basics:

- Milk
- Eggs
- Whole-grain cereals (freeze fresh bread and rolls)
- Pasta, rice, potatoes
- Quinoa
- Nuts and seeds and nut butters
- Canned tuna and salmon
- Frozen berries
- Frozen vegetables
- Boneless and skinless chicken thighs, frozen
- Beef, frozen
- Fish, frozen
- Variety of herbs and spices
- Low-sodium canned soups and vegetables
- Low-sodium canned beans and lentils
- Fresh fruit and vegetables, local and seasonal
- Low-sodium crackers
- Variety of oils: safflower, olive, canola (mix with butter when cooking)

Daycare nutrition

Working parents are a fact of modern life. It is a reality for approximately 30% to 40% of American households. And finding the right kind of care for your child can be a most stressful time. Once the daycare setting is selected, many parents assume that the nutritional needs of their children will be met by experienced individuals who have a good knowledge about nutrition. Although this may be

Meals at a minimum

Sample menu for a picky 3-year-old

BREAKFAST		
¼ cup	o-shaped oat cereal	50 mL
½ cup	whole milk	125 mL
¼	banana	¼
SNACK		
1	unsalted soda cracker	1
½	banana	½
LUNCH		
½	slice bread with 1 tbsp (15 mL) peanut butter	½
¼	raw carrot, shredded	¼
1 cup	whole milk	250 mL
SNACK		
2	unsalted soda crackers	2
1 oz	Cheddar cheese	25 g
DINNER		
2	fish sticks	2
¼	baked potato	¼
1 tbsp	mayonnaise-type dressing (for potato)	15 mL
SNACK		
½ cup	whole milk	125 mL
1	oatmeal cookie	1

Note: Provides approximately 1000 calories and 44 g protein, and meets more than 50% of iron requirements.

true in many instances, research indicates that it is not always so.

It is up to the parent to become familiar with the menus and other specific choices of foods offered to their child. This is important because, as parents in one study indicated, a childcare setting is equal to, if not more important than, home for establishing specific food likes and dislikes. Typically, where children are enrolled in a full-time program of 8 hours a day, a daycare facility provides about 50% to 60% of a child's daily energy needs. In other words, a majority of nutrients are consumed away from the watchful eye of the parent.

Children should be provided with a varied diet, and foods given at the daycare and at home must complement each other. If one food group is not taken well in one setting, then it should be encouraged in the other. Of course, it is possible to offer a variety of foods from all food groups if the nutrition program at the daycare and at home are balanced and well planned. Nutrition standards for daycare programs have been published by the American Dietetic Association and are required to meet licensing regulations.

Tips for monitoring daycare meals

Here are some things you can do to ensure that you are familiar with what your child consumes.

1. Check the menu each week. For the first few weeks, look at the menu and review the food choices offered, both at mealtimes and for snacks. If you have any questions about why certain foods are not offered, ask the director of the daycare. Find out how the menu selection was evaluated, and who was involved in the decision making.

2. Monitor your child's intake. If you are concerned about your child's intake, ask the daycare to keep a record of what he or she eats each day — at least for the first few weeks of care.

3. Ask about fruits and vegetables. Ensure that there are plenty of fresh fruits and vegetables offered, and that they are age-appropriate (for chewing and swallowing).

4. What are they drinking? Make sure that the daycare provides water as the main beverage of choice and that juice is limited. Where fruit beverages are served, make sure that they are fruit juices — not fruit drinks, which are not as nutritious and typically contain more added sugar.

5. Check out the snack menu. Evaluate the type and quality of the snacks provided. Are they nutritious?

6. Offer a complementary menu at home. Daycare facilities obviously can't tailor their menus to the needs of each child's family, so take the initiative and complement the foods offered at the daycare with the meals that you provide at home. If pasta was served at the daycare, try to provide something different for supper.

7. What is your child learning about nutrition? Find out if the daycare offers any type of education about nutrition and health. If so, what is being taught?

Dental care for kids

By the time children reach the age of 2 years, most of their teeth have come in, except for the second molars. Teeth do not begin to fall out until children are about 6 years of age, usually starting with the teeth that were first to come in. During this period, dental hygiene is important, even though many of the child's teeth are not permanent.

Keeping teeth clean

Dental hygiene involves brushing teeth at least twice a day — in the morning and evening — as well as after eating any foods that are sweet and sticky. Encourage your child to drink water after meals and snacks. This is a good habit to develop. It helps to clean out the mouth and rinses teeth of leftover food. If the mouth is not cleansed properly, bacteria in the mouth digest the carbohydrate from foods — which can come from many sources, including milk, juice or sweets — and create an acid that leads to tooth decay.

Nursing bottle syndrome

When an infant or child falls asleep with a bottle — typically containing milk or juice — in his or her mouth, it can lead to something called "nursing bottle syndrome." This is believed to occur in 3% to 6% of children under 4 years of age. The syndrome involves deterioration of the front teeth because of prolonged exposure to carbohydrates in the mouth, causing bacterial action that results in tooth decay.

While it's true that a bottle is helpful in soothing a child, it should contain water. Early exposure of an infant or child to water will encourage him or her to accept it as a replacement for milk at bedtime. Studies reveal that a child who wakes up crying more frequently at night is at higher risk of nursing bottle syndrome, because soothing techniques used by parents may include giving milk or juice in a bottle. Some parents are not aware of the syndrome, or believe it is only milk that can cause tooth decay.

tip
Frequent sipping of juice can cause cavities by providing a constant supply of carbohydrate, or sugar, to newly developing teeth. The American Academy of Pediatrics recommends limiting juice to 6 oz (175 mL) per day, while the Canadian Paediatric Society considers 4 to 8 oz (125 to 250 mL) an acceptable range. Both groups suggest offering water as the child's primary beverage.

Water? What's that?

Excessive juice consumption may seem like a relatively new phenomenon (about the same age as the juice box), but as early as 1957, a study reported that 29% of children between the ages of 6 months and 5 years had never had a drink of plain water! Since then the situation has not improved: A recent study in the UK of 2- to 7-year-olds showed that, over a 48-hour period, 50% to 70% never drank plain water, but consumed milk, juice, sweetened drinks and other beverages. The message to parents: Encourage your child to drink water!

Teaching children to brush

Children between the ages of 2 and 6 can learn to brush their own teeth, and brushing skills will improve with age. Only a small amount of toothpaste, less than the size of a pea, is needed. Once the child has finished brushing, parents should follow with a quick brush to ensure that cleaning is thorough. (Be sure to encourage your child to spit out the toothpaste.)

Finding fluoride

Toothpaste should provide all the necessary fluoride protection when combined with municipal water supplies that contain fluoride concentrations of at least 0.6 ppm (parts per million). If the drinking water contains less than this concentration, fluoride supplements are necessary. Your local water supply is just one source of fluoride. You can also find it in a number of commercial beverages and foods. Read the labels. If you are unsure about the fluoridation of your drinking water, check with your family doctor or dentist, or your local water company.

Too much fluoride can lead to a condition known as fluorosis. In severe cases, this can cause a brownish discoloration of the teeth — although it is not considered a health risk. Infants are more susceptible to fluorosis than older children. To regulate fluoride consumption, encourage children to limit the use of toothpaste to a pea size, not to swallow any, to spit out excess toothpaste and to rinse well with water after each brushing. Another option is to choose a children's toothpaste without fluoride.

Favorite recipes

Here are five of our favorite recipes for toddlers, which you will find in the recipe section in this book.

- Make-Ahead Breakfast Granola (page 153)
- Eva's Simple Chicken Fingers (page 237)
- Parmesan Quinoa (page 265)
- Edamame and Bean Salad (page 273)
- Tasty Potato Pancakes (page 288)

Top 10 Toddler Nutrition Questions

1 My daughter is 2½ years old, and now eats some meals away from home — either at daycare or at a friend's house for play group. How can I be sure that she is eating enough?

Normal growth and weight gain are the most important signs to watch for when assessing nutritional intake. Other indicators include your daughter's energy level and tolerance for exercise. At home, make every attempt to offer each of the four food groups at each meal to provide a balanced diet with a variety of vitamins and minerals. If you are really concerned, you could also ask your child's daytime caregiver to make a note of your child's food intake over a 3-day period. This will help you to determine if there are any types of food lacking in her diet.

2 Should I give my 3-year-old a vitamin supplement? I think he is eating a balanced diet, but I would like to be sure that he is getting all the nutrients he needs.

Vitamin supplements are costly and unnecessary for a young child who is growing normally and eating a variety of nutritious foods. In fact, these supplements often provide parents with a false sense of security, encouraging them to believe that less effort or attention is required to give their children a properly balanced diet. There are some exceptions, of course, such as those children who have iron-deficiency anemia and require a period of iron supplementation. Children with lactose intolerance may also require a supplement to provide the calcium and vitamin D that would otherwise be supplied by drinking milk (unless they are drinking a lactose-free fortified beverage). (See page 76 for more information on calcium.) Finally, keep in mind that children are especially vulnerable to vitamin toxicity when supplements are taken in excessive amounts. If your child requires a supplement, ask your doctor to recommend the appropriate type and dose.

3 I have a lot of difficulty getting my 3-year-old to drink plain milk — although she loves chocolate milk. Is it okay to give her this instead?

Chocolate milk provides the same important nutrients (including calcium and vitamin D) as plain milk. It is higher in sugar, however, and contains caffeine (from the chocolate), so you may want to dilute these ingredients by mixing some of the chocolate milk with plain milk. You might also try compromising with your child by alternating plain and chocolate milk with each snack or mealtime.

4 Getting my 3-year-old boy's teeth brushed each night is a constant battle. How often should we be brushing his teeth? Can we let him do it himself?

Children should have their teeth brushed at least twice a day — once in the morning and once in the evening — using only a small amount of toothpaste (about the size of a pea). Ideally, you should also brush your son's teeth after he eats sugary foods such as raisins or sticky candy. As well, drinking water, instead of juice, throughout the day helps to cleanse teeth. You should encourage your son to brush his own teeth — preferably by the example of brushing your teeth at the same time. After he has been given the opportunity to brush his own teeth, quickly brush them again.

5 My 4-year-old daughter seems to be eating less and less. Is there a safe appetite stimulant that I can give her?

No. Children have different growth stages, and each is accompanied by increases and decreases in appetite. Provided your daughter's growth is normal (ask your family doctor or pediatrician if you're unsure), there should be no reason to worry. Children are usually quite good at regulating their own intake when given a varied supply of nutritious and healthy foods. Appetite stimulants are not safe for children.

6 My 4-year-old daughter had a viral illness with diarrhea that lasted for a few days. I have read that the "BRAT diet" can help relieve diarrhea. What is this diet and how effective is it?

BRAT (an acronym for bananas, rice, applesauce and toast [or tea]) is not a balanced diet, because it is limited in protein, fat and calories — and may even promote more diarrhea. It has never been proven to help decrease diarrhea. Your child will be better off with her normal diet and adequate fluid. Check with your family doctor to see if a special electrolyte replacement fluid is necessary. (See page 125 for more information.)

7 My 3-year-old son seems to be much heavier than other children his age. Should I be putting him on a diet?

Placing a child on a diet — at least, in the adult sense of the word — is not appropriate at this age. Keep in mind that being heavier than other children does not mean he is fat. If your son has always been larger than most kids his age, this may be normal for him. Children typically grow into their weight and need a constant supply of the appropriate amount of energy and other nutrients required for normal development. So continue to give him three meals and snacks daily, and do not restrict foods. Snack foods should be healthy, including fresh vegetables and fruits. Try to limit snacks, such as chips or candy, which are high in fat or low in fiber and nutrients. (This

recommendation applies to all children.) Also, keep an eye on your son's juice consumption, because these calories can add up. Encourage him to drink water.

8 Should I be giving my 2-year-old son organic vegetables and fruits? Are they safer and more nutritious?

Although organic foods are promoted as being free of any pesticides or preservatives, existing government regulations are designed to ensure that conventionally produced foods are safe for consumption. Generally speaking, there is no evidence to support the use of organic over non-organic produce. Their nutrient values do not differ, although their prices do: Organic produce is usually more expensive than conventional fruits and vegetables.

9 Why should my baby daughter consume foods rich in omega-3 fatty acids?

For adults, there is good evidence to support that a diet rich in omega-3 fatty acids can have a positive effect on cardiovascular health. There is also good evidence to show that formula-fed preterm infants do benefit from the inclusion of both DHA and arachidonic acid (ARA) in infant formula throughout the first year of life. There have been studies to show that preterm infants fed a DHA-containing formula have improved mental and visual acuity, but the research for full-term babies has not been conclusive.

10 Should I buy vitamin water instead of plain water for the family?

This is a personal choice, but it is unlikely that the supplemental vitamins in the water will be of any added benefit to you or your family. This is an expensive way to provide fluids. Of course, the choice is yours to make, but there is no real health benefit.

CHAPTER 2

Feeding
Your 4- to 6-Year-Old

Between the ages of 4 and 6, a child's physical growth begins to slow down a little (although it probably won't seem that way!), while rapid changes continue in skill development and feeding behavior. It is at this stage that parents face a new set of challenges in educating their children and helping them to understand the essentials of healthy food, good nutrition and an active lifestyle.

The preschooler's progress

As children make the transition from toddlers to school-age, they typically become a little leaner-looking, losing some of the baby fat that was apparent when they were younger. This reflects their higher activity levels.

Eating habits also change as children get older. Since they have been introduced to a wider variety of foods, they become less likely to reject anything that is new or unfamiliar. Meal routines and self-feeding skills also become well established, so your children are able to assume a more active and independent role at the family dinner table.

Children between the ages of 4 and 6 will also gain new eating experiences outside the home — sometimes beginning in daycare and then, later, at school. The result is that children are often eating one or two meals, plus snacks, away from home each day. While this offers the benefit of exposing children to new foods and eating experiences, it also means that parents have a special responsibility to ensure that their child receives structured, nutritious meals and snacks, and develops the eating habits that will contribute to a lifetime of health.

tip
Let your kids help make decisions in the grocery store and let them help plan menus for the week.

Feeding milestones for children between 4 and 6 years

AGE	MOTOR SKILLS	SOCIAL/PERSONAL SKILLS
4 to 5 years	Uses knife and fork Good use of cup Good self-feeder	Would rather talk than eat Likes to help with food preparation Interested in the nature of food and where it comes from Peer influence increasing
5 to 6 years	Fully able to self-feed	Imitating Less suspicious of mixtures, but still prefers plain foods Social influence outside home increasing Food important part of special occasions

Note: This information is provided so parents and caregivers will understand what tasks most children should expect to have mastered by a certain age. It is important to remember that children grow and learn new skills at different rates.

ADAPTED FROM: Canadian Paediatric Society, *Little Well Beings*, 1994.

Setting an example

Young children learn from what they see, and this is reflected by imitating the people around them. Between the ages of 4 and 6 years, they especially love to copy their moms and dads. So it is parents who need to present a model of good eating habits to their children.

By eating with your children at the table during mealtimes, you can teach them to enjoy a variety of familiar foods, as well as the experience of trying out new ones. By making mealtime a pleasant place to be for your child, you can provide positive reinforcement for learning, and thereby contribute to his or her self-esteem.

Avoid weighty issues

Research shows that, in recent years, children have started to develop adult-like preoccupations with weight and dieting at increasingly younger ages. Part of this is no doubt attributable to endless coverage of these issues in the media (to which children are exposed almost from infancy), but parents still need to ensure that they avoid contributing to the problem. So try not to complain about your weight in front of your children.

Developing feeding skills

Every child develops self-feeding skills at different rates. Nevertheless, it is reasonable for parents to expect that their children achieve certain basic abilities when eating with the family.

Typically, between the ages of 4 and 5 years, children make real progress in being able to feed themselves efficiently. They become proficient in using a knife and fork to cut foods (provided that utensils are small enough for them to use). They make good use of a cup and, although they may still dribble and spill milk out the sides, it happens less often than it did when they were 2 or 3. These skills should continue to develop between the ages of 5 and 6 years.

Steps to healthy eating and living

Educate your children

Studies have shown that children are quick to absorb health and safety information, and that their ability to be "health smart" begins at a young age — as early as $3\frac{1}{2}$ years, according to a study from the University of Texas — with much of this information being mastered by their 6th birthday. For example, by the age of 4 years, many children are able to identify that drinking milk is better for you than drinking soda pop. By $5\frac{1}{2}$ years, many children can evaluate the relative health benefits of different food choices — an apple versus a piece of cake, for example, or a chicken dinner versus a pizza dinner. As a parent, it is important to understand that your children are capable of learning a great deal about food and health, and that much of this will come from your teaching and the example you set as a role model.

Explore the possibilities

It is important for parents to explore a variety of foods for themselves and their children. Look for foods with different colors, flavors and textures. Preschoolers are naturally curious and eager to learn about food. Use new ingredients or try new dishes from different ethnicities or cooking styles. For example, if you usually eat white bread for dinner, try substituting something different, such as a whole wheat baguette, pita bread, bannock, chapati or focaccia. When parents explore new types food, they encourage their children to do so as well.

Table manners

By the age of 4 years, a child should be capable of behaving pleasantly at the dinner table. You can encourage this by making the table a pleasant and privileged place to be. It should not be a place for punishment — for example, where children are made to stay until they finish their carrots.

Be active

An active lifestyle needn't involve strenuous exercise or punishing workouts at a gym. It can be something as simple as taking a stroll in the evening with your children or participating in recreational family sports, such as skiing or rollerblading. The key is to ensure that your children don't spend all their free time in front of the television or the computer screen.

Encourage vitality

Essentially this means living life to the fullest — enjoying good food, being active, feeling good about yourself and fostering these feelings in your children. Children enjoy eating and exploring food. Children like to feel good about themselves and need to have a positive body image fostered by their parents. It is important for parents to help build self-esteem by providing affection and attention. When parents feel good about themselves, they are more likely to have children who feel good about themselves as well.

Delegating mealtime authority

When children are very young, their role in the feeding process is essentially passive: It is their parents who decide what, when, where and how much they eat. As the child gets older and more independent, however, these roles change, and the child begins to assume greater responsibility for his or her eating decisions.

The concept of divided responsibility for childhood feeding has been put forth by Ellyn Satter, a registered dietitian, social worker and author of several books on child behavior as it pertains to eating. The basic premise here is that both the child and the parent have certain responsibilities at mealtime, and that parents should be aware of the child's obligations as well as their own. This idea of delegating responsibility is more evolutionary than revolutionary because the bulk of decision making remains with parents, who continue to be responsible for determining what, when and where the child eats. It simply becomes the child's responsibility to decide whether or not he or she will eat and, if so, how much to eat.

tip

For many parents who are accustomed to exercising control over every aspect of their children's lives, it may be difficult to accept the notion that a 4- to 6-year-old should be given any decision-making power at all — particularly with respect to eating. But give it a try.

To eat or not to eat...

If given the chance, children are remarkably good at determining whether or not, or how much, they need to eat. In fact, it is usually when parents interfere excessively with the child's eating decisions (or do not provide enough support for those decisions) that children end up consuming too much food or too little.

The important thing to remember is that between the ages of 4 and 6, a child's appetite does not remain consistent from day to day. It will increase during growth spurts or at times when your child is very active. Conversely, it will often decrease when a child is tired or over-excited. (These fluctuations become less frequent as children get older.)

Children should be allowed to eat as much food as they wish during mealtimes, but not between meals, until they are full. When children are not hungry at a given meal or snack time, they should not be forced to eat. Let them decide for themselves whether or not they are hungry. But make sure they understand the consequences of their decision — specifically, that if the child chooses not to eat now, he or she will not have another opportunity to do so until the next scheduled meal or snack. Do not feel guilty about saying this. It will encourage eating at designated meal and snack times, and will enable your child to trust his or her own sense of hunger and fullness.

Too young to diet

Some well-meaning parents attempt to restrict a child's food intake in an effort to control what they perceive as excessive weight gain. But research has shown that such restrictions can actually have the opposite effect, leading children to overeat and gain even more weight. When food is perceived as a carefully controlled commodity, children can become obsessed with it, eating more than they need to avoid the possibility of becoming hungry. (See Chapter 10 for more information on childhood obesity.)

How much to serve...

While children should ultimately decide how much they will eat, it is still the parent's responsibility to provide the structure in which these decisions are made. For example, you will need to decide how much food to offer your child, recognizing that overly large portions can be intimidating.

As a rule, it's best to provide children with smaller amounts of food, giving them the option of seconds if they wish. To determine the serving size appropriate for your 4- to 6-year-old, use the table opposite as a guide.

Suggested serving sizes for 4- to 6-year-olds

FOOD GROUP	FOOD ITEM	RANGE OF SERVING SIZES
Grain products	Bread	½ to 1 whole slice
	Cold cereal	½ to 1 cup (125 to 250 mL)
	Hot cereal	⅓ to ¾ cup (75 mL to 175 mL)
	Bagel, pita or bun	¼ to ½
	Muffin	½ to 1 whole
	Pasta or rice	¼ to ½ cup (60 to 125 mL)
	Crackers	4 to 8
Vegetables and fruit	Whole fruit or vegetable	½ to 1 medium
	Vegetables, fresh, frozen or canned	¼ to ½ cup (60 to 125 mL)
	Salad	½ to 1 cup (125 to 250 mL)
	Fruit, fresh or canned	¼ to ½ cup (60 to 125 mL)
	Vegetable or fruit juice	¼ to ½ cup (60 to 125 mL)
Milk products	Milk	½ to 1 cup (125 to 250 mL)
	Cheese	1 to 2 oz (25 to 50 g)
	Yogurt	⅓ to ¾ cup (75 mL to 175 mL)
Meat and alternatives	Meat, fish or poultry	1 to 2 oz (25 to 50 g)
	Egg	1 whole
	Beans, legumes	¼ to ½ cup (60 to 125 mL)
	Tofu	¼ to ⅓ cup (60 to 75 mL)
	Peanut butter	1 to 2 tbsp (15 to 30 mL)

Note: For each range of serving sizes, the lesser amounts are appropriate for 2- to 4-year olds.

Keep in mind that there are a number of variables to consider, including the child's age (younger children will eat less) and individual eating patterns.

When to eat...

Providing toddlers and preschoolers with structured meal and snack times helps to establish hunger and facilitates eating at mealtimes. Snacks should be well timed, and of appropriate size, so that children are hungry but not "starving" at mealtime. Snacking is an important source of energy and nutrients. However, if you find that you are having difficulty getting children to eat at the table, "grazing" should be limited between meals. When children are thirsty throughout the day, encourage them to drink water. If appetite at mealtime is a problem, you may wish to restrict consumption of milk, juice or beverages other than water to meals and snacks only.

Where to eat...

Meals should be eaten in a designated spot. For most families, this will be the kitchen table. Whenever possible, sit with your children and eat meals together as a family.

Keep in mind that eating with your child involves more than just sitting with your child while he or she eats. It is important to talk with children so that they appreciate mealtime as a time to interact with the family. The dinner table should not be a place for family arguments; instead, it should provide the kind of environment where your child can tell you about his or her day — or about anything at all. Try to establish the ritual of eating together when your children are young; it will be much more difficult to get into the habit once members of the family are older and have schedules of their own.

No TV dinners here

Meals should be a time for enjoying food and conversation, not watching television. So turn off the set. You'll find that it enhances family togetherness. Research has shown that children who eat in front of the television tend to eat more because they are not paying attention to their feelings of being full.

What to eat...

The final responsibility of parents is to provide their child with healthy meals and snacks. This task will be considerably easier if you have a basic understanding of the four food groups, the essential nutrients children need, and you use the recipes in this book.

Remember that growing children require energy-dense foods (such as peanut butter, cheeses and whole milk), as well as lower-energy foods (such as vegetables and legumes), and you should try to provide a balance of both types at meals. A sample menu, providing a well-balanced diet, is shown opposite.

Healthy school lunches

During the school day, a child will eat up to 30% of the recommended daily food energy intake. That's a significant portion. As kids go off to school, it is important to send nutritious lunches. Try to involve your kids in selecting foods for their lunches. This will help them learn the importance

Lunch toolkit

Here is a list of "must have" tools for packing your child's lunch and keeping it fresh until snack and meal time:

- Insulated lunch bag
- Mini ice packs
- Small Thermos (for hot foods)
- Refillable liquid container (for milk or water)
- Refillable stainless steel water bottle
- Washable cutlery (an inexpensive fork and spoon that won't be missed if it goes missing — try the dollar store)
- Reusable containers for vegetables, cheese, sandwiches and other foods

of eating from the different food groups and improve the odds they'll eat the lunch you packed. A healthy school lunch should include a choice from each of the four food groups. This includes a protein choice (meat or vegetarian), a vegetable or fruit, a dairy food (low-fat milk or yogurt) and a grain (preferably whole-grain). Don't be tempted to pack prepackaged foods ("lunchables") because they can contain additional fat, calories and sodium kids don't need. Avoid sending sweetened beverages, such as soda pop, iced tea or fruit punches (disguised as fruit juice).

Junior carte du jour

Sample menu for a 4- to 6-year-old

BREAKFAST		
1	slice whole wheat toast	1
1 tsp	margarine	5 mL
¾ cup	oatmeal	175 mL
1 cup	2% milk	250 mL
SNACK		
1	apple	1
1 oz	cheese	25 g
½ cup	water	125 mL
LUNCH		
¾ cup	Tuscan Bean Soup (see recipe, page 171)	175 mL
1	whole-grain roll	1
½ cup	2% milk	125 mL
½ cup	plain yogurt with ¼ cup (60 mL) blueberries	175 mL
SNACK		
2	banana oatmeal cookies	2
½ cup	apple juice	125 mL
DINNER		
1 serving	Beef Satays (see recipe, page 250)	1 serving
½ cup	steamed brown rice	125 mL
¼ cup	broccoli	60 mL
¼ cup	cauliflower	60 mL
½ cup	2% milk	125 mL
½ cup	peach slices	125 mL

Note: Provides approximately 1500 calories and 65 g protein, and meets over 100% of calcium and iron requirements.

Tips for packing some punch
in your child's lunch

Once children reach kindergarten, many parents provide them with a bag lunch to take to school each day — usually at the last minute and without giving its contents a lot of thought. Not surprisingly, children often complain that they "don't like what mom sends for lunch" or that they are "tired of peanut butter sandwiches." Here are a few healthy and nutritious suggestions that will add variety to your child's lunch bag.

1 Purchase a small stainless steel Thermos and fill it with hot soups or leftover stews and pastas. It can also be used to help keep milk or other beverages cold.

2 A small ice pack (or frozen juice or water container) is ideal for keeping cold foods cold and to protect them from spoilage (see Chapter 7 for more information on food safety). Use it with milk, cheese slices, yogurt or meat sandwiches.

3 If sandwiches are a family favorite, choose lower-fat deli meats (preferably nitrate-free), such as turkey, ham or roast beef. Avoid fatty deli meats, such as salami, mortadella and bologna.

4 A plain hard-boiled egg makes a great protein alternative for kids who don't like sandwiches.

5 Try making soup in large batches (we have lots of great recipe ideas) and freeze it in single servings for quick lunches in the weeks to come. If you use canned soups, choose reduced-sodium broth or tomato-based varieties.

6 Liven up sandwiches by using different types of bread, such as pita pockets, small submarine buns, raisin bread or whole-grain bread. Try mustard instead of mayonnaise.

7 Make sandwiches with a variety of fillings, such as sliced deli meats, tuna, ham, and salmon or egg salad. Other ideas include: hummus; nut butters (where not prohibited; many schools have declared themselves "nut-free" zones because of allergy concerns); refried beans; leftovers, including roasted chicken or meatloaf; soy alternatives, such as textured vegetable protein slices; and various types of cheese, such as Cheddar, cream cheese, Havarti, and Monterey Jack.

(8) Instead of ordinary sandwiches, try making one of the following alternatives: rice cakes with almond butter; hummus with flatbread; melba toast and cheese slices; bagel pieces with flavored cream cheese; muffins with apple butter; English muffin mini pizzas.

(9) When it comes to packing fruits and vegetables, the options are endless. Cut up fresh veggies at the beginning of the week and keep them in the refrigerator for easy access and quick snacks. Carrot and celery sticks can be kept fresh in water for a couple of days. Serve veggies plain or with a low-fat, yogurt-based dip. Any fresh fruit is a terrific choice. Other good fruit choices include fruit canned in its own juice and unsweetened applesauce. Try to avoid fruit canned in syrups because they have unnecessary sugar added.

(10) Yogurt and cubed or sliced cheese are good dairy choices. Commercial milkshake products are not great options because they often contain a lot of sugar and calories. Milk or water is the best choice for something to drink.

(11) Try to involve your kids in selecting a variety of foods for their lunches. This will help them learn the importance of eating from different food groups — and improve the odds they will eat the lunch you packed!

(12) Pack a combination of fruits and vegetables, such as: baby carrots and celery slices; vegetable pieces with low-fat salad dressing dip; fresh fruit pieces with flavored yogurt for dipping; and individual fruit cups.

(13) When in season, provide whole fresh fruit, including apples, pears, plums, grapes, bananas, melon pieces, mango or kiwi slices (the list is endless).

(14) Good dessert choices can include: cookies, such as arrowroot, chocolate chip, oatmeal; granola or other cereal bars; small serving of pudding or yogurt.

(15) Make sure you include a healthy treat in your kids' lunches every day. Ask them to help you choose it, but try to sneak in a surprise now and then just for fun. Healthy treats include a high-fiber cereal or granola bar, a small homemade muffin, trail mix with unsalted seeds or nuts (if your school permits) and dried fruit, or a couple of plain cookies.

(16) See the lunch recipes in this book for other terrific ideas!

100% fruit juice

We encourage kids to drink less juice and more water. Many fruit beverages are not actually fruit juice. Fruit punches and fruit drinks contain little or no actual fruit juice and contribute mainly sugar to a child's diet.

While these products may boast providing 100% of daily requirements for vitamin C in each serving, the major ingredient is actually sugar. When you do choose juice as a drink for your son's or daughter's lunch, make sure it says 100% fruit juice on the packaging. Also keep in mind, a serving size of 1 box or 1 cup (250 mL) of juice is more than enough juice in a day for any school-age child.

Tips for making green lunches

In response to our desire to be more environmentally friendly, we thought it would be a good idea to outline some ideas for reducing waste in school lunches. Many schools have adopted litterless or waste-free lunch days to encourage parents and students to reduce the amount of waste at lunchtime. Many of these ideas not only help save the planet, but are also easy on the pocketbook as well.

1. No more baggies or plastic wrap. Purchase reusable containers to store sandwiches and snack foods. Many plastic containers are now available free of bisphosphonates, but for those who would rather avoid plastics altogether, there are stainless steel lunch containers available.
2. Buy in bulk or multi-serving packages for yogurt, crackers, cookies and dried fruit. As a matter of convenience, many parents opt for prepackaged individual servings of many foods, including cookies, crackers, chips and other snack foods, but these products include wasteful packaging. Again, make a one-time purchase of reusable containers.
3. No more tetra packs or juice pouches or cans of soda. Again, reusable containers only.
4. Consider buying reusable cutlery (preferably stainless steel and not plastic). Inexpensive sets can be found at the dollar store so that mom's good flatware doesn't accidentally end up in the trash bin.
5. Try reusable cloth napkins instead of paper. These can be brought home and washed rather than thrown out.

Family food diary
Snack saviors

In our house, my 7-year-old twin daughters come home from school hungry for a snack. Their first impulse is to run to the pantry where I keep the cookies and other snack foods and ask me for one of these treats. I usually let them choose one small snack out of this stock, but after this the girls are aware that anything more before dinnertime must be a healthy snack. Ideally, they would wait until dinner, but in practical terms, my husband doesn't get home until 5:30, and I am a big believer in eating as a family.

At these times, having fresh fruit and prepared raw vegetables handy is a savior. The girls' favorites are sliced cucumbers or carrots and celery sticks or cubes of watermelon. This ensures that they get at least one serving of veggies or fruit, and then, when they complain that they are not hungry at dinner or that they are full when they have seemingly eaten very little, they can be excused from the table and I do not need to worry that they have not eaten well. (*Joanne*)

Favorite recipes

Here are five of our favorite recipes for preschoolers and youngsters 4- to 6-years old, which you will find in the recipe section of this book.

- Multigrain Waffles with Warm Berry Sauce (page 142)
- Mushroom and Broccoli Stromboli (page 177)
- Miso-Glazed Haddock (page 221)
- Mixed Bean and Vegetable Salad (page 272)
- Banana Bread (page 311)

Top 10 Preschooler Nutrition Questions

❶ My 5-year-old daughter won't eat any vegetables. What should I do?

While having an aversion to one or two vegetables is common, it is unusual for a child to dislike all vegetables. Try preparing a vegetable with which your child is unfamiliar. Take your daughter shopping and ask her to pick out a vegetable that appeals to her. Try frozen instead of canned vegetables. Prepare vegetables with ingredients that change or embellish their flavor — adding a small amount of butter to green beans, for example, or low-sodium soy sauce to bok choy. Also, make sure that you are setting a good example by eating vegetables yourself. Regardless of whether these strategies are successful, do not force your child to eat her vegetables. Instead, continue to place a small quantity on her plate each day. It may take many exposures, but there's a good chance she'll eventually give in and sample the food.

❷ Is brown sugar or honey more nutritious than white sugar?

White sugar is produced from sugar cane or sugar beets. Brown sugar is granulated sugar that contains some molasses (refiner's sugar), while honey is a sweet syrup produced by bees. Each type of sweetener is a simple sugar or carbohydrate. All provide some calories, but none is more "nutritious" than the others, since they contain no vitamins or minerals. Regardless of their form, these sugars are best consumed in moderation.

❸ When is it okay to give my child soda pop?

Nutritionally speaking, there is no reason ever to give soda pop to a child, because these sugary carbonated beverages offer nothing more than "empty" calories and an increased risk of tooth decay. As a practical matter, however, school-aged children enjoy the flavor of soda pop, which is why it is often served at birthday parties and other special occasions. Allowing your child a small amount of pop at these events is fine, although consumption on daily basis is not. While there are no specific recommendations on the subject, we suggest that soda pop not be given to children under the age of 5 years.

❹ Every day I pack my son a lunch for school, but he often brings much of it home uneaten. What should I do?

Young children often respond unenthusiastically to a bagged lunch. As a result, they may bring food home at the end of the day. But this does not mean they are not eating at all. Ask your son why he is not eating his lunch. Is he trading with friends? This is not unusual, although you may want to find out what he is eating instead. Another question to ask your son is whether his lunch is too large for his appetite. There is also the possibility that he simply doesn't like the food you've given him. If this is the case, see page 40 for packed lunch ideas.

❺ My 6-year-old daughter won't eat breakfast. How can I convince her?

Breakfast is often referred to as the most important meal of the day. For many people who are rushed for time in the morning, it often consists of a granola bar, milk or juice, muffins, or fresh fruit. But there's no rule that says you have to restrict your breakfast to traditional choices. For example, leftovers from dinner the night before with a glass of milk will provide your daughter with the calories and energy she needs to get through the morning. Another strategy is to take your daughter with you to the grocery store and encourage her to pick out foods that she would enjoy for breakfast. Above all, make sure that you are setting a good example for your daughter by eating breakfast yourself.

6 My 5-year-old won't drink milk. How can I be sure he gets the nutrients he needs?

While government food guides recommend that preschoolers have 2 to 3 servings of milk per day, there is nothing that says it has to be plain milk. Like many children, your son may enjoy chocolate milk instead of the white variety. Also, cheese or yogurt are healthy alternatives to milk. And if your son refuses to drink milk but puts it on his cereal (as many children do), keep in mind that this amount (typically 4 to 6 oz/125 to 175 mL) represents $\frac{1}{2}$ serving of milk products.

7 Should I be giving my 6-year-old extra vitamin C when she is sick with a cold?

While vitamin C is required to help keep the immune system healthy, almost all vitamins and minerals play an important role as well. Enough vitamin C for a child can be found in one orange — supplying her full day's needs. Extra vitamin C will not be any benefit, according to the numerous studies that have researched this. The same is true for zinc, selenium and other nutrients, which can all be supplied by a balanced diet — by choosing foods according to *Canada's Food Guide* or the USDA's *MyPyramid* food guide and ensuring that enough fruits and vegetables are consumed daily.

8 Does my 6-year-old need more protein if he plays competitive soccer?

No. If his diet is varied, and includes foods from all of the food groups, he is likely getting enough protein to meet the needs of his increased activity. Most children get more than double the protein they need through their diet, and even with competitive sports, that would be enough to meet their needs.

9 At Halloween, my 6-year-old daughter came home with a shopping bag full of candy. I don't want her eating that huge quantity. What do you suggest?

Without a doubt, a full bag or two of candy is not appropriate for a young child to be eating, even if spread out over many days or weeks. One option would be to choose the favorite chocolates or chips and discard the chewier, plain sugar candies that can be harmful to young teeth. You can choose to offer a few sweets every few days. As in so many situations, moderation is the key. Do not let kids keep candy in their bedroom. Keep candy in the kitchen for a few days, and then discard whatever remains. Have your kids go through the bowl and throw out less favorite treats right after trick or treating.

10 I'm confused. Should I increase my son's exposure to the sun to produce more vitamin D or protect him from the sun to prevent skin disease?

Yes, exposure to the sun helps produce vitamin D, but that same exposure may lead to skin disease later in life. The ultraviolet rays of the sun at certain latitudes convert a cholesterol-like substance in the skin into vitamin D, which is then used in the body in its active form. This conversion in the skin will not occur, however, if the skin is covered with sunscreen. Those with darker skin color are also unable to form as much vitamin D as those with fairer skin.

So what should parents do? Experts recommend moderate exposure of unprotected skin to the sun without the skin turning red — for example, 10 to 20 minutes about two to three times per week, with sun exposure to face, arms and legs — and before 11:00 a.m. and after 3:00 p.m. (not in the hottest time of the day). However, people living in a northern climate cannot get adequate vitamin D delivered from the sun in cooler, darker months, and must rely on foods, chiefly cow's milk and fatty fish (trout, salmon, herring, tuna, shrimp, sardines) or supplements as sources of vitamin D. It is best to speak with your family physician about the recommend dose, but research indicates that a range of 400 to 1000 IU per day may be required.

CHAPTER 3

Feeding
Your 6- to 10-Year-Old

By the age of 6, children should have some basic knowledge of why healthy eating is important to everyone's well-being. Parents play a very large role in this education, as do teachers and caregivers. Children can begin to understand why some nutrients are important for their health. For example, children should be aware of the role calcium plays in keeping bones strong and healthy. They should also be able to identify which kinds of foods provide the needed nutrients. Reviewing Health Canada's food guide (page 64) and the United States Department of Agriculture (USDA) food guide (page 66) with your child is an excellent way to illustrate the need for a variety of nutrients from key food groups (see page 63). Encourage children to talk nutrition with friends at school or at their sport events. Help them search the Internet at a trustworthy health website for a topic every month — they can then keep a journal on particular nutrition- or health-related topics.

tip

Take it one step further. Most schools have monthly newsletters. Suggest that a monthly nutrition column be written by students and endorsed by their health teachers.

I'll do it my way

As children become more independent, they begin making decisions about many things, including what they would like for snacks and lunches. When it comes to lunchtime, eating is not the only focus that children may have. This is a time for socializing for prolonged periods, sometimes preventing enough time for eating. They are on their own for the first time, without a parent or caregiver coaxing them to eat. This can be a concern for some parents, but persevere. If you keep teaching them about the value of good nutrition, they will gain the skills they need for lifelong healthy eating.

Starting the day off right

Without a doubt, young children at this age need to start the day off with a healthy breakfast. While mornings are often rushed, this should not be at the expense of a healthy meal. Try not to fall back on the same breakfast every day. Cereal and milk can become boring. Here are some great ideas for adding variety to this fundamental meal:

- Scrambled, poached or boiled eggs with a slice of whole-grain toast, bagel or English muffin
- Oatmeal with yogurt and toasted pumpkin seeds sprinkled on top
- Fresh sliced fruit, also with yogurt and seeds
- French toast, pancakes or waffles topped with fresh mashed fruit or yogurt mixed with maple syrup
- Variety of whole-grain cereals (try mixing two together) with milk but low on sugar content
- Leftover protein-rich foods and a grain from supper the night before

Untouched lunch

Be prepared; many lunches will come back untouched. This can be quite discouraging, but do not give up! Kids do love to eat, but at this age, they like to have a say in what they eat. Ask your children what their friends are eating that they would like to try. Listening to their ideas on what makes a great lunch is sure to help reduce the returns. As with breakfast, prepare a variety of lunches. Include some protein, which will give them energy for longer periods than if they eat carbohydrate food sources alone. Here are a few ideas for preparing lunches that will be enjoyed:

- Boiled eggs with fresh whole-grain bread and slices of tomatoes
- Egg or tuna salad sandwich on whole-grain bread, roll or bagel or in a pita

> ## Hot lunches
>
> A hot lunch is always a delight as it breaks the monotony of a cold lunch — and warms up your child on a cold day. Soups, stew and chili all make for great meals. But how do you keep this food hot until lunch? Purchase a reliable stainless steel Thermos. Fill it with hot water, cover and let stand for 2 to 3 minutes, then discard the water. Once the Thermos itself has been heated, you can add the hot food, and the Thermos will keep it hot. Talk to other parents about which type of Thermos they are using.

- Wraps of veggies, tofu or beans, diced chicken or turkey
- Cut-up veggies and whole-grain bread with hummus
- Leftovers from supper, which may include soup, meatballs, pasta with meat sauce, cut-up pizza, quinoa with egg and edamame, salad (with cheese, or beans or lentils) with dressing on the side
- Fresh fruit, cut up for younger children, whole for older children
- Fresh vegetables with a favorite dip in separate container

Drink up!

Fluids are very important, not only for kids but also for adults, because, like their kids, they probably don't drink enough fluids. Just how much do kids need very day?

These recommendations for fluids for children take into account fluids from all food, drinks and water.

1 to 3 years
- 5 cups, or 1.3 liters, per day

4 to 8 years
- 7 cups, or 1.7 liters, per day

9 to 13 years
- $8^1/_2$ cups, or 2.1 liters, per day for females
- $9^1/_2$ cups, or 2.4 liters, per day for males

If children are involved in a sports activity, such as hockey or soccer, it is recommended that they drink about 1 cup (250 mL) of water about 1 hour before the game or practice, and then about $1/_2$ cup (125 mL) each 20 minutes or half hour. If it is a hot day and the activity is outside, then more frequent water breaks and more fluid is required during the event. It is especially important for kids to drink before their event to prevent dehydration.

Caffeine and kids

Recent research indicates that caffeine can be harmful to children's health. While caffeine is a natural ingredient found in some plants — like cacao, kola and tea — excess intake can cause irritability, nausea, increased heart

Sports drink overdose

While studies have shown that sports drinks do help kids drink more because they are also sweet with some added electrolytes, water and salty snacks, such as pretzels, work just as well. Kids often drink an excess of the sports drinks, which come in large bottles and have a large amount of sugar. These beverages make their way into daily snacks, providing excess calories. It is not necessary for young children to be routinely consuming these sports drinks on or off the field.

rate, increased cholesterol, decreased bone mineral density (increasing risk of fractures), mood changes, and anxiety.

For this reason, Health Canada recommends not more than:

- 45 mg a day for children ages 4 to 6
- 62.5 mg for children ages 7 to 9
- 85 mg for children ages 10 to 12

One to two 12 oz cans (355 mL) of cola a day would be the maximum amount of caffeine for kids. When trying to reduce or restrict caffeine, take into account caffeine from all drinks and foods. These may include soft drinks, tea, chocolate and cold coffee beverages, which are sometimes popular with children.

Sporting nutrition

On your mark, get set ... Two working parents. Soccer practice at 4:30? Hockey game at 5:00? Ballet lessons at 6:00? Wait, when do you fit in supper? Many parents and

Arena foods aren't winners

A big reason to prepare food at home before heading out to a sports event is that most sports arenas simply do not offer healthy food choices. Food items in the arena or at the field tend to have limited nutritional value and are often high in sugar, fat and salt. Chocolate bars or tacos with loads of melted cheese are not the best choices for young athletes, before or after a healthy workout on the field or ice.

Tips for managing the evening meal

We are both working moms, both with two young children in this age group. We face the meal challenges so many moms face on a day-to-day basis. Here are some meal strategies we use.

1. Organize most of meals at the beginning of the week by buying groceries required.
2. Buy foods that are easy to prepare. For example, fresh or frozen fish cooks up quickly. Drizzle a piece of trout with a honey garlic glaze, or simply sprinkle with olive oil and lemon and bake in the oven for a few minutes. Serve with prepared rice or quinoa.
3. Prepare some meals in advance and freeze them so they are ready to go when needed. Take out some homemade frozen soup, reheat and serve with a whole-grain roll or fresh bagel or pita.
4. Prepare quinoa or brown rice the night before and serve with firm tofu chunks, leftover chicken or beef slices.
5. Consider some carefully chosen prepared-food options from your favorite grocery store or local market.
6. Provide bottled water at home and in the car ride to the planned activity.

caregivers today feel the same time pinch. Kids arrive home from school, with homework to be done and a quick bite before that practice, game or lesson. Despite the anxiety, with the right planning and organization, supper can be provided in a quick and healthy way. Don't forget the fluids.

School meal programs

Research indicates that students who eat breakfast and are well nourished do better academically. They have longer attention spans and have been shown to have fewer academic and behavior problems than children who are hungry.

A recent Minnesota State study demonstrated that children who ate breakfast had higher scores in math and reading. Other studies have shown that children who are not hungry demonstrate less irritability, anxiety and aggression. Such children are also less likely to be late or absent from school.

In Canada, although there are no federally funded school breakfast or lunch programs, many schools do have cafeteria-style facilities that offer food choices at economical prices. It is up to parents and the school system to ensure that children are educated about making healthy food choices for themselves.

In the United States, there are federally funded breakfast and lunch programs, which are administered by Food and Nutrition Services of the United States Department of Agriculture (USDA). The mandate of these programs is to provide nutritionally balanced meals and snacks at low cost (or no cost) to children in public schools, not-for-profit private schools and residential childcare facilities. Both programs must meet the recommendations of the Dietary Guidelines for Americans, which state that no more of 30% of the day's calories come from fat and no more than 10% of the day's calories come from saturated fat.

Critical nutrients

While all nutrients are important to a child's health, one study of children's intakes at daycare has suggested that the nutrients of greatest concern were iron, zinc and energy. See pages 74 and 84 for information on foods that contain adequate amounts of iron and zinc.

Lunch program

The US National School Lunch Program (NSLP) provides lunches and snacks to even more children than the school breakfast program. In 2000, the NSLP provided nutritionally balanced lunches and snacks to more than 27 million children each day. The lunches must provide at least one-third of the Daily Reference Intake (DRI) for energy, protein, iron and calcium, as well as vitamins A and C. Although these school lunches must meet federal nutrition requirements, the school boards or institutions themselves are able to make their own decisions about specific foods to serve.

Family food diary

Kids on the go!

Both of my children (ages 11 and 10) play a variety of sports. Whether we are off to a soccer field or driving across the city to a hockey arena, we need some "fast" food to keep energy levels up for the games or practices. Our version of fast food includes these mini meals on the go:

- Quinoa mixed with edamame and yellow peppers
- Hummus with pita bread
- Feta cheese and tomatoes
- Bagels with lox and cream cheese
- Homemade bean soup
- Smoothies made with berries and yogurt
- Fresh fruits and vegetables — sliced apples or pears, berries, cut-up peppers, carrots and cucumbers
- Water always accompanies the car ride to make sure the kids are well hydrated well before the sports event

(Daina)

The School Breakfast Program started in 1966 as a pilot project and has been a permanent program since 1975. It is currently available in more than 72,000 schools and institutions across the US. As mandated by the program, the breakfast must provide at least one-quarter of the recommended dietary allowances (RDAs) for energy, protein, calcium and iron, as well as vitamins A and C. In the year 2000, the School Breakfast Program provided a morning meal each day to an average of 7.55 million American children. In 2001, Congress appropriated US$1.5 billion for the school breakfast program.

Food to go

Traveling with a young child can be a wonderful experience, but it can also presents many challenges — not the least of which is ensuring that their nutritional needs are being met throughout the duration of the trip. The possible effects of food and water from unfamiliar sources may also cause problems. Still, you shouldn't let these things keep you at home. Here are some practical tips on how to feed your child when traveling.

Tips for eating while traveling

Water

Depending on your destination, you may have to purchase bottled water. Always check the water safety of any country you are visiting — and remember that the quality of water is not guaranteed just because it's in a bottle. Be sure to purchase bottled water from a reliable source. Even if the drinking water is considered safe, you may want to purchase bottled water. Your travel agent should be able to provide information on the water in the area. Keep in mind that water quality can vary even between different parts of the US and Canada.

Fresh fruits and vegetables

Traveling is a good opportunity to try different fruits and vegetables with your child. If you are unsure about the quality of the drinking water in the area, peel the fruit or vegetables before serving. Even in a restaurant, the vegetables used in a salad (for example) may not have been rinsed with "safe water." When in a foreign country where food contamination is a risk, be careful of the food choices you make when eating out.

Food for car trips

Ensure that you always have some snacks to offer, because mealtimes may not be as regular as they are at home. Try bringing containers of your child's favorite cereal mix or plain cookies. Offer plenty of fluids, especially in hot weather. (You may forget to drink adequate fluids yourself and not be aware of your child's fluid needs.) For younger children, provide fluids in a spill-proof cup. The best foods to bring are those that are easy to eat and not too messy, such as soft cheese, cookies and fruit pieces. To minimize the risk of choking,

---

Relieving the pressure

When the plane in which they are traveling is landing or descending, some young children may experience earaches as the pressure in the cabin is adjusted. Try to offer a beverage during this part of the travel so your child is swallowing constantly, which may help to prevent the pressure changes from causing any problems. Older children can be offered gum to keep them chewing and swallowing.

Gather round the table

Families who eat together tend to eat better. Studies show that when children and their parents sit down to a meal together, more vegetables and fruits are consumed. More healthy grains and calcium-rich foods are also eaten in greater amounts than when children eat alone. Given that the recent Canadian Community Health Survey (2004) and the Heart and Stroke Foundation Survey (2009) showed that 70% to 85% of children (and 50% of adults) do not eat enough fruits and vegetables (and take in more than double the amount of sodium and less than half the fiber needed), it seems that one solution would be to eat together to help improve intake of fruits and vegetables. An increase in fruits and vegetables would help to lower sodium intake and increase fiber intake, a benefit to the whole family.

Family food diary
Sit-down meals

I am a big believer in the family meal and its importance at the end of the school or work day. My husband and I make it a priority to eat as a family as often as possible during the week, and we schedule after-school activities so that they do not interfere with the family meal. The benefits of family mealtime include allowing time to connect with my kids and review what's been happening in their day, and ensuring that they are eating healthy, well-balanced meals without relying on fast food or takeout. My kids do have activities on average two nights a week, so on those nights I try to make sure that whatever we are eating is something quick and simple, usually a chili or a slow cooker meal that I can put together in a pinch. *(Joanne)*

make sure someone is observing your child while he or she is snacking. If possible, stop the car before consuming snacks. It is always handy to keep wet wipes in the car.

Shopping for food with your kids

One great way to engage kids in the food planning — and in discovering how to combine foods so that there is lots of variety and many choices at home — is to take them shopping. Label reading can be a part of this outing. Parents can suggest to their children to pick out their favorite cereals, crackers or nut butters and have them compare different products to see which have less sodium, more fiber, less sugar and the lowest calories. Challenge them to pick the healthier choice.

Favorite recipes

Here are five of our favorite recipes for children 6 to 10 years old, which you will find in the recipe section of this book.

- Best Breakfast Berry Scones (page 156)
- Tofu in Sesame Crust (page 201)
- Delicious Halibut in Fresh Cilantro Sauce (page 222)
- Best Chicken Curry (page 242)
- Quick and Easy Bok Choy Stir-Fry (page 282)

Top 10 Children's Nutrition Questions

1 What is a nutritious meal that I can give my daughter in the car on our way to her hockey game?

Try to include a protein and a carbohydrate source. Great options include warm soup or pasta in a Thermos, leftover pizza, a yogurt smoothie, nut butter on a pita, cheese slices on a whole-grain bagel, dried fruit and nut mixture or quinoa salad with tofu or chicken. Always include water and some fruit slices too, for both before and after the game.

2 How do I convince my 8-year-old son that he should eat his lunch every day? It seems to come back almost untouched most of the time.

This is a common concern that many parents may face. Often children have limited time to eat because they are very busy socializing and sharing stories. You can discuss what happens in the lunch room with your children, and ask if they have any preferences for lunches, finding out which foods that their friends are eating appeal to them. Try sending half of a sandwich or a smaller portion of pasta or grain salad along with sliced-up fruits and vegetables and homemade desserts for snacks. Try colorful reusable cutlery and containers. Fun notes in the lunch bag from mom or dad always bring a smile to kids' faces, and gives them another reason to open that lunch bag with anticipation. Variety is important. Let your child help choose what goes in the lunch.

3 How much water should my 8-year-old be drinking every day?

Children between the ages of 4 and 8 years need a total of 7 cups (1.7 L) of fluid per day from all fluid sources and foods. To ensure that fluid intake is adequate, provide 3 to 4 cups (750 mL to 1 L) of water daily, but in hotter weather or during increased exercise or activity, offer water before, during and after the event.

4 How can I get my 7-year-old daughter to try a new food?

Trying new foods can be an exciting adventure, opening up possibilities for many more food choices. Encourage your daughter to at least lick or take a small bite of a new food. While she won't enjoy every food, encouraging a taste will help her discover different flavors.

5 I would love to get my child to help me more in the kitchen, but I think that at 6 years of age he is too young. What do you suggest?

You can certainly have your son start to help measure out proportions in a measuring cup or using measuring spoons. You can also get him to help slice a cucumber or a soft pear with your close supervision. One simple meal that your child can help with is scrambled eggs. He can mix the eggs and milk, and pour the mixture into the pan with supervision. Rules should be made about allowing this only in the presence of an adult or another caregiver.

6 I have read that probiotics can help my child recover from diarrhea. Is this true? Should I buy foods that contain probiotics for my child?

Treating diarrhea in children, especially if more severe, requires special attention to replacing fluids and electrolytes. Special solutions are available for this purpose, and you should get guidance from your physician on which products to use.

But yes, there is some evidence to suggest that probiotics may help decrease the duration of diarrhea and help restore normal bowel habits. These kinds of studies are done with known amounts of probiotics in a study setting, but the products that are found on store shelves are not yet regulated, so there is no way to know if they contain the amounts described on the package. More research is needed to help ascertain which type of probiotics can help improve health issues such as diarrhea, and how much of them is appropriate. For now, you can safely include food products to which probiotics have been added in your child's regular diet. Yogurts fortified with probiotics contain other important nutrients, such as calcium and protein, so this is a healthy choice overall.

7 What's the difference between a milk allergy and lactose intolerance? The terms seem interchangeable.

Although these conditions are both associated with cow's milk and milk products and present similar digestive symptoms, most notably gastrointestinal upset, they are distinct. Like all food allergies, cow's milk allergy is an immune reaction to a protein, whereas lactose intolerance results from a deficiency of the lactase enzyme. Cow's milk allergy is relatively common, while lactose intolerance is rare. The allergy can be treated by avoiding cow's milk products and substituting other food sources of calcium and other essential nutrients. Lactose deficiency can be managed by consuming lactose-free milk, taking lactase enzyme supplements or avoiding cow's milk products. If you suspect your child has one of these conditions, see your doctor for a proper diagnosis and treatment management.

8 Which foods will provide more fiber for my 9-year-old son? I hear that kids are not getting enough in their diet.

Many children and adults are not getting enough fiber in their diet. Offering the following foods in meals and snacks will help ensure an adequate intake of fiber, but remember, drinking fluids at each meal and snack and during active sports events is important as well. Foods that are high in fiber include berries, whole-grain cereals and breads, and beans, lentils, nuts and seeds. See page 59 for more information on fiber.

9 I am trying to get my 9-year-old daughter to gain weight, as her pediatrician mentioned that she is about 5 pounds (2.5 kg) lighter than she should be for her height and her age. What suggestions do you have?

Recommendations for increasing energy in a diet in a healthy way include using whole milk instead of lower-fat varieties, offering nuts and seeds with snacks, adding extra butter or oil to vegetables or pasta or other dishes, offering cream soups instead of clear ones, and offering dips with vegetables and fruits, such as higher-fat yogurts for fruit and cheesy dressings for vegetables. Spreads mixed with avocado or higher-fat hummus dips are also healthy higher-energy snack options.

10 Are video games that involve activity good for my child?

While video games that get your kids moving around are better than those that do not require movement, they are still no replacement for actual physical activity. A real game of tennis, for example, will increase your child's heart rate far more than the video game version of a tennis game can ever do.

CHAPTER 4

Essential
Foods and Nutrients

What we eat and drink provides us with the essential elements of life and health. They provide us with the raw materials that our bodies need to function and, particularly in the case of young children, to grow. In this chapter we look at the basic components of food and how each is important to your child's well-being.

Food as fuel

For children, calories are a measure of the energy their young bodies need to grow and develop normally. Energy is required by the body for a variety of reasons. It is used for muscular work, to fuel the brain and nervous system, and to make and repair body tissues. The nutrients in food — specifically, carbohydrate, protein and fat — are metabolized by the body to release usable energy.

We all need a constant supply of food to meet our body's energy needs for survival. Compared to adults, children require more energy per unit of body weight. This is because energy is needed not only for basic body functions (as it is for adults), but for growth as well. Factors that affect total energy needs include sex, age, overall body composition (relative proportions of fat and muscle in the body), nutritional status (for example, normal weight, underweight or overweight), levels of physical activity, hours of sleep, fever — even climate. All of these energy needs must be met by the food we eat.

If the supply of food energy matches the body's requirements, we achieve an energy balance. But if the food

Measuring metabolism

How do we know how many calories a child requires daily? There are a variety of techniques for determining energy requirements, most of which involve measuring the process of metabolism itself. For example, we know that in order to metabolize a given quantity of energy, the body will take in a certain amount of oxygen and release a certain amount of carbon dioxide. By measuring the quantity of these gases inhaled/exhaled over a specific time, and by performing these measurements on a number of subjects within a particular group (selected by age or sex, for example), the average energy requirements can be determined for that group.

How much energy does your child need?

Daily energy requirements per unit of body weight

AGE (YEARS)	ENERGY (KCAL/KG)	ENERGY (KCAL/LB)
0 to 2	101	46
2 to 3	94	43
4 to 6	100	45

energy is greater than our needs, the excess is stored in the body as fat. This is why exercise is such an important factor in helping children to achieve an energy balance.

To calculate your child's energy requirements, use the table shown above. For example, an average 4-year-old child with a weight of 16.5 kg (36 lbs), requires about 16.5 kg x 100 kcal/kg, or 1600 calories, to meet his or her daily energy needs. (Boys and girls have about the same energy needs per unit of body weight until they reach the age of 7 years.)

Powerful proteins

Proteins are part of the living tissue in the body. Built from long chains of amino acids, they serve as the building blocks from which components of cells are constructed, as well as for antibodies, enzymes and hormones.

Most protein is found in muscle tissue, with the remainder found in the soft tissues, bones, teeth and blood. Certain components of protein can only be delivered to the body through the diet. The quality of the protein, then, is of great importance. Once proteins are broken down by the body's digestive system, they are absorbed as amino acids into the body and are used for many different body functions, including building and repair of tissues, fighting infections, providing a source of energy and transporting other substances.

During growth, protein needs per unit of body weight are high for infants and children. If protein intake is very low, fat and carbohydrate (assuming an adequate supply) can act to spare the need for protein as energy.

Good protein sources

- Eggs
- Chicken
- Fish
- Beef
- Beans
- Tofu
- Quinoa
- Nuts
- Seeds
- Milk
- Cheese

Protein endurance

Protein is not only important for growth and cell maintenance, but protein also helps someone feel full longer, providing lasting energy. This is especially important for children in school where they need sustained energy for learning, such as developing math and language skills. Including a source of protein at all meals and some snacks will enable a child to sustain energy for longer periods.

How much protein does your child need?

Daily protein requirements

AGE	PROTEIN (TOTAL GRAMS PER DAY)
1–3 years	13
4–8 years	19
9–13 years	34

Generally, the typical diet of North American children provides more than double the amount of protein they actually require. Vegetarians are a possible exception, however, particularly in terms of the quality (if not quantity) of protein they consume to meet their needs. (See Chapter 6 for more information on vegetarian diets.)

Do athletic children need more protein?

Athletic children need more energy than those who are less active. Their protein needs are slightly higher as well. However, the majority of all children receive more than enough protein daily for growth and activity.

Fats and essential fatty acids

Fat is an important source of energy for growing children, and should provide a minimum of 30% to 35% of their total calories. (See page 129 for more information on fat requirements.) The fats we get from our food include many compounds that are required for maintaining the structure and function of cells in the body. Fatty acids are the smallest part of fat. They are a vital source of energy and provide most of the calories from dietary fat. Fat is an important source of energy for growing children and should provide 30% to 35% of their total daily calories.

Depending on their chemical structure, fatty acids are generally classified as either saturated or unsaturated. Most saturated fats come from animal products and are solid when they are at room temperature. Polyunsaturated fats are liquid at room temperature, and are derived from vegetable sources, as well as from fish.

Short on omega-3

Research shows that some children in North America are not eating enough foods that contain omega-3 fatty acids. Only 16% to 22% of children receive an adequate amount in their diet. Having adequate amounts of omega-3 fatty acids may be protective against asthma and may help decrease symptoms of asthma in children. One way to get more of these important fatty acids is by serving up fatty fish at least twice a week. Salmon, trout and sardines are great options.

Linolenic acid (or omega-3) and linoleic acid (or omega-6) are "essential" fatty acids, which means that they cannot be synthesized by the body and have to be provided in the diet. Both are unsaturated fatty acids.

Omega-3 fatty acid is relatively well known by most health-conscious adults, since it has the effect of lowering levels of LDL cholesterol (the bad cholesterol). But what about children?

A diet that includes fish (such as salmon and tuna) and vegetable oils (such as soy and canola), as well as leafy vegetables, will meet all their requirements for omega-3 fatty acid. Children may benefit later in life if they get in the habit of eating these omega-3-rich foods and following a healthier diet.

Carbohydrates

Carbohydrates from food are a main source of energy for children and adults. They make up about 45% to 65% of total energy intake. Carbohydrates are found in breads, grains and cereals, legumes, fruits and vegetables, and milk. Simple carbohydrates, or sugars, found in candies, soda pop and cakes and pastries provide shorter-lasting energy than more nutrient-rich, complex carbohydrates like polysaccharides.

Increasing dietary fiber

Dietary fiber is a component of plant-based food that is not completely broken down in the digestive tract. This happens because we do not have all of the enzymes necessary to digest fiber (as we do for other parts of the foods we eat, such as protein, fat and other carbohydrates). Fiber is contained in many foods, and includes cellulose, pectin, lignins and other undigestible carbohydrates.

Dietary fiber is categorized as either soluble or insoluble. Soluble fiber is found in fruits, some legumes, and grains such as oats, rye and barley. This type of fiber dissolves in water to form a gel. This gel

Are there disadvantages to a high-fiber diet?

High fiber intakes may decrease the amount of certain minerals available for absorption. This is because high-fiber foods often contain phytates — compounds that can bind with minerals, such as iron or calcium, and make them less available to the body. That being said, the risks of vitamin or mineral deficiency are vastly outweighed by the potential health benefits of eating a diet high in fiber. In fact, adults who live a vegetarian lifestyle (and who consume a diet very high in fiber) typically don't suffer from vitamin or mineral deficiencies.

helps to slow the rate at which food passes through the digestive system and helps to increase the absorption of certain nutrients in the foods we eat. Soluble fiber is also known to help lower LDL cholesterol levels.

Insoluble fiber is found in vegetables and wheat bran. This type of fiber absorbs water and helps to increase the volume of stool. It also helps to increase the movement of material through the colon and makes stool easier to pass.

Why kids need fiber

Most adults understand the need for fiber in their own diets, but dietary fiber has important health benefits for kids as well. A fiber-rich diet can help prevent constipation, which is a frequent cause for referral to a pediatrician. Studies have shown that children who consume sufficient quantities of fiber also have better intakes of vitamins and minerals, including vitamins A and E, folate, iron and magnesium. On the other hand, where their diet is low in fiber, children have been shown to have higher intakes of dietary fat and cholesterol. A low-fiber diet may also increase a child's risk of developing in later life chronic conditions such as obesity, hyperlipidemia (a risk factor for cardiovascular disease) and adult onset (type 2) diabetes.

Yet the fact is that a great many North American children — about 50%, according to some studies — are not getting enough dietary fiber. So how much fiber should your child be eating?

tip

To prevent childhood constipation, make sure your kids are getting enough fiber in their diet. Choose foods that contain 4 grams or more of fiber per serving.

How to meet the daily fiber requirements of a 6-year-old

MEAL	FOOD	SERVING SIZE	FIBER (GRAMS)
Breakfast	Bran cereal with raisins	3/4 cup (175 mL)	5
	Whole wheat toast	1 slice	3
Lunch	Roasted red pepper hummus	1/4 cup (60 mL)	3
	Whole wheat pita	1	2
	Pear	1	4
Dinner	Chili	1 cup (250 mL)	6
	Blueberries	1/2 cup (125 mL)	2
Total			25 g

How much fiber does your child need?

AGE	FIBER (TOTAL GRAMS PER DAY)
1–3 years	19
4–8 years	25
9–13 years male	31
9–13 years female	26

How to increase the fiber in your child's diet

In many cases, if your child isn't getting enough fiber, then neither is the rest of the family. So start taking steps to increase everyone's fiber consumption by serving more fiber-rich fruits and vegetables, as well as legumes, cereals and other grains.

As always, of course, be sure that you keep your diet in balance. Consult the USDA's or Canada's food guide for suggestions about choosing the foods that will provide enough fiber to meet the recommendation without sacrificing calories or other nutrients. (See pages 64 and 66.) Remember that although milk, milk products and meats are low in dietary fiber, they remain an important source of other nutrients, including energy, protein, calcium, vitamin D, iron and zinc.

Start by adding one or more servings of fiber-rich foods per day. The key here is to increase the amount of fiber gradually. Keep in mind that while fresh fruits and vegetables are great sources of fiber, fruit and vegetable juices are not. Try switching from white breads and processed cereals to whole grains, breads and cereals. Legumes (such as dried peas and beans) are also a great source of fiber. See if you can include them in your family's diet at least once a week.

No quick fiber fix

A number of commercial products claim to provide a quick and easy way to add more fiber to your diet. But these supplements — whether pills or powders — are no substitute for the fiber contained in foods. This is particularly true for children.

Kid-friendly fiber-containing foods

Offer your children whole-grain cereals and breads, as well as vegetables and fruit. A diet with adequate fiber for children should not exclude energy-dense foods (such as cheese or milk, which are low in fiber) or exclude any one particular food group.

- Whole-grain breads
- Whole-grain pasta
- Legumes (black beans, black-eyed peas and kidney beans)
- Vegetables
- Fruit (especially berries, pears and apples with the skins on)
- Dried fruit (raisins or apricots)
- Whole-grain cereals
- Nuts and seeds

Finally, in order to avoid gas, bloating or the other complaints occasionally associated with high-fiber diets, be sure that your child consumes more water (or other fluids) as the amount of fiber in his or her diet increases.

Probiotic and prebiotic protection

Probiotics are live organisms (usually bacteria) found in fermented foods, particularly in yogurt, that can affect the growth of "good" bacteria in the intestinal tract. The most common probiotics come from two different families of bacteria, known as lactobacilli and bifidobacteria.

Everyone has trillions of gut microorganisms in their intestines. These microorganisms enter the intestines soon after birth and provide a strong defense mechanism against harmful microbial pathogens entering our bodies and blood stream. In other words, probiotics enhance this defense system.

Prebiotics are undigested parts of fiber called oligosaccharides that nourish probiotics. The most common examples of prebiotics include inulin (from chicory root) and FOS (fructooligosaccharide). Inulin is found naturally in many fruits and vegetables, but chicory root is an especially rich source. Fructooligosaccharide (FOS), also known as oligofructose or oligofructan, is synthesized enzymatically from sucrose.

Prebiotics are now being added to foods such as yogurts, infant cereals and breads. Many popular brands of infant cereals are now adding inulin and/or FOS to their infant cereals.

Storing probiotic foods

If you are going to try foods that contain probiotics, such as yogurt, here are some tips to ensure that these living organisms do not die prematurely:

- Refrigerate the product after opening
- Use the product as soon as possible after opening
- Use the product as close to the manufactured date as possible

Good for kids?

In children, probiotics may help in reducing or preventing viral diarrhea, in helping decrease incidence of allergy and in helping reduce antibiotic-associated diarrhea. Probiotics may also promote regularity and restore the "balance of the digestive bacteria." There is some evidence that probiotics may reduce stool frequency and duration of diarrhea. In some studies, young infants who were not breastfeeding benefited from probiotic-containing formula. Probiotics have been used in infant formula in Europe for many years, and there are several research studies looking at the use of probiotics to treat colic in infants. However, there is no substantive research that suggests probiotics should be used on a routine basis for children, and there are no recommendations from pediatric societies on how much probiotics children need or what amount is considered safe.

Using the food guides

In both the United States and Canada, health authorities have devised charts that recommend a range of servings from each of the four food groups. Whether it's *MyPyramid* in the United States or *Eating Well with Canada's Food Guide*, the message is very much the same: Enjoy a variety of healthy foods every day, and keep high-sugar and other non-nutritious foods to a minimum.

The four food groups are described briefly below, followed by the charts themselves.

- **Grains** are an essential source of carbohydrates, vitamins and minerals, and provide fiber as well.
- **Vegetables and fruits** provide another variety of carbohydrates, vitamins (particularly vitamin C) and minerals, as well as fiber.
- **Milk and alternatives** provide a balance of proteins, carbohydrates and fats, and are an important source of calcium and vitamin D.
- **Meat and alternatives** are an important source of proteins, fats, vitamins and minerals (particularly iron).

Understanding food labels

When you buy commercially prepared food, how do you find out what's in it? Chances are you'll look at the nutritional information printed on the label or package. Most of us take this information for granted today, but it wasn't many years ago that food manufacturers were only required to list ingredients. Now we're provided with the number of calories per serving, as well as the amount of carbohydrates, protein and fat. Micronutrients, such as vitamins and minerals, are also listed. This allows consumers to choose foods that are lower in salt by checking the amount of sodium per serving.

tip
Take time to sit down with your kids to review food guides. They are available online and are interactive, making it fun to learn about nutrition.

Look for the daily value (DV)

The % DV on food labels gives consumers an idea of how much of a specific nutrient is available in a serving of the packaged food.

Eating Well with Canada's Food Guide

Recommended Number of *Food Guide Servings* per Day

		Children		Teens		Adults			
Age in Years	2-3	4-8	9-13	14-18		19-50		51+	
Sex		Girls and Boys		Females	Males	Females	Males	Females	Males
Vegetables and Fruit	4	5	6	7	8	7-8	8-10	7	7
Grain Products	3	4	6	6	7	6-7	8	6	7
Milk and Alternatives	2	2	3-4	3-4	3-4	2	2	3	3
Meat and Alternatives	1	1	1-2	2	3	2	3	2	3

What is One Food Guide Serving?
Look at the examples below.

Fresh, frozen or canned vegetables
125 mL (½ cup)

Bread
1 slice (35 g)

Bagel
½ bagel (45 g)

Milk or powdered milk (reconstituted)
250 mL (1 cup)

Cooked fish, shellfish, poultry, lean meat
75 g (2 ½ oz.)/125 mL (½ cup)

The chart above shows how many Food Guide Servings you need from each of the four food groups every day.

Having the amount and type of food recommended and following the tips in *Canada's Food Guide* will help:

• Meet your needs for vitamins, minerals and other nutrients.
• Reduce your risk of obesity, type 2 diabetes, heart disease, certain types of cancer and osteoporosis.
• Contribute to your overall health and vitality.

For the full guide, please contact Health Canada or visit their website.

SOURCE: Health Canada. Used with permission.

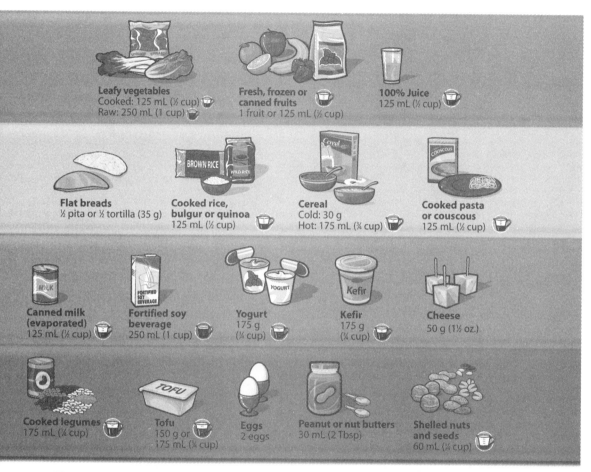

Leafy vegetables
Cooked: 125 mL (½ cup)
Raw: 250 mL (1 cup)

Fresh, frozen or canned fruits
1 fruit or 125 mL (½ cup)

100% Juice
125 mL (½ cup)

Flat breads
½ pita or ½ tortilla (35 g)

Cooked rice, bulgur or quinoa
125 mL (½ cup)

Cereal
Cold: 30 g
Hot: 175 mL (¾ cup)

Cooked pasta or couscous
125 mL (½ cup)

Canned milk (evaporated)
125 mL (½ cup)

Fortified soy beverage
250 mL (1 cup)

Yogurt
175 g
(¾ cup)

Kefir
175 g
(¾ cup)

Cheese
50 g (1½ oz.)

Cooked legumes
175 mL (¾ cup)

Tofu
150 g or
175 mL (¾ cup)

Eggs
2 eggs

Peanut or nut butters
30 mL (2 Tbsp)

Shelled nuts and seeds
60 mL (¼ cup)

Oils and Fats

- Include a small amount – 30 to 45 mL (2 to 3 Tbsp) – of unsaturated fat each day. This includes oil used for cooking, salad dressings, margarine and mayonnaise.
- Use vegetable oils such as canola, olive and soybean.
- Choose soft margarines that are low in saturated and trans fats.
- Limit butter, hard margarine, lard and shortening.

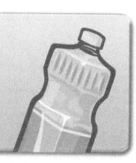

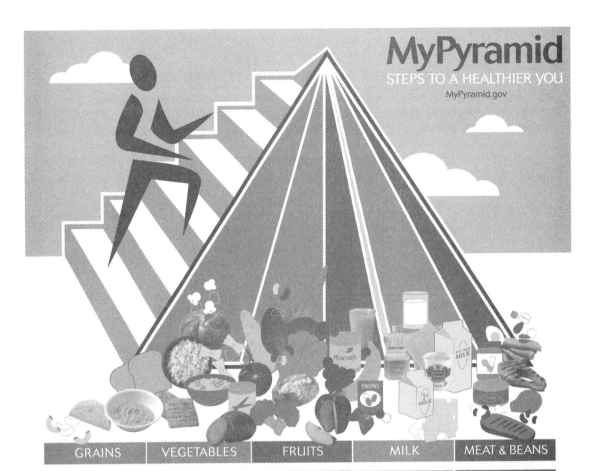

MyPyramid
STEPS TO A HEALTHIER YOU
MyPyramid.gov

GRAINS	VEGETABLES	FRUITS	MILK	MEAT & BEANS
GRAINS Make half your grains whole	**VEGETABLES** Vary your veggies	**FRUITS** Focus on fruits	**MILK** Get your calcium-rich foods	**MEAT & BEANS** Go lean with protein
Eat at least 3 oz. of whole-grain cereals, breads, crackers, rice, or pasta every day 1 oz. is about 1 slice of bread, about 1 cup of breakfast cereal, or ½ cup of cooked rice, cereal, or pasta	Eat more dark-green veggies like broccoli, spinach, and other dark leafy greens Eat more orange vegetables like carrots and sweetpotatoes Eat more dry beans and peas like pinto beans, kidney beans, and lentils	Eat a variety of fruit Choose fresh, frozen, canned, or dried fruit Go easy on fruit juices	Go low-fat or fat-free when you choose milk, yogurt, and other milk products If you don't or can't consume milk, choose lactose-free products or other calcium sources such as fortified foods and beverages	Choose low-fat or lean meats and poultry Bake it, broil it, or grill it Vary your protein routine — choose more fish, beans, peas, nuts, and seeds

For a 2,000-calorie diet, you need the amounts below from each food group. To find the amounts that are right for you, go to MyPyramid.gov.

Eat 6 oz. every day	Eat 2½ cups every day	Eat 2 cups every day	Get 3 cups every day; for kids aged 2 to 8, it's 2	Eat 5½ oz. every day

Find your balance between food and physical activity
- Be sure to stay within your daily calorie needs.
- Be physically active for at least 30 minutes most days of the week.
- About 60 minutes a day of physical activity may be needed to prevent weight gain.
- For sustaining weight loss, at least 60 to 90 minutes a day of physical activity may be required.
- Children and teenagers should be physically active for 60 minutes every day, or most days.

Know the limits on fats, sugars, and salt (sodium)
- Make most of your fat sources from fish, nuts, and vegetable oils.
- Limit solid fats like butter, stick margarine, shortening, and lard, as well as foods that contain these.
- Check the Nutrition Facts label to keep saturated fats, trans fats, and sodium low.
- Choose food and beverages low in added sugars. Added sugars contribute calories with few, if any, nutrients.

MyPyramid.gov
STEPS TO A HEALTHIER YOU

U.S. Department of Agriculture
Center for Nutrition Policy and Promotion
April 2005
CNPP-15

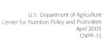

The % daily value (DV) indicates what percentage of the recommended daily amount of a given nutrient (iron, for example) is contained per serving. (Note that the % daily value is based on adult requirements, not on children's needs.)

Health claims

Food labels provide nutrient information in a standardized format, and will allow certain health-related claims where warranted (and backed by research). For example, a product containing a good source of calcium (along with vitamin D) may be allowed to display the health claim that calcium is good for bones and may help prevent osteoporosis. Other approved nutrition claims include "a low-sodium diet reduces the risk of high blood pressure"; "a diet that includes plenty of fruits and vegetables reduces the risk of some types of cancer"; and "diets low in saturated and trans fats reduce the risk of heart disease." Manufacturers of food products cannot make claims about their products unless they are proven to be true.

Not listed

A standard nutrition label appears on all suitable food products, with 13 nutrients listed, in the nutrition facts label, that have been determined by government health authorities to be most important to our health. However, there are many other nutrients in foods not listed on food labels that contribute to overall health.

Foods that do not require a label include fresh fruits and vegetables, and fresh meats, poultry and fish. Because regulations do not require these fresh foods to be labeled, consumers are not given the opportunity at the store to see what rich nutrients are found in these foods.

Other foods prepared for takeout, such as salads and sandwiches, also do not require labeling, nor do foods prepared in a bakery or by a restaurant.

Orders of magnitude

When reading the list of ingredients in a product, remember that they are listed in decreasing order of quantity used in the product. This is a good way to judge which cereals, for example, have a higher proportion of sugar relative to other (more healthful) ingredients.

Government regulation

The Food and Drug Administration in the United States and the Canadian Food Inspection Agency have strict labeling guidelines regulating the kind of information that must be included on a food label.

What if an orange had a label?

So what if an orange had a label? This is what it would look like:

NUTRITION FACTS PER 1 MEDIUM ORANGE		
Calories	69	
Fat	0.21 g	
Cholesterol	0 g	
Sodium	1 mg	0% DV
Potassium		
Carbohydrate	18 g	
Fiber	3.1 g	12.4% DV
Sugars	12 g	
Protein	1.3 g	
Vitamin A	346 IU	10% DV
Vitamin C	82.7 mg	138% DV
Calcium	60 mg	5.5% DV
Iron	0.18 mg	1% DV

Note: The orange is low in calories but is a good source of fiber and an excellent source of vitamins A and C. While the orange does have sugars listed, that does not mean that they are "bad" sugars. They are naturally occurring in the orange, providing a healthy source of energy along with other nutrients. The label does not reveal all the other phytonutrients (chemical components of plants that have many health benefits) and other possible elements that make it a nutrient-rich food choice.

Nutrient claims

Manufacturers in Canada and the United States are permitted to make specific nutrient claims, but they sometimes differ. For example:

Low sodium = 140 mg or less per serving (both countries)

High fiber = 4 mg (Canada) and 5 mg (America) or more

These nutrient claims help consumers identify foods that are higher in nutrients that should be restricted, such as sodium and cholesterol, and foods with nutrients that should be increased, such as fiber and vitamin C.

% daily value

The % daily value (DV) presented on labels is based on Daily Reference Intake (DRI) values for adults. For example, the reference used for sodium is 2400 mg per day, which is the upper limit for adults. If a product has 500 mg per serving, the % DV would be 500 divided by 2400, or 21%. That product would provide 21% of the maximum recommended level of sodium that adults should consume daily.

However, the reference for sodium for children is quite different. For example, the amount of daily sodium intake for a 3-year-old should be no more than 1000 mg. So that same product with 500 mg would provide that 3-year-old with 50% of the daily sodium need.

Child-friendly label conversions

Here we have charted the % daily value (DV) of key nutrients for adults and the age-graduated Dietary Reference Intake (DRI) values for children.

NUTRIENT	% DV ADULT	DRI FOR CHILDREN 2–3 YEARS	DRI FOR CHILDREN 4–8 YEARS	DRI FOR CHILDREN 9–13 YEARS
Sodium	2400 mg	1000–1500 mg	1200–1900 mg	1500–2200 mg
Iron	14 mg	7 mg	10 mg	8 mg
Calcium	1100 mg	500 mg	800 mg	1300 mg

Quick recipe nutrient calculation

You can use this conversion principle to calculate the % of a specific nutrient provided by our recipes. Simply look up a recipe and divide the nutrient by the recommended value, multiply by 100 and you get the % daily value of that nutrient our recipe provides per serving for your child.

Comparison of DV reference values in Canada and America

Note the difference for reference values for calcium, iron and vitamin A between these two countries.

NUTRIENTS	CANADIAN REFERENCE VALUE	AMERICAN REFERENCE VALUE
Sodium	2400 mg	2400 mg
Fiber	25 g	25 g
Calcium	1100 mg	1000 mg
Iron	14 mg	18 mg
Vitamin A	3333 IU	5000 IU
Vitamin C	60 mg	60 mg

Restricting salt

While we tend not to recommend restricting any food groups or items, salt (sodium) is an exception. Today, young children, adolescents and adults are getting more than double the amount of sodium required through the foods they eat. Approximately 75% to 80% of the salt that people consume comes from processed or convenience foods, with the remainder coming from the salt shaker and the salt found naturally in foods they eat. High sodium intake is associated with high blood pressure, heart disease and hypertension.

Food labels tell the story. Check packaged foods to see just how much sodium one serving provides. Condiments and sauces are usually very high in sodium. Teach your children to look for products that have a lower sodium content, for example by comparing two different brands of cereal or crackers, and restrict intake to within the total recommended daily amount (see table at top of page 69). Low sodium on a label means that one serving will have less than 140 mg.

More or less

A good rule of thumb is to

- Eat fewer foods that are high in saturated fat, cholesterol and sodium
- Eat more foods that are high in fiber, vitamins A and C, calcium and iron

Tips on how to reduce sodium intake for your family

One teaspoon, or 5 mL, of salt has 2400 mg sodium. About ¹/₂ tsp, or 2.5 mL, of salt would contain the recommended daily amount of sodium for a child.

1. Remove the salt shaker from the table and enjoy most foods fresh or with as little salt as possible.
2. Reduce the salt you use in cooking or eliminate it completely.
3. Try sea salt, which has the same flavor as regular table salt, but less is required for the flavor.
4. Check labels for the sodium content of foods. Choose foods that have less than 100 to 140 mg per serving (when it comes to food labeling, low sodium means less than 140 mg sodium per serving).
5. Purchase salt-free butter.
6. Look for lower-sodium crackers, chips and sauces.
7. Replace convenience or processed foods with fruits and vegetables as snacks.

Sodium content of common foods

FOOD ITEM (SERVING SIZE)	SODIUM (GRAMS)
Bacon, 3 oz (90 g) (4 slices)	1442
Lean ham, 3 oz (90 g)	1194
Canned soup, 1 cup (250 mL)	1000–1200
Soy sauce, 1 tbsp (15 mL)	1029
Soy sauce, 40% reduced salt, 1 tbsp (15 mL)	600
Pickle, 1 medium	833
Wieners, pork or beef, 1 medium	638
Cheeseburger	500
Pizza slice	481
Processed sliced cheese, 1 slice	406
Potato chips, salted	230–350
Canned tuna or salmon in water, 3 oz (90 g)	340–470
Feta cheese, 1 oz (30 g)	335
Ketchup, 1 tbsp (15 mL)	120–190
Peanut butter, salted, 2 tbsp (30 mL)	150
Regular salad dressing, 1 tbsp (15 mL)	100–220
Mozzarella cheese, 1 oz (30 g)	130
Mayonnaise, 1 tbsp (15 mL)	75–110
Milk or yogurt, 1 cup (250 mL)	125
Butter, 1 tbsp (15 mL)	124
Chicken breast, no skin, 3 oz (90 g)	67
Egg, 1 medium	63
Fish, fresh, 3 oz (90 g)	50–95
Soy milk, 1 cup (250 mL)	29
Tofu, firm raw, 3 oz (90 g)	13
Legumes, boiled without salt, 1 cup (250 mL)	less than 12
Fresh fruits, 1 cup (250 mL)	0–20
Fresh vegetables, 1 cup (250 mL)	0–100
Oatmeal, cooked, 1 cup (250 mL)	2
Air-popped popcorn, 1 cup (250 mL)	0

Family food diary
Kids keen on recipes

What we find so very satisfying is when friends of our children are over and ask us to share with their moms our recipes, like potato pancakes or biscotti. It shows they have an appreciation for homemade, good-tasting foods, and this will only help them form life-long habits of sharing homemade foods with others. To encourage your children to take part in reading and preparing recipes, try preparing a recipe a month together. Shop for the food needed and let them select unknown or unusual produce just for fun. *(Daina)*

Salt content of common foods

Use the list on page 71 of common foods and their approximate salt content to choose foods. The sodium content of packaged and processed foods will vary depending on the food manufacturer. Notice the foods at the bottom of the list, where sodium content is less or minimal. They are typically fresh foods — fruits and vegetables, poultry, fish and meat before cooking.

Favorite recipes

Here are five of our favorite recipes for providing essential nutrients, which you will find in the recipe section in this book.

- Breakfast Fruit Smoothie or Strawberry Banana Smoothie (page 140)
- Mix and Match Stir-Fry (page 245)
- Mixed Bean and Vegetable Salad (page 272)
- Broccoli and Quinoa Salad (page 275)
- Couscous Pilaf (page 291)

CHAPTER 5

Important
Vitamins and Minerals

In terms of quantity consumed, vitamins and minerals represent only a tiny fraction of what we eat. Yet they are absolutely essential to our health. In this chapter we take an in-depth look at the most critical of these substances — iron, calcium, vitamin C, vitamin D and zinc — and how they relate to children's nutrition.

Children need their iron

Iron is essential for the normal growth and development of children. Yet in North America this nutrient is often deficient in a child's diet — thereby increasing the risk of iron-deficiency anemia.

Iron is found in hemoglobin, a component of the blood that carries oxygen to different parts of the body. Since this oxygen is used to form energy, children with iron-deficiency anemia may appear to be pale and more tired, and have a decreased tolerance for exercise. Iron deficiency can also affect a child's behavior, appetite and ability to learn. In fact, according to one well-publicized study, iron deficiency in infants affected their learning ability well into childhood.

How serious is this problem? Serious enough: It is estimated that 9% of young children (1 to 2 years) are deficient in iron (although not anemic), while about 3% actually have iron-deficiency anemia (where the hemoglobin levels in the blood fall below the normal range). About 3% of children aged 6 to 16 years are iron deficient, and a much higher percentage of iron deficiency is found in adolescent girls, with 9% being deficient, according to the US National Health and Nutrition Examination Survey III.

tip

How can we get our kids interested in the nutrient content of the food they eat? Try having a debate. Assign each family member a nutrient to describe and defend as the most important. Select a judge to decide the winner.

Food sources of iron

FOOD	SERVING SIZE	IRON (MG)
Cream of wheat, iron-enriched, cooked	¾ cup (175 mL)	11.3
Infant cereal	8 tbsp (120 mL)	8.0
Infant formula, fortified with iron	8 oz (250 mL)	5.0
Spinach, cooked	½ cup (125 mL)	3.2
Liver, beef, pan-fried	1.75 oz (45 g)	3.0
Potato, baked, skin on	6.5 oz (190 g)	2.6
Beef, lean, broiled	3.5 oz (100 g)	2.8
Raisins	⅔ cup (150 mL)	2.2
Beans, navy, canned	½ cup (125 mL)	2.4
Avocado	1 medium	2.0
Prune juice	½ cup (125 mL)	1.5
Chicken, light/dark, no skin	3.5 oz (100 g)	1.2
Strained infant meat	4 tbsp (60 mL)	0.9
Halibut	3 oz (75 g)	0.8
Whole wheat bread	1 slice	0.8
White bread	1 slice	0.7
Broccoli, cooked	½ cup (125 mL)	0.7
Apricots, raw	3 medium	0.6
Rice, wild, cooked	½ cup (125 mL)	0.5
Tofu, firm	3 oz (90 g)	2.1

Preventing iron deficiency

One reason for the disturbingly high incidence of iron deficiency may be that the diet of young preschoolers is unbalanced, with an excessive intake of juice or milk, which can displace the intake of other foods that contain iron. Not surprisingly, the American Academy of Pediatrics (AAP) and the Canadian Paediatric Society (CPS) suggest limiting juice to a maximum of 4 to 8 oz (125 to 250 mL) per day (CPS) or 6 oz (175 mL) per day (AAP) in order to encourage children to eat a greater variety of foods.

Math scores make the grade

In one study, a group of children who were iron deficient had lower math scores than did those children with normal levels of iron. This indicates just how important this mineral is for learning, and how important it is to ensure that foods containing iron are part of a child's daily diet.

How much iron does your child need?

The Dietary Reference Intake (DRI) for iron is 7 mg per day for children from 1 to 3 years of age, 10 mg per day for children from 4 to 8 years of age and 8 mg per day for children 8 to 13 years of age. In order to calculate what percent of a child's intake one serving of a recipe in this book provides, simply divide the total mg of iron in one serving by the amount of iron that your child needs. Take the example of a 9-year-old eating our beef satays on page 250. One serving provides 1 mg iron, so 1 mg divided by 8 mg (DRI for a 9-year-old) = 12.5% of the daily value of iron for that child. This same calculation can be done for calcium (see page 69), fiber (see page 61) and sodium (see page 69).

How much iron are your kids getting?

Looking at the table on page 74, you can see that some foods contain more iron than others. But the amount of iron in a food is often less important than the *type* of iron.

There are two types of dietary iron: heme iron, which is most easily absorbed by the body; and non-heme iron, which is less easily absorbed.

Heme iron is found in meat, fish and poultry. Especially high in this type of iron are organ meats, such as liver, as well as red meat. Non-heme iron is found in plant foods such as nuts, vegetables and grains, in dairy products such as milk and cheese, and in eggs.

> ### Iron regulation
>
> As with calcium, the body adjusts its absorption rate for iron according to how much the body needs. So if your child's iron supply is low, the rate of iron absorption increases.

Because non-heme iron is not as well absorbed as heme iron, it is important to know which type is contained in your child's diet. For example, a vegetarian child's diet contains only non-heme iron, so he or she will need more of it (provided by foods such as tofu) to get the amount of iron required. To enhance the absorption of non-heme iron, it is a good idea to accompany meals with a serving of fruit or vegetables that contain vitamin C, such as mangos, oranges or yellow peppers. Vitamin C helps iron absorption. Eating sources of heme iron, such as red meat, also increases the absorption of non-heme iron.

Treating iron-deficiency anemia

If your child is diagnosed with iron-deficiency anemia, your pediatrician or family doctor will prescribe an iron supplement. These supplements may darken the color of your child's stool.

Of course, it's much better to avoid this condition in the first place. So encourage your child to eat iron-rich foods — and limit excess milk and juice intake — to maintain iron stores at healthy levels.

Calcium for bones and teeth

While calcium is an essential mineral for people of all ages, it is especially crucial for growing children. And while daily calcium intake is important at every age, it is especially important for girls age 10 to 15 and boys age 12 to 15 to ensure a good intake of calcium-rich foods. These are the ages when a large amount of adult bone is accumulated (between 25% and 40% of adult bone). If calcium intake is insufficient or low in the teen years, there is a higher likelihood of osteoporosis later in life.

Calcium is a main component of teeth and bones (99% of the body's calcium is located in bones and teeth). Calcium also has a very important role in the blood, where it is carried to different parts of the body to serve in many cell functions. The essential role of calcium in a young child's diet has been stated by the American Academy of Pediatrics as follows: "Of most importance in this age group is the development of eating patterns that will be associated with adequate calcium intake later in life."

All in the family

Adults may not be setting the best example for their children in terms of meeting calcium needs. Surveys suggest that 70% of Canadian women do not get enough calcium in their diet. To ensure that the whole family is meeting their calcium needs, provide calcium-rich foods at meals and in snacks.

How much calcium is enough?

The Dietary Reference Intake (DRI) for calcium is

- 500 mg per day for children from 1 to 3 years of age
- 800 mg per day for children from 4 to 8 years of age
- 1300 mg per day for children 9 to 13 years of age

This is the equivalent of 2 to 4 servings of milk or milk products daily.

Calculating calcium

If you want to calculate the amount of calcium that a serving of one of the recipes provides, simply divide the amount of calcium per serving by the DRI that is recommended for your child's age, and multiply by 100. That way, you can see how much of the daily amount of calcium required is provided by that recipe.

Finding calcium you can use

As shown in the table on page 78, the best dietary sources of calcium include milk and milk products, salmon and sardines, bok choy, almonds and molasses. Moderate sources (not listed in the table) include broccoli, oranges, beans and legumes. A food's calcium content is only part of the story, however; the critical factor is how much of that calcium your body is able to absorb.

Certain factors can increase or decrease the absorption of calcium:

- **Lactose.** A sugar found in milk, lactose enhances the absorption of calcium.
- **Fiber.** The fiber content of foods may decrease calcium absorption. Fiber increases the bulk of food in the intestines, which speeds its travel through the digestive tract and reduces the time during which calcium can be absorbed. However, fiber is not something that should be cut from a child's diet. It is better to compensate for fiber's effects by increasing the amount of dietary calcium.
- **Phytates and oxalates.** Phytates are minerals found in some plant foods, and oxalates are found in vegetables and some berries. Both compounds can reduce calcium absorption.
- **Protein.** A high-protein diet can increase urinary losses of calcium. However, foods that are high in protein also contain phosphorous, which can offset the calcium loss.

Non-dairy caution

Sometimes children who have an allergy to milk and milk products or who are vegetarian are offered almond milk as a main source of calcium. Parents need to check the amount of calcium in the alternatives to milk they choose and how that compares to cow's milk. There is a case study reported of a child who was fed only almond milk as the milk of choice from about 2 to 4 years of age and then developed rickets (decreased bone mineral) due to lack of sufficient calcium in the diet. Ensure a varied intake of calcium-rich food sources if milk or milk products are not offered in a child's diet. Supplements of calcium may sometimes be required.

How kids absorb calcium

When children eat foods that contain calcium, about 75% of the mineral is actually absorbed. (Adults do not absorb calcium as well.) This figure varies with the amount of calcium being consumed at any given time. If the amount is relatively high, less is absorbed; where smaller amounts are consumed, then more is absorbed. This regulating mechanism helps to maintain an adequate calcium supply.

Bone-friendly foods

Foods that provide at least 300 mg calcium per serving

MILK AND MILK PRODUCTS	SERVING SIZE
Milk: skim, 1%, 2%, whole, lactose-reduced, buttermilk, chocolate	1 cup (250 mL)
Milk, powdered	6 tbsp (90 mL)
Yogurt, plain or flavored	3/4 cup (175 mL)
Yogurt, frozen	1 cup (250 mL)
Cheese, firm (e.g., brick, Cheddar, Colby, etc.)	1.5 oz (45 g)
Grated Parmesan cheese	4 tbsp (60 mL)
Ricotta cheese, regular/light varieties	1/2 cup (125 mL)
Puddings made with milk (e.g. rice, instant, baked custard)	1 cup (250 mL)
NON-DAIRY BEVERAGES	**SERVING SIZE**
Soy beverage, calcium-fortified	1 cup (250 mL)
Rice beverage, calcium-fortified	1 cup (250 mL)
Orange juice, calcium-fortified	1 cup (250 mL)
Almond milk, calcium-fortified	1 cup (250 mL)
CANNED FISH	**SERVING SIZE**
Salmon (with bones)	1/2 (7.5 oz/213 g) can
Sardines (with bones)	7 medium
SOY-BASED FOODS	**SERVING SIZE**
Tofu, firm or extra-firm, set with calcium*	1/2 cup (125 mL)
Tofu, silken or regular, set with calcium	1 cup (250 mL)
Soybeans, cooked	2 cups (500 mL)
Soybeans, roasted	1 cup (250 mL)
VEGETABLES	**SERVING SIZE**
Bok choy (pak-choi), cooked	1 cup (250 mL)
Turnip greens, cooked	1 cup (250 mL)
Kale, mustard greens, turnip greens, cooked	1 1/2 cups (375 mL)
Seaweed, dry (hijiki, arame, wakame)	1 oz (25 g)
OTHER	**SERVING SIZE**
Almonds	3/4 cup (175 mL)
Blackstrap molasses	2 tbsp (25 mL)

* Where calcium is the ingredient listed immediately after "soy milk" or "soybeans and water"

SOURCES: *Bowes & Church's Food Values of Portions Commonly Consumed*, 6th edition, 1994; Jan Main, *Bone Vivant! Calcium-Enhanced Recipes and Bone-Building Exercises*, 1997; Osteoporosis Society of Canada, *Building Better Bones: A Guide to Active Living*, 1996.

Non-dairy sources of calcium

If your child is unable to drink milk — because of allergy or lactose intolerance, for example — it will be necessary to find alternative sources of calcium. These may include some of the high-calcium foods of non-dairy origin, such as fortified soy or rice drinks and almond milk, which are listed in the table on page 78.

When substituting cow's milk with an alternative product for a child, parents need to exercise caution in choosing the appropriate beverage. Many soy or rice drinks, even when fortified with added calcium, do not contain adequate amounts of other nutrients, such as protein or vitamin D, or they may not provide sufficient calories. Since children typically derive a lot of their nourishment from milk, such deficiencies can have a serious effect on nutrition. If you are unsure about the ingredients and nutritional composition of a milk substitute, check with a dietitian or family doctor before giving it to your child.

If non-dairy food sources are inadequate for your child's calcium needs, you may be advised to provide a calcium supplement. These are available in many different forms, and your doctor will choose the one that is best for your child. Calcium carbonate, for example, is one of the most widely used supplements (it is also used in antacid tablets), with an absorption rate of 39%. Other alternatives, with their respective absorption rates, are shown below.

> ### Calcium-added O.J.
>
> As awareness of its nutritional importance has grown, calcium is now being added to an increasing number of products. Of these, calcium-fortified orange juice is one of the most popular, and you may be wondering whether it is worth buying for your child. First, keep in mind that it is not a substitute for milk, which contains vitamin D and other important nutrients not found in fortified orange juice. However, between 30% and 35% of the calcium added to this type of juice can be absorbed (which is similar to cow's milk), so it is a good choice if calcium intake needs to be increased.

Absorption rates of calcium supplements

CALCIUM COMPOUND	ABSORPTION
Carbonate	39%
Acetate	32%
Lactate	32%
Gluconate	27%
Citrate	30%

The sunshine vitamin

While calcium is essential for the normal development of bones and teeth, it cannot be used properly without vitamin D. Exposure to the ultraviolet rays of the sun in summer months for those of us living in northern latitudes, and specific foods, such as cow's milk and some fatty fish, are natural sources of vitamin D. Ultraviolet light converts a cholesterol-like substance in the skin into a form of vitamin D the body can use.

However, research studies indicate that many children and adults are just not getting enough vitamin D, in part because of the need to prevent sunburn in fair-skinned people. Sunscreens block the ultraviolet light needed to produce vitamin D. People with darker skin color are also unable to form as much vitamin D. This may be affecting our health in a negative way. Blood levels of this vitamin are in a range that is believed to be inadequate for prevention of certain illnesses, but there is no final word yet on what the right amount of vitamin D supplementation is for children.

Eating vitamin D

What does an 8-year-old need to eat in order to get enough vitamin D based on current recommendations, given no sun exposure? Cow's milk and fish are the chief sources of vitamin D in the diet.

3 cups (750 mL) of milk = 300 IU vitamin D
or
4 oz (125 g) of salmon = 410 IU vitamin D

Children who have limited milk and fish intake may be at risk, especially in the winter months, of developing vitamin D deficiency. In those cases, a supplement of 400 to 1000 IU per day may be recommended.

What does vitamin D do?

Vitamin D is not just needed to help get calcium into the body. Vitamin D receptors are all over the body, indicating that this vitamin has many roles to play. Vitamin D is important for maintaining a healthy immune system and may be protective against immune diseases, such multiple sclerosis. Other studies indicate adequate levels of vitamin D in the blood are associated with a reduced risk of certain types of cancer.

More studies needed

The DRI for vitamin D is 200 IU per day for children over 1 year of age, though some studies indicate the need for higher intake. One study found that supplementation with 2000 IU vitamin D per day for 1 year was safe and resulted in improved blood levels of vitamin D.

While current studies show no negative short-term effects of vitamin D supplementation, increasing the amount of one nutrient may have an effect on another nutrient, or on another mechanism. High vitamin D intakes may, some suggest, decrease the ability of the body to form vitamin D naturally from the sun. More research is needed in order to determine the right amount of vitamin D required for children living at different latitudes relative to the equator, and considering skin color.

Check with your family doctor or pediatrician for the latest research regarding vitamin D in order to keep current with what the latest vitamin D recommendation is for your child. Keep up with the latest research by checking out reliable sources, such as Health Canada, the Food and Drug Administration (FDA), the Canadian Paediatric Society, the American Academy of Pediatrics, Dietitians of Canada and the American Dietetic Association.

Essential vitamin C

Humans need to obtain vitamin C from the foods they eat. This distinguishes us from most other mammals, which are able to manufacture their own vitamin C from sugar (glucose) in their diet. Vitamin C has many functions in the body, including

- **Dietary antioxidant.** Vitamin C helps to reduce the damage done to the body's cells by "oxidizing free radicals." As a dietary antioxidant, it converts these free radicals into harmless substances that the body can eliminate. It has been suggested that vitamin C (and other antioxidants) can help prevent cancer or cardiovascular disease, but this has yet to be confirmed definitively by research.
- **Collagen formation.** Vitamin C plays an important role in the formation of collagen — a type of protein found in connective tissue, bones, teeth and skin. This why a vitamin C deficiency can result in conditions such as scurvy or wounds not healing properly, or bones becoming weakened and eventually distorted.

Vitamin C in history

Descriptions of scurvy — a severe form of vitamin C deficiency that results in dry, cracked skin, aching bones and joints, and bleeding gums — were recorded as early as 1500 BC. Throughout history, it caused many deaths among soldiers and sailors (whose rations consisted largely of preserved meats and bread), often proving more lethal than swords and guns. It was not until the 1600s that the link between scurvy and diet was recognized. Today, with the widespread availability of fruit and vegetables, scurvy is extremely rare.

Where to get your vitamin C

Per 1/2-cup (125 mL) serving unless otherwise indicated

FOOD	VITAMIN C (MG)
Orange juice, fresh	62
Broccoli, cooked	58
Cantaloupe	34
Cauliflower, cooked	34
Orange, 1/2	34
Honeydew melon	21
Spinach, cooked	9
Frozen peas, cooked	8
Prune juice	5*
Apple, 1/2	4
Carrots, cooked	3
Apple juice	1*
Grape juice	0.12*

* 18 to 50 mg per 1/2 cup (125 mL) if fortified

SOURCE: Food Smart Professional Edition 2.0, Sasquatch Corp., © 1994–1996.

Can you have too much vitamin C?

The maximum amount of vitamin C recommended for 1- to 3-year-olds is 400 mg per day and 650 mg per day for children 4 to 8 years old. Beyond these levels, studies suggest there is the potential for negative effects from excess vitamin C. It is estimated that between 20% and 25% of the US population takes vitamin C supplements, in doses that range from 100 mg to 10 g (or 10,000 mg!) daily. Regardless of whether you think such large doses contribute to adult health, it is generally unwise to give supplements of vitamin C (or any other vitamin) to children. Most children do not need any more vitamin C than they get from eating half a fresh orange every day.

- **Improves absorption of other nutrients.** Vitamin C helps the body absorb non-heme iron (the iron found in plants) and calcium. Vitamin C also helps convert folic acid into its active form, so that it can do its job in the body.

How much vitamin C does your child need?

The Dietary Reference Intake (DRI) for vitamin C is 15 mg per day for children from 1 to 3 years of age, 25 mg per day for children from 4 to 8 years of age and 45 mg per day for children from 9 to 10 years of age. While this may seem like very little — particularly to adults who are accustomed to taking megadoses of this vitamin (see "Can you have too much vitamin C?" on page 82) — it is all that's required to prevent vitamin C deficiency.

Children can get all the vitamin C they need from plant foods, especially citrus fruits and their juices, broccoli, spinach and melon. The vitamin C content of food can be enhanced by eating fruits when they are ripe, by refrigerating fruits and vegetables, and by not overcooking foods.

The mineral to grow with

Because of its role in growth and development, zinc is a particularly important mineral for children. The requirement for zinc increases during periods of growth spurts. In girls, the growth spurt occurs between ages 10 to 15 years, and for boys, the growth spurt is between 12 to 15 years. Even after these growth spurts, zinc requirements are increased as tissues continue to grow.

While zinc is only needed in very small amounts and is found in many different food sources, deficiencies of this important mineral can occur in children. We do not know exactly what the incidence of zinc deficiency is in our developed countries, as it is very hard to get a good measure of zinc status, but it can affect growth by causing stunting and by increasing risk of infections.

Does vitamin C cure the common cold?

In 1970 the Nobel prize–winning scientist Linus Pauling stirred up considerable debate with his book *Vitamin C and the Common Cold*, in which he suggested that vitamin C could offer protection against the common cold and relief from its symptoms. Since then, much research has been done on whether this theory holds true. Most of the current literature does not support the idea that vitamin C reduces the incidence of colds, although it may help people to recover faster and suffer less severe symptoms.

Where to find zinc

FOOD	SERVING SIZE	ZINC (MG)
Oysters	1 medium	12.7
Lean ground beef, cooked	3½ oz (100 g)	6.3
Chicken breast, cooked	3½ oz (100 g)	1.0
2% milk	1 cup (250 mL)	0.9
Oatmeal, cooked	½ cup (125 mL)	0.6
Egg, boiled	1 large	0.6
Halibut, cooked	3 oz (90 g)	0.5
Whole wheat bread	1 slice	0.4
Broccoli, cooked	½ cup (125 mL)	0.3
Apple	1 medium	0.06

SOURCE: Food Smart Professional Edition 2.0, Sasquatch Corp. © 1994–1996.

What does zinc do?

Zinc is involved with the function of every cell in the body, particularly in cell division and multiplication (hence its importance for growing children). It also plays a role in our ability to fight infection, which is especially important for the sick or elderly. It helps to maintain a healthy appetite, and is involved with the sense of taste. Zinc is also required for adequate night vision.

How much zinc does your child need?

The Dietary Reference Intake (DRI) for zinc is 3 mg per day for children from 1 to 3 years of age, 5 mg per day for children from 4 to 8 years of age and 8 mg per day for children 9 to 10 years of age. The body is very good at controlling its own zinc level, adjusting its absorption rate according to the amount of zinc present in the diet. This being said, when a child's diet is too low in zinc, there may still be some risk of deficiency.

While we do not know how many children are zinc deficient in North America, studies have shown that intake of zinc can fall below recommended amounts and some children may be at risk of zinc deficiency. This can affect growth and immune function, as well as cognitive development.

The best food sources for zinc include beef, chicken, milk and eggs. (The protein in these foods helps to improve zinc absorption.) Moderate amounts of zinc are also contained in some vegetables and cereals, although these foods contain high amounts of fiber and phytates, which inhibit zinc absorption.

Juice limit

Juice intake should be monitored so that the energy from juice does not decrease a child's appetite or displace other nutritious foods from being consumed. While providing some vitamins and minerals, juice does not have the same nutritional value as the whole fruit, which contains much needed fiber and phytonutrients, or phytochemicals, which help our immune system stay strong.

Vitamins and minerals

What they do, where to find them

VITAMIN/ MINERAL	TYPE	ASSISTS IN	SOURCES
Vitamin A (from beta carotene)	Fat-soluble	Vision, growth, bone development, healthy skin	Liver, eggs, whole milk, dark green leafy vegetables, yellow and orange vegetables and fruit
Vitamin B_1 (thiamin)	Water-soluble	Enzyme activity, metabolism of nutrients	Oatmeal, enriched breads and grains, rice, dairy products, fish, pork, liver, nuts, legumes
Vitamin B_2 (riboflavin)	Water-soluble	Growth, metabolism of nutrients	Dairy products, eggs, organ meats, enriched breads and grains, green leafy vegetables
Vitamin B_3 (niacin)	Water-soluble	Tissue repair, metabolism of nutrients	Organ meats, peanuts, brewer's yeast, enriched breads and grains, meats, poultry, fish, nuts
Vitamin B_6 (pyridoxine)	Water-soluble	Metabolism of nutrients (primary role)	Brewer's yeast, wheat, germ, pork, liver, whole-grain cereals, potatoes, milk, fruits and vegetables
Folate (part of B vitamin group)	Water-soluble	Growth, enzyme activity, prevents neural tube defects	Liver, lima and kidney beans, dark green leafy vegetables, beef, potatoes, whole wheat bread
Vitamin B_{12}	Water-soluble	Metabolism of nutrients, prevents anemia	Liver, kidneys, meat, fish, dairy products, eggs
Biotin (part of B vitamin group)	Water-soluble	Enzyme activity; deficiency can lead to a type of dermatitis	Liver, milk, meat, egg yolk, vegetables, fruit, peanuts, brewer's yeast
Vitamin C	Water-soluble	Many cellular functions, promotes healthy teeth, skin and tissue repair	Citrus fruits such as oranges and grapefruits, leafy vegetables, tomatoes, strawberries
Vitamin D	Fat-soluble	Essential for normal growth, development, bones and teeth	Liver, butter, fortified milk, fatty fish (fish liver oils), exposure to sunlight
Vitamin E	Fat-soluble	Antioxidant function protects cells; assists neurological function, prevents anemia	Vegetable and fish oils, nuts, seeds, egg yolk, whole grains
Vitamin K	Fat-soluble	Blood clotting	Green leafy vegetables, liver, wheat bran, tomatoes, cheese, egg yolk
Zinc	Mineral	Growth and development, immune system	Meat, poultry, eggs, dairy products
Calcium	Mineral	Bone and tooth formation, heart functions, muscle contraction	Meat, cheese, yogurt, calcium-soaked tofu, dark green leafy vegetables, oats, sesame seeds, almonds, canned sardines, salmon, navy beans
Iron	Mineral	Formation of hemoglobin which carries oxygen in the blood to every cell of the body	Organ meats, chicken, tofu, dried fruit, fortified cereals, molasses, dried beans, lentils

SOURCES: JL Groff, SS Gropper and SM Hunt, eds., *Advanced Nutrition and Human Metabolism*, 1995; MV Krause and LK Mahan, *Food, Nutrition and Diet Theory*, 6th edition, 1979.

Family food diary
Brain food

My kids enjoy their fish, but when occasionally only a few bits are eaten, a gentle reminder from Mom about fish being "brain food" often prompts them to finish up their trout, especially when there is a math test coming up! Why eat fish? There are studies suggesting that kids are not getting enough of the essential omega-3 fatty acids — found in fish — that are important for the growth and development of a healthy brain in children. Fish is also a great source of protein, which provides even more brain power. *(Daina)*

Favorite recipes

Here are five of Daina's kids' favorite recipes, which you will find in the recipe section of this book.

- Tofu in Sesame Crust (page 201)
- Beef Satays (page 250)
- Simple Parmesan Zucchini (page 281)
- Tasty Potato Pancakes (page 288)
- Rindy's Ginger Chews (page 303)

CHAPTER 6

Vegetarian
Diets

About 2.5% to 4% of adults in North America follow a vegetarian diet. Such dietary decisions are typically made by adults, but often affect children within the same family. And since children have special nutritional needs, it is important to make sure they follow a well-balanced vegetarian diet.

What is a vegetarian?

Vegetarians are generally defined as people who consume mainly plant foods, including vegetables, fruits, legumes, grains, seeds and nuts. However, there are actually many types of vegetarians in North America, and their diets can differ greatly. Within these sub-groups of vegetarianism, there can be many variations in diet.

- **Semi- or partial vegetarians** generally avoid red meat, but may continue to eat some poultry and fish while primarily consuming vegetarian fare.
- **Pesco-vegetarians** avoid red meat and poultry but continue to consume fish and/or seafood.
- **Lacto-ovo vegetarians** avoid all animal flesh, including meat, poultry and fish. However, they still include dairy (lacto) and egg (ovo) products as part of their diet. It has been estimated that 90% to 95% of all vegetarians in North America consume dairy and/or eggs.
- **Vegans** avoid all foods of animal origin, including meat, poultry, fish, eggs, dairy, gelatin and honey. Many vegans also extend this prohibition beyond what they eat, eliminating from their lifestyles other animal-based products such as leather, wool and tallow candles.
- **Macrobiotic vegetarians** often follow highly restrictive diets that can involve eliminating entire food groups. These diets are not recommended for children.

tip

Vegetarian diets can be healthy but must be carefully planned so that they provide all the required nutrients. This is especially important for children who are vegetarians.

Vegetarianism and health

What's behind the growing popularity of vegetarianism? While a number of people become vegetarians for reasons of principle (ethical, environmental, economic or religious), for many others it's simply a matter of believing that a vegetarian diet is healthier. And there's some justification for this belief: Although vegetarianism is not for everyone, it can provide a number of potential health benefits, including a lower incidence of several chronic diseases.

It's a way of life

In addition to dietary considerations, vegetarians tend to be healthier because they often make positive lifestyle choices, including weight maintenance, regular exercise and abstinence from smoking, alcohol and drugs.

- **Heart disease.** Vegetarian diets tend to be "heart healthy." They are typically lower in total and saturated fat, as well as dietary cholesterol. They are also generally higher in fiber and polyunsaturated fat, which helps to lower LDL (popularly known as "bad cholesterol") levels in the blood. Vegetarians are statistically less likely to have high blood pressure or to die from coronary artery disease.
- **Certain types of cancer.** Vegetarians have lower rates of certain types of cancer. The precise reason for this is unknown, although one suggestion is that vegetarians consume more antioxidants, such as vitamins C and E. Other possible factors include lower fat consumption and increased fiber intake.
- **Obesity and diabetes.** Vegetarians are also less likely to suffer from obesity and non-insulin-dependent diabetes.

Energy boost

Because many plant foods are not concentrated sources of calories, vegetarian diets have the potential to be low in energy. It is important that vegetarian children, especially vegan children, receive adequate energy for growth and health. This is less of a challenge in the case of lacto-ovo vegetarian children, because milk and eggs are concentrated sources of energy. Vegan children need to boost their energy intake by including high-calorie plant foods — such as avocado, nuts and nut butters — as a part of their daily eating regimen.

Where's the protein?

Sources of protein for vegetarians

FOOD TYPE	EXAMPLES
Grains	Wheat, oats, brown rice, quinoa, bulgur
Legumes	Chickpeas, lentils, peanuts, kidney beans, black beans
Nuts and seeds	Walnuts, sesame seeds, almonds, nut butters

Notes: Few vegetables contain significant amounts of protein, but they do provide essential amino acids needed to help complement the amino acids in other plant-based proteins.

For vegetarians who consume them, milk and eggs are good sources of protein.

Complete protein

Proteins consist of amino acids. There are 20 different amino acids, and they can be found in a variety of the foods we eat. The body can make many of these (called *non-essential* amino acids) on its own, so we don't need to obtain them from our diet. But there are nine amino acids that our bodies cannot make, and we must get them from the foods we eat. These are called *essential* amino acids.

Amino acids perform many different jobs in our bodies, and it is important to ensure that we consume an adequate amount of all nine essential amino acids daily. For meat eaters this is not a concern, because meats contain all nine essential amino acids and are therefore described as *complete* proteins. Because plant proteins are missing one or more essential amino acids, they are called *incomplete* proteins. Consequently, vegetarians need to eat plant proteins in combination, consuming a variety of foods that, together, make the proteins complete.

This is not difficult. We do it inadvertently every day by consuming plant foods in pairs — like toast and peanut butter or split pea soup with a roll. Mixing different types of plant proteins together often makes a complete protein. Eating a variety of plant-based proteins over the course of the day provides all the essential amino acids an individual needs.

Too much of a good thing

Fiber is found only in plant foods and has many benefits for children and adults alike. It helps to maintain regular bowel movements and to lower cholesterol. Fiber may help in the prevention of certain types of cancers. (See page 59 for more information.) For vegetarian children, however, there is a risk that they may be getting too much of a good thing. Because high-fiber diets have the potential to be deficient in the energy (calories) needed to ensure proper growth, and are high in "bulk" (which can make you feel full more quickly), it is important to balance a child's diet with foods that are concentrated sources of calories and fat, such as nuts, cheese and eggs.

Iron

Because this mineral plays an important role in the function of blood cells, vegetarian children need to ensure they receive sufficient iron. There are two types of dietary iron (see page 75). Heme iron is found in meats and is generally well absorbed by the body. Non-heme iron is found in plant foods and is not as readily absorbed. For children consuming a plant-based diet, it is important to ensure that they obtain enough iron.

Plant sources of iron include tofu, prunes, legumes and dark green leafy vegetables. Fortified cereals and cream of wheat are other options. Infant cereal is also a terrific source of iron that can be added to pancakes, cereals and other foods. Enhancers of iron absorption can affect the percentage of non-heme iron that the body receives. Vitamin C, for example, helps with iron absorption. Try offering fresh fruit with all vegetarian meals and cooking with tomatoes.

Adequate zinc

Because zinc is important for growth and development (see page 83), it is important to ensure that vegetarian children (and non-vegetarians too, of course) receive adequate amounts of this mineral. This is rarely a problem for vegetarians, because zinc can be obtained from grains, legumes and nuts.

Vitamin B$_{12}$

Like iron, vitamin B$_{12}$ is essential to the proper functioning of red blood cells. It also helps in nerve conduction by maintaining the protective sheath that surrounds nerve fibers. Because it can only be found in animal products, vegans need to be particularly concerned about this vitamin. Lacto-ovo vegetarians should receive adequate vitamin B$_{12}$ from milk and eggs. Vegans need to take a supplement or consume reliable food sources of vitamin B$_{12}$, such as fortified commercial breakfast cereals, soy beverages or nutritional yeasts. Alternatively, children's multivitamins generally contain enough vitamin B$_{12}$ to avoid deficiency.

Calcium

Getting enough dietary calcium is especially important for children to help maximize bone mass during growth and to minimize the bone loss that occurs later in life. Calcium is generally less of a concern for lacto-ovo vegetarians who consume adequate amounts of milk and milk products. For others, it takes some planning to ensure adequate calcium intake. While many plant foods contain calcium, it is often difficult for the body to absorb because the plant also contains phytates and oxalates, which inhibit the absorption process. Of those plant foods that do contain bioavailable calcium — such as kale, broccoli, bok choy and soybeans — the calcium content is so low that they must be consumed in very large amounts to meet a child's dietary requirements of between 500 and 800 mg per day. (See page 78 for information on the calcium content of selected foods.) For children who do not consume dairy products, it may be necessary to add calcium-fortified foods or supplements to their diet.

At risk

Babies of vegan mothers are particularly at risk of vitamin B_{12} deficiency. A reduced amount of this vitamin crosses the placenta during pregnancy and decreased amounts are present in the break milk of vegan mothers.

Terrific tofu

One of the best plant-based sources of protein is tofu. Manufactured from soybeans (which is why it's sometimes called "soybean curd"), tofu is a soft, cheese-like food that, when fortified (as it usually is), can also be a source of calcium. Tofu is quite bland on its own, but has an amazing ability to soak up the flavors of whatever food it is cooked with.

There are three main types of tofu available:

- **Firm or extra-firm.** Dense and solid, this type of tofu is great in stir-fries, soups or on the grill. It will maintain its shape as it cooks. This type of tofu also contains the most protein and fat (see below).

How they compare

Nutrients per 4-oz (125 g) serving for different types of tofu

	FIRM TOFU	SOFT TOFU	SILKEN TOFU
Calories	120	86	72
Protein (g)	13	9	10
Carbohydrate (g)	3	2	3
Fat (g)	6	5	2
Calcium (mg)	120	130	40

SOURCE: United States Department of Agriculture, Human Nutrition Information Service, *Composition of Foods: Legumes and Legume Products*, Agriculture Handbook 0-16, Revised December 1986.

Key Vegetarian Nutrients and Good Food Sources

NUTRIENT	FOOD SOURCE
Protein	Milk, eggs, grains, legumes, nuts and seeds
Calcium	Fortified-cow's milk, soy milk, rice milk
	Calcium-fortified fruit juice
	Calcium-set tofu
	Yogurt
	Almonds
	Canned salmon with bones
Vitamin D	Sunshine (not a food but still the best source)
	Margarine
	Fortified soy milk or milk alternatives
Vitamin B_{12}	Red Star Vegetarian Support Formula nutritional yeast
	Fortified soy milk, milk, eggs, yogurt
	Fortified meat analog
Iron	Iron-fortified cereals
	Dried fruits (e.g., apricots)
	Beans (e.g., chickpeas)
Omega-3 fatty acids	Fortified eggs, milk, margarine
	Ground flaxseed, flaxseed oil
	Walnuts
Zinc	Chickpeas
	Whole wheat bread, whole grains
	Dried beans
	Yogurt and cheese

- **Soft.** Less solid than the firm variety, this type of tofu is often used in Asian-style soups.
- **Silken.** With its creamy, custard-like consistency, silken tofu works well in puréed or blended dishes, and is often used in tofu desserts or soups.

Vitamin D

Like calcium, vitamin D also plays a role in bone health, and is an important vitamin for all growing children. The most common food source of vitamin D is milk, so lacto-vegetarian children who drink an adequate amount of milk need not worry about getting enough vitamin D. However, children who do not drink fortified cow's milk or an acceptable fortified alternative — or who do not receive 10 to 15 minutes daily exposure to sunlight (which the allows the body to manufacture its own vitamin D) — may require a vitamin D supplement. Vitamin D drops are now available, which may be easier to administer to some children than tablets.

Tips for healthy vegetarian eating for kids

1. At each meal, be sure to include a variety of foods from all six "vegetarian food groups": calcium-rich foods (milk and milk alternatives); grains; legumes and beans; vegetables and fruit; nuts and seeds; and fats.

2. Preschoolers should receive 16 to 20 oz (500 to 625 mL) daily of whole cow's milk or a nutritionally acceptable replacement. School-age children should receive 16 oz (500 mL) daily. Milk is a valuable source of energy, calcium, vitamin D and riboflavin. For vegan children ages 2 to 5 years, a fortified soy infant formula will provide all the vitamins and minerals necessary to prevent deficiency.

3. Include protein-rich foods with every meal. Lacto-ovo vegetarian children can obtain high-quality protein from milk and eggs. High-quality vegan sources of protein include fortified soy infant formula or milk, tofu, quinoa or legume and grain combinations. Non-dairy beverages, such as rice milk or potato milk, are very low in protein. They should not be used for vegetarian children until they are 6 years old and are consuming a wide variety of other foods.

4. Balance high-fiber foods with those that are concentrated sources of energy and fat, such as cheese or yogurt (for those who consume dairy products) or, for vegan children over the age of 4, nuts and nut butters. A vegan diet can be very high in fiber and bulk, making it difficult for children to meet their daily caloric requirements.

5. Provide plant foods each day that are good sources of iron and zinc.

6. Include 6 or more servings of vegetables and fruits each day. These foods are great sources of vitamins and minerals, including vitamin A, vitamin C and folate. Try to eat at least one serving of fruit or vegetables at each meal.

7. Include a reliable source of vitamin B_{12} in the diet. Lacto-ovo vegetarian children can meet their daily vitamin B_{12} requirements from about $1\frac{1}{2}$ glasses of milk or from 1 glass of milk and 1 egg. Because this vitamin is not found in plant foods, vegan children must obtain it from fortified foods such as soy infant formula, or by taking a vitamin B_{12} supplement.

ADAPTED FROM: V Melina, B Davis and V Harrison, *Being Vegetarian*, 1994.

Family food diary
Helping hands
Our kids love to help with food preparation. Joanne's daughters enjoy chopping vegetables for fresh and delicious salads, and Daina's kids have fun measuring out ingredients for their favorite quinoa recipe and grating the Parmesan cheese, not to mention mixing the batter for their favorite chocolate chip cookies! (*Joanne and Daina*)

Favorite recipes
Here are five of our favorite vegetarian recipes, which you will find in the recipe section of this book.

- Tuscan Bean Soup (page 171)
- Tofu with Hoisin Sauce (page 203)
- Spinach and Mushroom Lasagna Roll-Ups (page 214)
- Chickpea and Potato Curry with Spinach (page 264)
- Quinoa with Tomatoes, Herbs and Cheese (page 266)

CHAPTER 7

Avoiding
Food Contamination

There are hundreds of microorganisms present in our everyday lives. Many of these are harmless to humans, while others, such as the bacteria that ferment cheese and yogurt, are actually beneficial. But some of these "bugs" are harmful and, when they get into our food, are capable of causing serious illness. As a parent, you need to be aware of what these microorganisms are, and how to prevent them from making your child sick.

The bugs in our food

The microorganisms that cause illness are known as pathogens. These are mostly bacteria, which are responsible for more than 90% of all food-poisoning cases.

Food-borne bacteria can cause illness in two ways:

- **Infection.** This is caused by bacterial growth in the food itself. Generally, cooking foods thoroughly can prevent infections.
- **Intoxication.** Here it is not the bacteria that cause harm, but rather the toxins produced by the bacteria. In most cases, these toxins are unaffected by heat and cannot be destroyed by cooking.

Bacterial contamination occurs primarily in cases where products or ingredients are eaten raw, or where food is improperly handled or stored.

Hamburger disease

Named for the undercooked ground beef that is often its source, "hamburger disease" is caused by a particularly nasty strain of E. coli, called verotoxigenic E. coli, or VTEC. In addition to hamburger, it is also found in unpasteurized milk or contaminated water, as well as cheese, yogurt or cold cuts. This bacterium produces a toxin that breaks down the lining of the intestines and, in severe cases, can damage the kidneys. Symptoms include severe stomach ache and bloody diarrhea. In severely affected children, a specific kind of kidney failure can develop, called hemolytic uremic syndrome (HUS). Hamburger disease can be prevented by observing standard rules of safe food preparation and by never eating undercooked meat or unpasteurized milks and cheeses.

Food poisoning

Which bacteria cause food poisoning? There are many different varieties, but here are some of the worst offenders.

- *Staphylococcus aureus.* Although this common bacterium is found in the nose, throat, hair or skin of about 50% of healthy people, it is also responsible for about 1 in 4 cases of all food-borne illness in North America. Staph aureus contamination is found in foods such as meat, fish, poultry, dairy products and salads.
- *Escherichia coli* 0157:H7. This is a rare but dangerous type of E. coli found in the intestinal tract of both animals and humans. It is occasionally found in raw meats or poultry, but can be eliminated by thorough cooking. Other potential sources of E. coli 0157:H7 include unpasteurized milk, juice and cider, as well as contaminated water.
- *Salmonella enteritidis.* Most commonly found in raw or partially cooked eggs, as well as raw or undercooked chicken. Salmonella poisoning often results when foods containing uncooked egg ingredients (such as Caesar salad dressing) have not been properly refrigerated.
- *Listeria monocytogenes.* Unusual for its ability to survive in the cold (in fact, it thrives at normal refrigerator temperatures), this bacterium can be found in cooked meats or seafood, prepared salads and soft cheeses, as well as unpasteurized milk and milk products. Listeria is also very resistant to heat, requiring a minimum of 2 minutes at 160°F (70°C) to significantly reduce its numbers.
- *Clostridium botulinum.* Found most often in canned goods, usually where the can has been damaged slightly, allowing the bacteria to enter. In this oxygen-free, low-acid environment, the bacteria grow, producing a dangerous neurotoxin, which can only be destroyed by exposure to temperatures of 180°F (85°C) or greater for at least 10 minutes. To avoid C. botulinum, do not purchase goods in dented cans. The bacteria have occasionally been found in unpasteurized honey, which is why this sweetener should not be given to infants less than 1 year of age.

Cider caution

The next time you are visiting a fall farm at harvest time and they are serving apple cider, be sure the cider is pasteurized. *Escherichia coli* 0157:H7 (E. coli 0157:H7) is a rare but dangerous type of E. coli bacteria typically found in the intestinal tract of animals. It is occasionally found in raw beef, but can be eliminated by thorough cooking. Other potential sources of E. coli 0157:H7 include contaminated water and unpasteurized milk, juice and cider.

Keeping it clean and safe

The following are some suggestions to help minimize the risk of food-borne illnesses in your home:

- Always wash your hands before preparing or serving foods.
- Avoid breathing, coughing or sneezing on foods, especially if you have a cold.
- Keep your preparation area and utensils clean.
- Keep high-chair trays clean. Wash them down with hot soapy water after each meal. Once a week, be sure to clean with a diluted solution of bleach and water.
- Always keep raw foods and cooked foods separate. Use separate cutting boards or clean the boards thoroughly between uses.
- Never place cooked foods on a plate that held raw food unless that plate has been thoroughly washed.
- Store uncooked meats, poultry or fish on the lowest refrigerator rack to avoid juices spilling onto other fresh foods.
- Wash fruits and vegetables thoroughly under running water.
- Thaw frozen foods overnight in the refrigerator or use a microwave. Foods thawed on the counter are at risk of microbial contamination.
- Cook meats thoroughly to kill bacteria.
- Always keep hot foods hot (over 140°F/60°C) and cold foods cold (less than 40°F/4°C).
- Do not eat food from any can that is swollen or dented.
- Always check the expiration date on foods. Do not consume foods beyond the expiration date.
- Don't eat raw eggs or fish.
- Do not eat moldy or spoiled foods.
- Do not give foods that contain raw eggs (uncooked cookie dough, homemade Caesar salad dressing, homemade mayonnaise) to young children. Raw eggs may contain salmonella.
- Do not give children raw meats or poultry, raw fish or sushi or unpasteurized milk, juice or cider products.

Signs of sickness

Symptoms of food poisoning can include stomach cramps, diarrhea, vomiting, sweating or chills. They usually commence within 12 to 18 hours of eating the contaminated food.

If in doubt, throw it out

A refrigerator slows down the rate of bacterial growth but doesn't stop it. So don't keep foods in the fridge too long. Fresh poultry should be stored for no longer than 2 days, and other fresh meats no longer than 3 to 5 days. Cooked leftovers can be kept for up to 4 days. If you're unsure how long food has been in the refrigerator, it's better to throw it out than risk illness.

Safe internal food temperatures

To be safe, be sure you cook meat, poultry and eggs until they reach these internal temperatures. Hold the thermometer for at least 15 seconds.

Beef, medium	160°F	71°C
Beef, well done	170°F	77°C
Ground beef	160°F	71°C
Pork	160°F	71°C
Poultry, whole	185°F	85°C
Poultry, other than whole	165°F	74°C
Fish	158°F	70°C
Egg Dishes	165°F	74°C

SOURCE: canfightbac.org

Guide to storing and thawing frozen foods

You can preserve food by freezing it to eat at another time, but only for a limited period of time. Follow these guidelines for eating frozen food safely. Remember to defrost frozen foods in the refrigerator or microwave oven, not on the counter.

FOOD ITEM	FREEZE SAFELY FOR
Leftovers (meat and vegetables)	2–3 months
Soups	4 months
Breads	2 months
Milk	6 weeks
Ground meat	2–3 months
Beef (roasts and steaks)	10–12 months
Chicken pieces	6 months
Fatty fish	2 months
Most vegetables and fruit (except potatoes, lettuce, radishes, green onions, celery and tomatoes)	12 months

SOURCE: www.eatrightontario (Freezing 101)

Tips for packing a safe lunch

Many school-age children take a lunch to school in the morning, where it remains for several hours, usually at room temperature, before being eaten. To minimize the risk of bacterial contamination and growth, there are a number of steps you can take when packing the lunch.

1. **Put something cold in the bag.** A frozen juice box or small water container will act like a freezer pack to help prevent against food-borne illness. (By lunchtime, the drink will have thawed, but still be cold and refreshing.)

2. **Freeze those sandwiches.** This works better with coarse-textured breads that won't get soggy when they thaw. Veggies or mayonnaise will need to be packed separately.

3. **Insulate your food.** An insulated lunch bag with a freezer pack inside will keep foods cold. This is especially helpful when packing highly perishable foods, such as cold cuts, poultry, fish or egg sandwiches. Use an insulated container (Thermos) to keep liquids hot or cold.

4. **Find someplace cool.** Keep your lunch in the coolest part of the room — or at least away from warm places, such as hot air vents or sunny window sills. If the school has a refrigerator available, use it.

5. **Keep it clean.** Wash the inside of lunch boxes and bags with warm soapy water every night. Once a week, clean with a diluted solution of bleach and water.

6. **Wash your hands.** While you're at it, remind your kids to wash their hands before eating.

Meals for microbes

Foods that carry a high risk of contamination

FOOD TYPE	EXAMPLE(S)	CONTAMINANT
Raw or undercooked eggs	Caesar salad dressing, soft-cooked eggs, meringue pies, some puddings and custards, mousse, sauces made with raw eggs	*Salmonella enteritidis*
Raw dairy products	Unpasteurized milk; some soft cheeses, such as Brie and camembert	*Listeria monocytogenes* E. coli Salmonella Campylobacter
Raw or rare meat	Hamburger	E. coli Salmonella
Raw fish	Sushi, tuna	Parasites

Note: For an expanded list of high-risk foods, see information at www.foodsafety.gov.

Tainted tuna

Tuna is one of the most widely consumed fish in the world, but more recently there have been concerns about the amount of mercury in tuna. Mercury is a naturally occurring element in the environment, but it is also the by-product of industry and is released into the air as a pollutant. The mercury in the air then falls from the sky in the rain and pollutes the lakes and oceans as it turns into methylmercury. Fish absorb methylmercury as they feed in polluted waters. Because tuna is a predatory fish (that is, it eats other smaller fish), it is more likely to accumulate mercury than other species.

Guidelines for eating tuna

In Canada, canned tuna (including albacore) is tested to ensure that mercury levels are below an acceptable minimum (0.5 parts per million). Tuna harvested for sale as fresh or frozen fish are subject to an acceptable minimum of 1.0 parts per million, which is one of the most stringent guidelines worldwide. Albacore tuna (white tuna) contains higher amounts of methylmercury than light (skipjack, yellowjack or tongol) tuna. Young children, as well as pregnant and nursing women, should limit their intake of fish high in methylmercury.

In 2004 the US Food and Drug Administration (FDA) along with the Environmental Protection Agency (EPA) released a joint statement on methylmercury in fish. They suggest that young children avoid fish high in methylmercury, including shark, swordfish, tilefish and king mackerel. They also recommend that young children eat up to two average servings of fish and shellfish lower in mercury per week, including fish such as salmon, sole, shrimp, scallops, haddock, halibut and canned light tuna. It is recommended that young children have no more than one meal per week of canned white (albacore) tuna.

Health Canada (2007) recommends that Canadians should eat at least two servings of fish per week, preferably fish that are high in omega-3 fatty acids (which are also low in mercury), such as salmon, Atlantic mackerel and rainbow trout. Young children between the ages of 1 and 4 should limit their intake of

---

Toxic fish

Predatory fish that should not be consumed by young children include king mackerel, shark, swordfish, tilefish and fresh or frozen tuna.

---

predatory fish that are higher in mercury to a maximum or 75 g ($2^{1}/_{2}$ oz.) a month. Children between 5 and 11 should eat no more than 125 g (4 oz) a month.

The American Dietetic Association and the Dietitians of Canada recommend that children regularly consume fish as part of a healthy diet.

Environmental concerns

Many parents are concerned about the environment — particularly about the use of pesticides and other chemicals in the production of our food. While regulatory agencies in both the United States and Canada have declared the levels of these substances in food to be safe for human consumption, some parents still worry that chemicals may be having (as yet unknown) effects upon their children. In fact, the presence of these agents in food is often blamed for the overall increase in child allergies and asthma.

Modern agricultural practices have helped farmers to make huge gains in the quantity and quality of food they are able to produce, which has made that food much less expensive and more widely available to a larger number of people. But questions of safety still persist.

Pesticide scare

Agricultural pesticides (including herbicides and other chemicals) control many different types of pests, including insects, rodents, weeds and microbial pests such as bacteria, fungi and viruses. Pesticides can be chemical, biological, natural or synthetic. The widespread use of insecticides began in the 1950s with the introduction of DDT (dichlorodiphenyltrichloroethane).

While often effective in eradicating specific problems, pesticides can have larger effects that are not intended. As most people now realize, we need to consider the entire ecological system in which the pests live. Because all pesticides are made to kill some organism, no single agent is considered to be "completely" safe. Indeed, safety is always a relative term, in which minimal risks are weighed against major benefits. For this reason, the effects of pesticides (which are widely speculated about in the media) have alarmed many consumers, even though most of the scientific community consider the risks from pesticide use to be minimal.

Hormone exposure

The FDA restricts the amount of hormones that can be given to livestock to produce larger, leaner animals. Consumers should be aware that different countries have different regulations on use of antibiotics and hormones for their food safety, such as for beef and milk.

In the Canadian dairy industry, there are very strict regulations and standards on the use of hormones. Dairy farms and the milk produced are checked routinely and must be certified. The milk must be free from antibiotics and growth hormones, such as BST and rBGH. If a cow is treated with antibiotics, then the milk is tested until it is free from them. The only ingredients added to milk are vitamins D and A, as required by Canadian law. Regulations for milk are different in the United States, where hormones and antibiotics are permitted.

Beef boosters

When it comes to beef, the regulations on use of hormones are different between countries. Certain growth hormones are permitted to be used in beef in Canada and America in order to produce larger and leaner products, but the European Union does not permit the use of growth hormones in their beef supply. The amount of hormones used raising beef cattle in the United States and Canada is considered to be so small that it poses no risk to human health.

Antibiotic enhancement

Antibiotics are chemicals that inhibit the growth of harmful microorganisms. Originally used in medicine to fight infection in humans, they are now used in agriculture — typically in relatively small doses added to feed to promote or enhance growth in animals.

Antibiotic safety

There is much public concern about the safety of antibiotics and the effects of possible antibiotic residue in the foods we eat. One major concern is that the use of antibiotics in animals may cause certain microorganisms to develop a resistance that could make them difficult to control in humans, or that antibiotic residues could trigger human allergic reactions. To minimize this risk, Food and Drug Administration (FDA) regulations specify maximum allowable doses and minimum times before slaughter that administration of antibiotics must be stopped. The FDA limits antibiotic residues permitted in animal products.

Environmental contaminants

While not used deliberately (in the same way pesticides are, for example), environmental contaminants can enter the food supply by various means, including exposure to air, water or soil that contains industrial wastes and other environmental pollutants. Many of these chemicals are not biodegradable, so once they enter the food chain they can accumulate in parts of the body (human or animal), including the liver, brain or fatty tissue. Examples of environmental contaminants include increased levels of mercury in tuna or swordfish (see page 100), contaminated water from lead pipes or increased cadmium levels in soil.

Avoiding bisphenol A

Bisphenol A (BPA) is a chemical used in the production of polycarbonate plastics and epoxy resins formed into infant bottles, water bottles and food and beverage packages. BPA gets into our bodies mainly through food and beverages. Canned foods may contain BPA as epoxy resins used to coat the metal on the inside of the can.

While some animal studies suggest that BPA can cause developmental disorders and cancer, the evidence is not clear whether there are any health effects of BPA on humans at current exposure levels. However, many people have taken this to be true, lobbying governments and manufacturers to remove BPA products from the market. Today, bottles and containers are often marked "BPA free." Some countries have banned BPA for certain products, such as infant bottles, but other countries do not yet have similar restrictions on BPA-containing products.

PCBs in food

Polychlorinated biphenyls (PCBs) are dangerous compounds that, in sufficient quantities, damage the immune system, rendering it less capable of fighting infection. While they are no longer allowed to be used in products (such as insulation), they are still found in our environment, where they persist in the soil and water. PCBs typically enter our food supply through dairy products, meat and other processed foods.

Young children and infants are especially vulnerable to PCBs. Breast milk can be a major source of PCBs in infants if their mothers have consumed a lot of fatty fish (such as salmon) that have been harvested from contaminated waters. It is prudent for pregnant women (as well as infants and young children) to limit their consumption of fatty fish harvested from fresh waters where contamination is either known or suspected.

Tips for minimizing your family's exposure to BPAs

1 Do not microwave plastic food containers. Microwaves will release BPAs.

2 Do not add hot liquids to plastic containers. While BPA is a strong material, it may break down with time.

3 Look for BPA-free products

4 Reduce the use of canned products. BPA can be found on the inside of the can as a coating on the metal.

5 Use glass, porcelain or stainless steel containers more often, instead of plastic ones.

Organic foods

Conventional agricultural techniques have helped to make farming more efficient, so you might expect that organic farming — which does not use pesticides, antibiotics or hormones — would be less efficient, with higher costs for each unit of production. For these reasons, costs for organic foods are higher than conventional choices.

Are these foods worth their cost? Many studies have been conducted on the levels of chemicals and pesticides found in conventionally produced foods, and these have been determined to be safe for human consumption. Food production is also strictly regulated by government. Organic and conventional foods are not completely isolated from the environment, and may still contain traces of pollutants beyond the farmer's control. When it comes to nutritional value of foods, organic and conventional foods are similar, though depending on soil and other conditions, some nutrients, such as vitamin C, may be higher in organic than in conventional food.

When it comes to feeding their children, many parents take comfort from offering organic foods to their children. For those undecided or unsure whether organic foods are worth the extra cost, a compromise may be to purchase in bulk organic foods that are consumed in large quantity by their children. When possible, visit farms or farmers' markets. This would be a valuable education for all family members, providing an opportunity for communication between consumers and farmers where specific questions about farming methods can be answered.

Scrub that food

To remove chemicals that may be deposited on the surface, wash all fruits and vegetables thoroughly under running water.

Is it certified?

To qualify as organic food, the originating farm or processing facility must meet the requirements of (and be inspected by) a government-recognized certification body.

Food science

Technology is continuously advancing to make it possible to produce more and more food for the world's population. For example, genetic manipulation has created crops that are resistant to pests, thereby reducing the need for chemical pesticides. This is desirable, of course, but often leads consumers to trade one worry for another — in this case, about the possible hazards of changing plant genetics.

Novel foods

Also known as genetically engineered foods, novel foods are typically those where a gene from one food has been inserted into the genetic make-up of another food. In some cases, this is done to make the food more resistant to damage from pests or disease; in others, it is done to increase its nutritional profile. These foods are always tested thoroughly before they reach the consumer. For example, genes from Brazil nuts were used to enhance the protein content of soybean meal (feed for animals) a few years ago. However, it was discovered that the genetically modified soy contained a nut protein that caused allergy, so the product was never brought to market.

Novel, or genetically modified, foods have not been shown to be any less safe than traditional foods. Governments in North America regulate the types of foods that are allowed to appear on grocery shelves. For example, it is the responsibility of the FDA and Health Canada to ensure that, in their respective countries, products derived through biotechnology are assessed for their potential impact on human health. (For information on probiotics, see page 62.)

Irradiation

How do you keep food fresh and safe for human consumption? One technique is irradiation — where food is subjected to gamma rays from radioactive cobalt 60 or cesium-137. This process kills most bacteria, insects and mold that are normally responsible for causing both decay and many food-borne illnesses.

Irradiation does not cause the food to be radioactive and does not form harmful compounds in the food. In fact, the FDA and Health Canada both consider it to be a safe, effective and economical way of preserving food. But the general public has not responded well to the idea of eating anything that has been in contact with radioactive materials, and food retailers have had trouble promoting irradiated foods in the US, where irradiated foods must be identified as such. In Canada, there are currently no means of identifying foods that have been treated with radiation.

Additives and behavior

Studies looking at the effect of food additives and colorings on children's behavior have reported conflicting results. In some cases, parents may want to eliminate suspect foods as long as their child's nutritional needs are met by the foods permitted.

Sweet nothings

Many artificial sweeteners have been approved by the FDA and Health Canada for use in our food supply. Sweeteners are found in a variety of food products, including baked goods, puddings, frozen desserts, yogurts, soft drinks and chewing gum. They are also available in the form of tabletop sweeteners as alternatives to sugar.

However, the safety of artificial sweeteners has not been studied in growing children. It is important to remember that children of all ages need sufficient calories to grow and develop normally. Children generally do not need to eat lower-calorie foods containing artificial sweeteners, although there is no harm in a child consuming a yogurt or the occasional beverage containing sweetener. The key is the amount of sweetener eaten daily. The FDA and Health Canada set "Acceptable Daily Intakes" (or ADIs) for all sweeteners, and normal consumption of the occasional sweetened product should never reach these limits.

Approved sweeteners

There are a number of sweeteners on the market, each of which has different characteristics.

- **Aspartame** (sold as NutraSweet® or Equal®) is a non-nutritive sweetener that is composed of two amino acids (the building blocks of protein): phenylalanine and aspartic acid. Many foods naturally contain these two amino acids. Aspartame is 200 times sweeter than sugar. It is safe to eat by virtually all individuals except those who have a rare disorder called phenylketonuria, or PKU, and need to control their phenylalanine intake. The acceptable daily intake for aspartame in the United States is 50 mg per kilogram of body weight per day (40 mg/kg/day in Canada). This means a 15 kg, or 33 lb, child can safely consume up to 750 mg (600 mg) of aspartame daily, or the equivalent of 10 (8) cans of diet soda every day.

Sweet safety

Most health authorities do not recommend artificial sweeteners for children under the age of 2 years because they do not provide calories in the diet. Very young children should never have their caloric intake compromised. In addition, the safety of artificial sweeteners has not been determined for children under the age of 2.

- **Cyclamate** (sold as Sugar Twin®) is 30 times sweeter than table sugar. Cyclamate has no aftertaste and can be used in both hot and cold foods. In Canada, cyclamate is available only as a tabletop sweetener.

- **Sucralose** (sold as Splenda®) is a calorie-free sweetener created from ordinary sugar. It looks and tastes just like sugar, but the body is not able to break it down and use it as energy. Sucralose is 400 to 800 times sweeter than sugar, and is available in a wide variety of products, including hot and cold drinks, as well as other commercial foods.

- **Acesulfame potassium**, or Ace K (sold as Sunett®) is about 200 times sweeter than sugar. People who are on restricted potassium diets or who have sulfa allergies should talk to their doctor before using Ace-K.

- **Sugar alcohols** (sold as Xylitol or Dentec®) are different from other artificial sweeteners in that they contribute calories to the diet. However, they are endorsed for use in chewing gum by the Canadian and American dental associations because they help prevent cavities. Sugar alcohols are also used in hard candies jams and cough lozenges.

It is important to remember that although artificial sweeteners are safe for use in foods and beverages, there is no need for healthy children to consume them. Artificial sweeteners, if enjoyed, should be used as a part of a healthy, well-balanced diet.

Functional Foods

Everywhere you look these days, there are advertisements calling out to parents, telling them that the manufacturer's food is supplemented, enriched or fortified with a variety of nutrients. These functional foods are processed with omega-3 fatty acids (DHA), vitamin D, probiotics, prebiotics, fiber, beta carotene, lycopene, calcium, antioxidants and isoflavones, to name just a few nutrients now added to food. Parents want what is best for their

Saccharin scare

Saccharin (sold as Sweet'N Low®) was one of the first artificial sweeteners available. It is 300 times sweeter than table sugar, but has a slightly bitter aftertaste. Saccharin has received much media attention over the years because of its alleged connection with cancer; however, research has not been able to determine a direct association.

tip
Functional foods have been supplemented with a specific nutrient to enhance their health benefit. Look for omega-3-enriched eggs or high-fiber white breads.

Fiber content of functional foods

The following chart provides examples of foods aimed at children that contain added fiber. High-fiber foods have at least 4 g of fiber per serving (keeping in mind that young children in particular will eat smaller serving sizes).

FOOD	SERVING SIZE	FIBER (G) PER SERVING	SOLUBLE/INSOLUBLE
Macaroni and cheese (whole wheat)	¼ box	3	Insoluble
Whole wheat pasta	85 g dry	7	Insoluble
White enriched pasta	85 g dry	9	Soluble
White enriched bread	2 slices	4	Insoluble (whole wheat variety) Soluble (white variety)
Instant oatmeal with fiber added	1 package	4	1 g insoluble 3 g soluble

children, but do our kids need all of these additives? If so, do these foods contain good-quality sources of the additives they are claiming will ensure good health for all kids?

Dietary fiber example

Let look at the possible health value of adding dietary fiber to food. Dietary fiber is a non-digestible component of plant products and can be referred to as soluble or insoluble. Soluble fiber dissolves in water to form a gel. It can help lower cholesterol and blood sugar levels. Insoluble fiber promotes the movement of stool through the body and increases stool bulk. These added functional fibers may be synthetic (such as polydextrose) or naturally occurring (such as inulin).

As childhood obesity levels rise, there will be more interest in the use of fiber in controlling cholesterol and blood sugar levels, but for most children the primary purpose of dietary fiber is to promote regularity. American and Canadian children do not get the recommended amount of fiber daily. Constipation is one of the most frequent reasons for referral to a pediatrician. For this reason, children should increase their consumption of total fiber, with a focus on insoluble fiber. Functional foods may contribute to meeting this need.

Food sources supplemented with omega-3 fatty acids

The following chart highlights a selection of the foods targeted at kids available on the market.

FOOD FORTIFIED WITH OMEGA-3 EFAS	ALA (MG) ~ VALUES	DHA + EPA (MG) ~ VALUES
Infant formula	23–56	10–12 DHA only
Homogenized milk (1 cup/250 mL)	30	70
Eggs (1 egg)	270	130
Orange juice (1 cup/250 mL)	50	50
Yogurt (3.5 oz/100 g)	60	40
Bread (2 slices)	85	15

Functional fats

"Omega-3 fatty acids" is an umbrella term for three different essential dietary fatty acids (EFAs): DHA (docosahexanoic acid), EPA (eicosapentaenoic acid) and ALA (alpha-linolenic acid). Although the body can convert ALA into DHA and EPA, it is not done very efficiently, so DHA and EPA must be obtained directly through dietary sources. The best dietary source of DHA and EPA is fatty fish, but North Americans tend not to eat the recommended amounts of fish. To address this deficiency, manufacturers have started adding omega-3 EFAs to many different foods, including yogurt, breads, pasta, infant cereal and formula, eggs, orange juice, cookies and even pork.

There are still no specific recommendations about the requirements of omega-3 fatty acids or DHA. The American Dietetic Association and Dietitians of Canada released a position paper on dietary fatty acids in 2007, suggesting that children over the age of 2 years receive 20% to 35% of energy intake as fat. They should decrease saturated and trans fat intake and increase omega-3 polyunsaturated fatty acid intake. No specific target values are given.

Family food diary

Moderation

I have always been a big believer in everything in moderation. Recently, some of my friends who now have young children of their own have been big proponents of organic foods. While I do believe that organic foods have their place in the market and I am all for considering organic fruits, vegetables and meat, I question whether there is a significant benefit to purchasing organic snack foods, such as cookies, "rice treats" and crackers. Prepackaged or boxed snack foods, whether organic or not, should be used in moderation and may still contain excessive sugar or salt that children do not need. I still maintain that fresh fruit and vegetables, organic or non-organic, make better options as snacks than any boxed snack. (Joanne)

Favorite recipes

Here are five of Joanne's kids' favorite recipes, which you will find in the recipe section of this book.

- Roasted Chicken and Vegetables (page 231)
- Fajita-Style Chicken (page 235)
- Pork Tenderloin Stir-Fry (page 246)
- Greek Pasta Salad (page 276)
- Chocolate Banana Pudding (page 321)

CHAPTER 8

Food Allergy
and Intolerance

One of the most worrying aspects of feeding a child is the possibility of a food allergy (which involves an immune response) or a food intolerance (which does not). Reactions to food can be serious, and it is important for parents to be knowledgeable about this subject — particularly where there is a family history of allergy or intolerance.

Immune responses to food

Food allergy, or "hypersensitivity," is defined as an immune system response to a food protein that the body identifies as foreign. It has been estimated that approximately 3% to 6% of children have an allergy to at least one food.

One predictor of whether or not a child may develop an allergy is a strong family history of allergy. If a parent or sibling has a food allergy, the child's risk of developing an allergy to a food is increased.

Allergies in general are inherited, although specific allergies are not. For example, if one parent has allergies, then the child may have a 50% to 75% chance of also having an allergic problem, even though the specific allergy or allergies may be different from those of the parent. Breastfeeding may also protect against certain allergies.

How to diagnose a food allergy

If you suspect your child may have a food allergy, speak with your doctor. Remember that you should always seek professional assistance in cases of suspected allergy.

Signs and symptoms

Signs and symptoms of allergy generally fall into the following categories:

- **Skin:** rash, hives, eczema
- **Digestive:** nausea, vomiting, stomach cramps, diarrhea
- **Respiratory:** runny nose, nasal congestion, difficulty breathing, wheezing
- **Cardiovascular:** increased heart rate

Don't attempt to eliminate multiple foods from your child's diet unless advised to do so by a physician. An unbalanced diet due to elimination can cause poor weight gain and/or vitamin or mineral deficiencies, depending on the kind and number of foods eliminated. If there is a strong family history of food allergy, your doctor may recommend that your child's blood be tested. There are other, less invasive tests commonly used.

Elimination diet: With this technique, highly allergenic foods are eliminated from the diet for a period of time (usually about 2 weeks). The eliminated foods are then slowly reintroduced, one at a time, to attempt to identify which foods are causing symptoms. This diet should only be followed under medical supervision because it can lead to nutritional deficiencies if too many foods have been removed from your child's diet.

Skin test: A "prick test" is commonly used to diagnose food allergy. A small amount of food allergen is placed under the skin by pricking the skin with a small needle. The skin is then monitored for a reaction. Skin tests are not 100% accurate and false positives (a positive reaction in the absence of a true allergy) can happen.

RAST/ImmunoCAP: This blood test can be done when a skin test cannot be completed because the child has severe eczema or is on medications that may interfere with a skin test. This test should not replace the skin test, as studies have shown that properly performed skin testing is more reliable than RAST testing. The newer CAP-RAST is more comparable to skin testing but is also more invasive.

Emergency action

Anaphylaxis is an immediate, life-threatening response involving several organ systems. Symptoms can include hives, swelling of any part of the body (such as the mouth and face), itching, difficulty breathing, nausea and diarrhea. Severe cases can lead to anaphylactic shock or even death. Anaphylactic symptoms usually occur within minutes of food ingestion, although they may take as long as 1 or 2 hours. Because of these dangers, parents of a child with anaphylactic reactions should take strict measures to avoid the offending foods, and carry with them (or have older children carry themselves) an injection containing epinephrine (such as Epipen®) at all times. (Epinephrine is a drug that will help to keep the airways open if an allergen has been ingested.) A prescription can be obtained through your physician, pediatrician or allergist. If the injection is used, it is still important to go to the nearest hospital after the drug has been injected.

Oral food challenge: In this test, a small amount of the suspected food is given under controlled conditions. The patient is then monitored for a reaction. This is the gold standard for confirming a food allergy but comes with significant risk and should only be performed in an allergist's office.

Types of allergies

There are many types of food allergies prevalent in children. In North America the five most common allergies involve milk, soy, eggs, peanuts and wheat. Here we provide some general information about these common allergens.

Milk allergy and cow's milk colitis

It has been estimated that between 2% and 3% of infants have an allergy to cow's milk protein. The good news is that most of them will grow out of it by the time they are 3 years old. Milk allergy is much more common in children than adults.

Cow's milk allergy is the traditional form of milk allergy and is an immune system response to the protein in milk. Health-care professionals call this an IgE-mediated allergy. Children with this type of allergy may break out in a rash or hives when exposed to cow's milk.

There are more than 30 proteins in milk, and most children with a milk allergy will react to more than one of these proteins. Since many milk proteins are not broken down when heated, a child will generally be as allergic to cold milk as to cooked milk or cooked products containing milk. Many of these children are able to tolerate soy milk or other soy products as an alternative to cow's milk.

Food allergy labeling

In the United States, food manufacturers are required by the FDA to list the eight most common food allergens if a specific product includes them. These eight foods include milk, eggs, peanuts, tree nuts (such as almonds and walnuts), fish (such as cod and bass), shellfish (such as crab and shrimp), soy and wheat. If a prepackaged product contains one of these ingredients, it will be clearly labeled "Contains milk," for example. This includes domestic and imported food packaging. Of course fresh fruits, vegetables and meats do not contain these warnings. At this time, Canadian regulations do not require that these eight allergens be listed on food labels, although labeling regulations are currently being updated. It is important to always double check and reread labels.

Allergy or intolerance?

It is important to differentiate between a cow's milk protein allergy, which is an immune response to the protein in milk, and lactose intolerance, which is an inability to digest the sugar in milk (lactose). Lactose intolerance does not involve an immune response. For more information on lactose intolerance, see page 121.

Cow's milk colitis

Cow's milk colitis is an intolerance to cow's milk not related to an immune response. These children often have blood in their stools. Many children with cow's milk colitis are also intolerant of soy protein and must avoid all foods containing cow's milk as well as soy.

Once a child has been diagnosed with a milk allergy, it is important to avoid all milk and foods containing milk or milk products. This includes

- All liquid and evaporated milks
- Yogurt, buttermilk
- Cream
- All cheeses, including hard cheeses, soft cheeses, cottage cheese and cream cheese
- Ice cream and ice milks
- Foods containing milk solids, such as butter and many margarines

Milk alternatives

Milk and milk products are an important source of energy, protein, calcium and vitamin D for non-vegetarian infants and toddlers. Therefore, if these foods need to be eliminated from the diet due to cow's milk allergy, it is important to replace them with acceptable alternatives in order to ensure adequate growth. Energy and protein can be found in many other foods, including meats, poultry, fish, grains, vegetables and fruit. And provided we have adequate exposure to sunlight, our bodies can produce sufficient vitamin D. It is more challenging, however, to find another source of dietary calcium.

Milk protein disguises

When you have young children with milk allergy, it is essential to read all food labels carefully for milk or words indicating milk protein ingredients. Some of these are not obvious, as the following list demonstrates. Help your child find these ingredients on packaged food labels, and circle the ingredient when you "detect" it.

Ammonium caseinate	Hydrolyzed milk protein	Milk derivative/protein/fat
Calcium caseinate	Lactalbumin	Modified milk ingredients
Casein/caseinate	Lactalbumin phosphate	Potassium caseinate
Curds	Lactate	Rennet casein
Delactosed whey	Lactoferrin	Sodium caseinate
Demineralized whey	Lactoglobulin	Whey
Dried milk	Lactose	Whey protein concentrate
Hydrolyzed casein	Magnesium caseinate	

SOURCE: Health Canada. Used with permission.

Fortified milk alternatives: These contain calcium and vitamin D. Acceptable choices include

- *Fortified soy milk.* This may not be appropriate for all children with cow's milk allergy, since some children may also be intolerant of soy protein. Check with your doctor to see which is the best choice for your child. Remember, too, that while all infant soy formulas on the North American market are fortified, all soy milks are not. Check the label to make sure that a soy milk has been fortified with calcium and vitamin D, and that it is a good source of energy (since some varieties are low in fat).
- *Some rice beverages.* It is important to ensure that a rice beverage has been fortified with calcium and vitamin D. Rice beverages are also low in calories and protein, so ensure that the child's diet contains adequate energy and protein from alternative sources.

Unacceptable choices include

- *Goat's milk:* Between 70% and 80% of children with cow's milk protein allergy will also be allergic to goat's milk.
- *Nut milks (such as almond milk):* Many children with cow's milk allergy may also be allergic to nuts. In addition, many nut milks are not fortified.
- *Fruit juices:* Nutritionally speaking, fruit juices are no substitute for milk.

Green leafy vegetables: Broccoli, spinach and kale provide some calcium, although it is not easily absorbed by the body. They will probably not provide adequate dietary calcium on their own.

Canned fish with the bones included: Canned salmon with bones may be a good source of calcium for milk-allergic children. To reduce choking risk, make sure that the bones are well mashed before serving.

Fortify!

It is difficult to consume enough calcium in the diet if your child is not consuming a fortified alternative beverage. For these milk-allergic children, a calcium supplement may be recommended. Speak with your physician for more information.

Tofu: Since this product is made from soy, it is clearly not suitable for a child with soy allergy. Otherwise, tofu is a good source of calcium, although the silken variety is less so.

Legumes: These may contain some calcium.

Soy protein allergy

The symptoms of soy protein allergy are similar to those of an allergy to cow's milk protein. In infants and young children these may include abdominal pain, loose stools or diarrhea, vomiting, respiratory symptoms, such as a cough or wheeze, and eczema or hives.

Many unlabeled products — including bulk foods, unwrapped breads and baked goods — contain soy, especially when flour is an ingredient. If your child has been advised to follow a soy-free diet because of a soy allergy, it is important to also avoid these foods.

Although pure soy oil should not cause an allergic reaction (technically, it contains no protein), there is a risk that it could have been contaminated with soy

Best alternative

For children over the age of 2 years on a milk-free, soy-free diet, it is essential to find an acceptable milk alternative. We recommend a rice beverage fortified with calcium and vitamin D as the best alternative when cow's milk or fortified soy milk cannot be used.

Hidden soy

Because soy and soy products are found in so many commercially prepared foods today, it can be very difficult to follow a soy-free diet. With adequate education and information, however, it is possible to maintain a well-balanced diet that is free of soy proteins. Read food labels carefully for ingredients that indicate the presence of soy protein; many are not obvious. Help your child find these ingredients on packaged food labels, and circle that ingredient when you "detect" it.

Edamame	Soya, soja, soybean, soyabean	TSP (textured soy protein)
Miso	Soy protein (isolate/concentrate)	TVP (textured vegetable protein)*
Monodiglyceride	Tempeh	Vegetable protein
Natto	Tofu (soybean curds)	Yuba
Okara	TSF (textured soy flour)	

*Textured vegetable protein may come from different vegetable sources, including soy. If the source is not identified, it may contain soy protein.

SOURCE: Health Canada. Used with permission.

protein during the manufacturing process. To be safe, it makes sense to avoid soy oil in cases of soy allergy.

Egg allergy

Eggs are a terrific source of many nutrients, including energy, protein, fat and vitamins, such as riboflavin and vitamin B_{12}. However, there are many different types of protein in eggs — found primarily in the whites — to which some children may be allergic. Cooking can break down some of these proteins, in which case a child who is allergic to raw eggs may tolerate eggs when they are cooked. Keep in mind, however, that some egg proteins are not broken down during the cooking process and can still cause an allergic reaction.

Cooking without eggs

While an egg allergy can make it unsafe to eat commercially prepared foods (since so many egg ingredients are not clearly identified on food labels), it need not be a problem if you prepare the food yourself. For example, there are many recipes that call for eggs, but can be made egg-free by using egg substitutes. This allows children with egg allergies to enjoy foods (baked goods, say) that might otherwise be too risky for them to eat.

What's in that vaccine?

Some vaccines for common illnesses contain traces of egg protein. If your child has an egg allergy, be sure to check with your doctor that a vaccine does not contain egg.

Egg-free eggs

Check out your local health food store for some of the "egg replacer" products that are now available. These products do not contain egg protein, which allows children with egg allergies to enjoy "eggs" for breakfast. Be sure you don't confuse these specialized egg replacers with the low-cholesterol egg products commonly sold in grocery stores; they may be healthier, but they are not egg free.

Egg hunting

Avoiding eggs on their own is fairly simple. But eggs or egg proteins may be hidden in many prepared foods, including baked goods, salad dressings and sauces. The following is a list of words that indicate the presence of egg protein in food.

Albumin	Egg white	Mayonnaise	Ovovitellin
Baking powder	Egg yolk	Ovalbumin	Pasteurized egg
Egg	Frozen egg	Ovoglobulin	Simplesse®
Egg powder	Globulin	Ovomucin	Vitellin
Egg protein	Livetin	Ovomucoid	

SOURCE: Health Canada. Used with permission.

Egg substitutions

For egg-free baking and cooking, try some of the following substitutions for eggs in recipes.

1 Where egg is used as a leavening agent. For each egg required, use 1 tbsp (15 mL) egg-free baking powder + 2 tbsp (25 mL) liquid

OR

2 tbsp (25 mL) flour + $\frac{1}{2}$ tbsp (7 mL) egg-free baking powder + 2 tbsp (25 mL) liquid

You can make your own egg-free baking powder (see below) or buy an egg-free commercial variety (such as Magic brand). Use whatever liquid is appropriate for the recipe (water, vinegar, fruit juice, stock, etc.).

For recipes that call for only 1 egg and a relatively large amount of baking powder (for example, 2 tsp/10 mL baking powder or $1\frac{1}{2}$ tsp/7 mL baking soda), try replacing the egg with 1 tbsp (15 mL) vinegar.

2 Where egg is used as a binder. For each egg required:

In a saucepan, combine $\frac{1}{3}$ cup (75 mL) water and 3 to 4 tsp (15 to 20 mL) brown flaxseeds. Bring to a boil; reduce heat and simmer for 5 to 7 minutes or until a slightly thickened gel begins to form. Strain through a sieve, discarding seeds. Use gel for egg in recipe.

OR use

$\frac{1}{3}$ cup (75 mL) water + 1 tbsp (15 mL) arrowroot powder + 2 tsp (10 mL) guar gum

OR use

2 oz (50 g) tofu

3 Where egg is used as a liquid. For each egg required, use:

$\frac{1}{3}$ cup (75 mL) apple juice

OR

4 tbsp (60 mL) puréed apricot

OR

1 tbsp (15 mL) vinegar

To make egg-free baking powder, combine 1 part baking soda + 2 parts cream of tartar + 1 part cornstarch. Mix well and store in airtight container.

SOURCE: J Vickerstaff-Joneja. Dealing with Food Allergies in Babies and Children, 2007.

Peanut allergy

Of all food allergies, peanut allergy is one of the most dangerous, because it can trigger anaphylactic reactions. Peanut allergy affects 1% to 2% of the population. Unlike milk and egg allergies, most children do not outgrow it.

Symptoms of peanut allergy may not necessarily be as serious as anaphylaxis, but can include skin rash, eczema and hives; respiratory symptoms, such as wheezing; nausea or vomiting; and itching. Where the risk of anaphylactic reactions does exist, children with peanut allergies (or their parents or daycare providers) should carry an Epipen® — and should know how to inject the epinephrine — in case of emergencies.

Children with peanut allergy are not necessarily allergic to all nuts, and may be able to eat other tree nuts — such as pecans, walnuts and cashews — without effect. However, if your child has a peanut allergy, it is safer to avoid all nuts. Even when nuts are identified as being something other than peanuts (or, in the case of nut mixtures, as not containing peanuts), trace amounts may still exist. Also, be sure to read labels carefully for foods that "may contain" peanuts.

Dining out caution

Avoid pure peanut oil, which, although theoretically free of peanut protein, may also contain trace amounts. This type of oil is often used in Thai and Chinese cooking, so you may wish to avoid restaurants that serve these foods. In fact, whenever dining out with an allergic child, it makes sense to call ahead and ask about any ingredients that may cause a reaction.

A.K.A. peanuts

Peanuts can go by many other names, and parents should be able to recognize that many words on a label may indicate the presence of peanuts. Help your child find these ingredients on packaged food labels, and circle that ingredient when you "detect" it.

Arachide	Goober nuts/goober peas	Nu-Nuts®
Arachis oil	Ground nuts	Nut meats
Beer nuts	Kernels	Valencias
Cacahouète/cacahouette/ cacahuète	Mandelonas	

SOURCE: Health Canada. Used with permission.

Wheat allergy

The most common grain allergy in North America is to wheat. This allergy is an adverse reaction to the protein component of wheat. It is different from celiac disease, in which affected people cannot tolerate gluten (a protein found in many grains, including wheat, rye and barley). Gluten is found in breads and cereals (even rice crispies), pastas and cakes, cookies and candies, as we would expect, but it is also found in luncheon meats and sausages — in fact in any food that contains flour (made from wheat).

Because wheat flour is fortified with vitamins (riboflavin, thiamin and niacin) and iron, eliminating it from an allergic child's diet can result in nutritional deficiencies. Alternative flours, such as corn, rye or rice flours, can be used for cooking and baking for the wheat-allergic child, but these flours are not usually fortified. Other foods high in B vitamin content will need to be added to the child's diet to ensure adequate nutrient intake.

Wheat by many other names

All of the following words indicate the presence of wheat in the food item. Help your child in finding these ingredients on packaged food labels, and circle that ingredient when you "detect" it.

Atta	Enriched white/whole wheat flour	Semolina
Bulgur	Farina	Seitan
Couscous	Gluten	Spelt (dinkel, faro)
Durum	Graham flour	Triticale (a cross between wheat and rye)
Einkorn	High gluten/protein flour	Triticum aestivum
Emmer	Kamut	Wheat bran/flour/germ/starch

SOURCE: Health Canada. Used with permission.

Multiple food allergies

The majority of children allergic to food are allergic to one food only, although some may be allergic to two, three or four foods. Allergies to five or more foods are highly unusual and are more likely to be the result of incorrect diagnoses. The most common food reactions in infancy and childhood are·those to milk and dairy products, eggs, soy, peanuts, nuts, wheat, fish and shellfish.

While it is important to eliminate all allergens from the child's diet, it is also necessary to ensure that proper alternatives are provided to meet the child's nutritional needs for growth. The elimination of many foods without cause can be dangerous.

Food intolerances

While there are different types of food intolerance (which is distinguished from food allergy by its not involving an immune response), one of the most common among children is lactose intolerance.

Lactose intolerance

Unlike a milk allergy (where the immune system reacts to cow's milk protein), lactose intolerance is caused by a deficiency of lactase. This enzyme (located in the small intestine) is responsible for breaking down the sugar lactose, which is found in milk and milk products.

When lactose is not broken down, it builds up in the digestive system, causing excess water to be drawn into the intestines, which can cause diarrhea. Other symptoms include abdominal pain and discomfort. Bloating and gas are caused by the fermentation of lactose by bacteria in the digestive tract.

The good news for anyone suffering from lactose intolerance is that there are many products available to make your life easier. By taking lactase supplements at mealtime (usually in pill form), you can enjoy dairy and other foods containing lactose without discomfort. Lactose-free milks are also available for those who are lactose intolerant.

Medical caution

Allergy to a specific food should be confirmed before eliminating it from a child's diet, and should only be done under a physician's supervision. Occasionally, supplements may be required, and dietary counseling may be beneficial for some families.

Lactose loss

Lactose intolerance in infancy is extremely rare (since lactose is present in breast milk). However, many people lose the ability to produce lactase later in life. This is most common among people of Asian, African-American and Mediterranean descent, up to 80% of whom lose the ability to digest lactose starting at around age 5 (compared to only 20% of people with Northern European ancestry).

CHAPTER 9

Disturbances
in Bowel Function

Any parent will tell you that the bowel habits of their children have caused concern at some point in their lives. Indeed, the main point of discussion during routine visits to the family doctor or pediatrician is often focused on whether a child's bowel movements are too infrequent or too frequent. The information presented here may help parents to understand more (and worry less) about this subject.

Establishing patterns

During infancy, there is great variation in the frequency, color and consistency of bowel movements. This continues from the first few weeks of life to later months, when a wider variety of foods is introduced. By the age of 2, bowel patterns usually become established, with more regular and predictable consistency and number of movements per day. After this age, normal stools are soft and usually occur one or two times per day, although frequency may be less in some children. With the commencement of toilet training, however, and with other new routines — for example, when starting daycare — a change in bowel habits may be observed.

How digestion works

When food is chewed and swallowed, it is mixed with juices in the stomach and ground down to very small particles. This mixture is then released into the small intestine, where digestion and absorption take place. Once it reaches the large intestine, or colon, the mixture moves much more slowly, and much of the water is "pulled" out. Fiber, an undigested part of food, reaches the colon and helps to keep stools soft by holding water, making the stool softer and easier to pass.

Coping with constipation

Constipation is defined as a delay or difficulty in passing stool, lasting for 2 or more weeks, causing distress to the child. Constipation affects 5% to 10% of school-age children. Constipation occurs when there is reduced water content in the stool. This can lead to difficulty in passing stool and cause distress to the child. When children are constipated, their stools, which are normally soft, become harder, usually larger in volume and less frequent. It is estimated that this prompts some 3% of all visits to the general practitioner and 15% to 25% of pediatric gastroenterology consultations.

Constipation may start out with only one or two episodes of withholding stools due to painful stooling. But if left untreated, the condition may become chronic and last for years. Chronic constipation is believed to be one of the main causes of repeated abdominal pain in children.

Causes of childhood constipation

Only a very small percentage of children become constipated as a result of disease or other "medical" factors. Rather, the causes are much more likely to be dietary or behavioral. Your family doctor will be able to evaluate the cause and sort out the best treatment for your child.

The most common causes of childhood constipation are dietary, behavioral (deliberately withholding stool), toilet training and change in daily routine. When children begin to be toilet trained, they may "hold in" their stool so that they do not have to try to use the toilet, or sometimes they are "just too busy" to make the trip to the bathroom. When held in, the stool stays in the colon (the last part of large intestine) for a longer period, with the result that more water is drawn out of the stool and reabsorbed into the colon, thus making the stool drier and harder to pass. (Sometimes children who are constipated will have soiling in their underwear, which occurs when loose stool passes around the hard stool mass. Children are unable to withhold or control this loose stool.) The size of the stool becomes larger, and this also makes it more difficult to pass. This is naturally distressing for the child, who may have already experienced a hard stool that was pushed out with great effort, resulting in both pain and, occasionally, a small amount of blood (from a small tear in the bowel wall). Constipation can result in abdominal pain and create a decrease in appetite that, in extreme cases, may result in weight loss.

High-fiber diet

Children with constipation generally have a diet that is lower in fiber than is recommended. A high-fiber diet will alleviate constipation in the majority of children.

Family ties

In addition to its other causes, the tendency to become constipated may also have a genetic component. As a result, parents who have had problems with bowel movements may find that their children have the same difficulty.

Tips for treating childhood constipation

Experts agree that a number of factors can help relieve or reduce constipation.

1. Make sure the child's diet is rich in fiber and fluid. If the child is not eating the recommended number of fresh vegetables and fruits, these should be increased (see page 59 for more information on sources of fiber). Encourage consumption of whole-grain cereals and breads, along with plenty of water. If the child prefers a cereal that is low in fiber, mix it together with a higher-fiber variety. A diet rich in fiber will help alleviate constipation in the majority of children.

2. Set a regular bowel routine to help improve training and decrease the straining. This involves setting a specific time each day to sit quietly on the toilet. If you wish, set up a system of rewards, such as a sticker chart to recognize successes, as well as other positive reinforcements.

3. Provide sorbitol-rich juices. Some fruit juices, such as prune and apple, contain higher-than-average amounts of sorbitol, a sugar that remains in the small intestine and moves to the large intestine (or colon), where it is broken down into smaller particles, which pull water back into the stool. This has the effect of softening the stool, making it easier to pass. It may be worthwhile to try giving a child juices that contain sorbitol in order to relieve constipation.

4. If constipation persists for a long period, consult your family doctor, who may recommend intervention with some form of laxative. Mineral oil is sometimes used for children older than 2 to 3 years. Lactulose and sorbitol are also considered to be safe and effective treatments. New formulations that contain polyethylene glycol powders mixed with water or juice are safe and can be effective for constipation. Drinking extra fluids is always encouraged. Always consult your family doctor before beginning any laxative treatment. Prolonged use of laxatives should be avoided, if possible, and then only under the supervision of your doctor.

5. If the stool is impacted (and the child is unable to pass it voluntarily), then an oral or rectal medication may be given, including an enema. Any non-dietary treatments should be given under the supervision of the family doctor. Prolonged use of any treatment should be evaluated on a regular basis by medical personnel. Once the stool is passed, encourage a regular bowel routine, as well as the regular consumption of adequate fluids and fiber.

6. If these therapies fail, or if it is suspected that the constipation is caused by factors other than behavioral or functional, or if management becomes complex, then the case should be referred to a specialist.

Dealing with childhood diarrhea

Childhood diarrhea is defined as a change in bowel pattern that can result in more frequent or looser, watery stools. It the most common of all reasons for seeing the doctor. Guidelines have been developed by a number of medical groups, including the American Academy of Pediatrics, on the appropriate treatment for diarrhea.

The most frequent cause of acute (or sudden) diarrhea is viral infection. Stools may be more mucusy and have a distinctly different odor than usual. Viral illness causing diarrhea may also be accompanied by vomiting. Since dehydration is typically the result (a particularly dangerous condition for infants because of their small size), the focus of treatment is on rehydration with fluids, such as an appropriate electrolyte solution. Your family doctor will tell you the volume required and the period over which they should be given (usually 24 hours).

After rehydration, a normal diet should be resumed, even with continued diarrhea. (Be sure to remain watchful for signs of dehydration; your doctor can tell you what to look for.) A child should not be offered only juices, for example, or plain cereals until the diarrhea subsides. This may only prolong their diarrhea and result in weight loss. If vomiting is severe, a return to normal diet may have to be delayed until symptoms subside.

Chronic diarrhea is less common, and may be caused by excessive juice intake. As an alternative to juice, children should be offered water between meals to quench their thirst. Daily juice consumption of more than 6 oz (175 mL) can result in a decreased appetite for foods that make up a varied diet, and this lack of variety can itself be a cause of diarrhea.

There are other causes of chronic diarrhea that may be medical. Your family doctor will investigate further if necessary.

Rehydration solutions

When children become dehydrated, they lose electrolytes (for example, sodium, potassium and chloride). To restore these compounds, a doctor may recommend using an electrolyte solution, which can be found in pharmacies and grocery stores.

Lactose intolerance

Sometimes diarrhea is caused by a carbohydrate or lactose intolerance (which itself may be the temporary result of viral illness). Lactose is a sugar found in milk that is normally broken down by an enzyme, called lactase, found in the wall of the intestine. When the supply of lactase is inadequate, the undigested lactose has the effect of "pulling" water through the intestine, causing watery and more frequent stools. In these cases, it may be advisable to give a child lactose-free milk. Your family doctor can advise you, if necessary, on the type of milk to choose.

CHAPTER 10

Childhood Obesity

For the first few years of life, weight gain is both healthy and desirable for children. But after the age of 3, a child who is significantly heavier than his or her peers may be heading for a weight problem. Children should never be put on a "diet" that restricts food intake in order to promote weight loss. Weight problems can be avoided by teaching your child the importance of healthy living (which includes eating and exercise) from an early age.

Global epidemic

Childhood obesity is the most common nutritional problem among children in North America today. It has been estimated that 26% of children age 2 to 17 years are overweight and 8% are obese. And the number of obese younger children is steadily increasing. To counteract this problem, the building blocks of good nutrition and exercise need to be established while children are young.

In 1998, the World Health Organization declared obesity a "global epidemic" for both adults and children. The WHO also stated that being overweight because of poor nutrition and lack of physical activity is one of the greatest health challenges of the 21st century. Obese children have an increased risk of developing childhood hyperinsulinemia (which may be a risk factor for the development of non-insulin-dependent diabetes mellitus), as well as high blood pressure and dyslipidemia (abnormal blood cholesterol levels).

Double the risk

With each year after the age of 3, the probability that an obese child will become an obese adult continues to increase. It is generally estimated that overweight children are twice as likely to be obese as adults when compared with children who are not overweight. This risk increases when one or more of the child's parents are also overweight.

The health risks of obesity in adulthood are well known. Obesity has been associated with high blood pressure, high cholesterol, non-insulin-dependent diabetes mellitus, some cancers (including colon, breast and pancreatic), skin disorders, orthopedic conditions and psychosocial illnesses, including depression.

Shorter lives

New research now shows these complications are increasingly affecting children and that it is no longer uncommon for children to have type 2 diabetes, high blood pressure or abnormal cholesterol levels. In fact it has now been predicted that this generation of children is the first who may live shorter lives than their parents. In an article in the *New England Journal of Medicine*, it was predicted that obesity may shorten the lifespan of today's youth by 3 to 5 years over the next 40 years. This may not seem like much, but when you consider that cancer currently reduces longevity by about $3\frac{1}{2}$ years, obesity's effect is enormous.

Prevention is the key

Once a child (or adult) becomes obese, experience has shown that treatment programs often prove ineffective for long-term weight management. Therefore, prevention is the key.

The early childhood years are the best time to establish healthy eating habits and an active lifestyle that can be maintained throughout a child's life. Poor dietary and exercise habits have not yet been formed, and parents continue to have an influence over the lifestyle of their children. Young children are naturally active, and it is only a matter of encouraging them and giving them opportunities to continue to be active. This is also a great opportunity for many parents to give their own diet and exercise routines an overhaul. We are often motivated to make changes for the benefit of our children that we wouldn't necessarily do for ourselves.

Managing weight

Successful weight management programs for children have in common a team approach, and incorporate exercise with dietary changes and family therapy. Setting specific goals is also a key to success.

Healthy eating habits

The hectic lifestyle experienced by today's families makes it challenging to develop healthy eating habits — for adults and children. Families dine out more than they did in previous generations, and may make less nutritious choices. When families dine in, they may often choose prepackaged meals or convenience foods because some parents have less time to cook and have busy schedules that continue once they get home from work.

All these things do not escape the notice of young children who, unlike infants (typically fed on their own schedules), are now joining the family for meals. Therefore, it is important for parents to set a good example and choose healthy foods and meals for the entire family.

Parents' eating habits and beliefs mold children's food preferences and eating patterns. If parents adopt healthy eating patterns, their children will likely follow. If parents have poor eating habits, then that is what children will accept as the norm. Children also pay attention to the foods that come home from the grocery store, so it is important that moms and dads make healthy choices when they go to the market.

Severe restrictions should not be placed on the consumption of high-energy and/or high-fat foods for young children. Turning any kind of food into a "forbidden fruit" may simply focus the child's attention on that food and make it more desirable. Nutrient-dense, high-energy or higher-fat foods play an important role in a growing child's diet. Nutritious food choices should not be eliminated or severely restricted in a young child's diet simply because of their fat content.

Born to eat junk food?

While it has been said that young children have an innate preference for high-sugar or high-fat foods, there is no evidence to suggest this. Children can learn to like healthy, nutritious foods just as easily as sweets or other junk foods.

Putting fat into perspective

Thanks to widespread media reports, it is now almost accepted wisdom that a high-fat diet is bad for your health and causes obesity. The fact is that no single nutrient causes obesity, although consuming an excess number of total calories (in relation to activity) certainly will.

Tips for preparing homemade meals

Most families have extremely busy schedules that can make eating healthy, nutritious meals difficult. One temptation is to eat prepackaged foods or dine out often, but this is a long-term recipe for complications of overweight and obesity. Better to prepare your own meals. Try planning your menu at the beginning of the week, choose favorite healthy recipes and use the ingredients list as a shopping guide. Taking a few extra minutes to plan meals at the beginning of the week before heading to the grocery store can save time during the week.

1. Decide which nights of the week you (or your partner) will be home and have time to cook dinner.

2. Start writing your shopping list by noting staples you may be running low on, such as low-fat milk and whole-grain bread.

3. Then decide on a couple of main courses for dinners and build around them. For example, chicken breasts on Tuesday can be served with couscous and broccoli. Salmon on Thursday works well with frozen mixed vegetables and roasted red potatoes.

4. Have some dinners prepared in advance that can be frozen for making dinners in a hurry, for example, Spinach and Mushroom Lasagna Roll-Ups (page 214), Speedy Beef Strogonoff (page 251) or Tuscan Bean Soup (page 171). Double recipes and freeze some for a second meal.

5. Buy lots of fresh vegetables to cut up and put in the refrigerator at the beginning of the week for quick and healthy snacks during the whole week. Good examples include carrots, celery, broccoli and cauliflower. This may seem like a simple thing to do, but it can significantly increase your child's vegetable intake and also cut down on the number of cookies or other unhealthy snacks your kids may be eating.

6. Include your children in food selection and preparation. At the grocery store, let your children help make decisions about what types of veggies and fruits they would like to eat. Take the time to let them help in the kitchen. This could be as simple as stirring a bowl of homemade pancake mix or helping to chop vegetables for a salad (with supervision, of course).

Nutrition experts suggest that healthy individuals should get no more than 30% of the calories in the diet from fat and no more than 10% of calories from saturated fat. But these figures are intended for older children and adults. Infants tend to have a higher-fat diet, in which approximately 50% of calories come from fat.

Many health authorities now recommend a slow, gradual transition from the high-fat diet of infancy to the lower-fat diet of an adult. This transition should take place from the age of 2 years until a child has reached his or her full height potential at the end of adolescence. During this transition period, energy intake should be adequate to support normal growth and development.

Food for thought

Consider this: A recent paper published in the *New England Journal of Medicine* discusses the negative effects that marketing food directly at children can have on children's eating habits and weight. Marketing food to children specifically entices children who may be too young to tell the difference between fact and fiction to eat junk foods that are high in calories and low in nutrients. The majority of a typical American child's spending money is used to buy soda pop, candy and chips — foods repeatedly advertised on television and elsewhere. It has been estimated that at least 30% of the calories in an average child's diet come from the sweet and salty processed foods.

Restricted advertising

In response to this problem, government agencies in North America have restricted the amount of commercial time available during children's programming but not the types of foods that can be advertised to children. In Australia, Sweden and the Netherlands, they have prohibited the marketing of certain types of food directly to children under the age of 12 to 14 years. What effect these restrictions have on the intake of unhealthy foods for the children living in these countries has not yet been determined, but some researchers suggest it could decrease the rates of childhood obesity by as much as 2.5% to 6%.

Physical activity

Young children tend to be naturally active and enjoy playing and running about. As they get older and start preschool or grade school, it is important that they continue to

No good or bad foods

As you help to develop healthy eating habits in your children, remember that there are no "good" or "bad" foods. It is the overall diet that is important. Kids need a variety of nutrient-rich foods throughout the day. These foods should include whole grains, cereals, fruit and vegetables, and lower- and full-fat milk products (or other calcium-rich foods), as well as protein-rich foods such as beans, lean meats, poultry or fish.

be active. Yet with technological advances and societal changes, today's children have become generally less active, spending more time participating in sedentary activities, such as watching television or playing computer games. In fact, it has been estimated that young children in North America today expend about 25% fewer calories than current recommendations for caloric intake. And when more energy is consumed than expended, it is stored as fat.

Apart from television and computer games, there are other societal factors that contribute to the decline in children's activity levels. Today's parents are generally more safety conscious (or risk averse) than those of previous generations. As a result, children who were once free to play outdoors at every opportunity now have their activity restricted to supervised recreational activities and playgrounds — which may or may not be available for much of the time. Some school-age children may come home after school to an empty house until mom or dad comes home from work. These "latch key" children are often forbidden to play outside by parents because of safety concerns.

A family that plays together...

Spontaneous physical activity should be a part of daily life for children. These lifestyle activities are easier to sustain than regimented exercise programs. Children are more likely to continue with an activity if they are allowed to choose an activity in which they are interested, rather than having one chosen for them. Forcing children to exercise can decrease chances of success.

Children do not exercise the way adults do. When they are physically active, they "exercise" in short bursts of activity; for example, when playing tag or a game of hide and seek. They do not exercise like adults with regimented exercise programs because it is good for them to do so. They are active because it is fun. They play and have a good time but do not generally "exercise." This type of physical activity is much easier to sustain because it is enjoyable.

Activity for life

Encouraging physical activity does not mean embarking on an ambitious fitness program. Instead, it should be seen as a program of maintenance — taking familiar activities (such as walking and bike riding) and making them part of your (and your child's) life. Maintaining an active lifestyle is always easier than trying to make big changes to lifestyle habits.

Parents should participate in activities with their children. This provides a wonderful opportunity for parents to spend time with their children and increases the physical activity of the entire family. Activities may include things such as family walks or bike rides. Research has shown that parents who are inactive tend to have children who are inactive. Likewise, parents who enjoy an active lifestyle tend to have children who also enjoy being active.

Other strategies for maintaining physical activity may include encouraging children to reduce time spent in sedentary pursuits. Limits should be set on the amount of television watched and computer games played. Research has shown that setting these limits can be just as (or more) effective as trying to get kids to go outside and exercise.

Overcoming the power of television

It has been estimated that the average North American child watches approximately 3 hours of television per day. When combined with computer games and other physically undemanding activities involving other media (watching movies, for example), this figure may be in excess of 6 hours a day.

Studies have shown a significant link between television watching and the prevalence of obesity. The time spent watching television or other media can displace other activities that are more enriching for the mind and body, including reading, exercise and playing with friends.

Television can also cause an increase in between-meal snacking. Children may snack on less nutritious foods while watching television and may not be aware of how much they are actually eating.

Commercials also affect a child's eating patterns by encouraging the consumption of foods advertised on television. Television advertising has been shown to influence a parent's grocery store purchases, often

Graduates of TV

The exposure of American children and adolescents to television is estimated to exceed the time they spend in the classroom. By the time they graduate, children will have spent an average of 12,000 hours in the classroom and 15,000 hours in front of a television set.

Tips for increasing family physical activity

1 Aim for 90 minutes or more of active play each day.

2 Limit screen time (this includes television and computers) to no more than 1 hour per day.

3 Have fun as a family — go for a bike ride or hike or kick a soccer ball around. This is fun for both your children and you.

4 Make sure that your kids have lots of opportunities for active play throughout the week.

because children make requests for specific foods. Even brief exposures to televised food commercials have been shown to have an influence on the food preferences of young children. Commercials typically aired during children's programming are often for calorically dense foods such as sugared breakfast cereals, chocolate bars, cakes, cookies and soda pop. One recent Australian study found that 63% of food advertisements during children's programming were for high-fat and/or high-sugar foods.

While there are some worthwhile, educational benefits of watching television — including the promotion of many positive social behaviors, such as sharing, manners and cooperation — there are also many negative health effects, apart from increasing the prevalence of obesity. These include the depiction (not always unfavorably) of violent or aggressive behavior, substance use and abuse, and sexual activity, as well as decreased school performance. A recent American study found that 32% of children between the ages of 2 and 7 years old have a television in their bedroom. In such cases, it is not surprising that parents are often not aware of what their children are watching, or that they do not limit the amount of television their children watch. Many young children are not able to distinguish between what they see on television and what is real, and children's programs can be some of the most violent on television.

Body and soul

Too much television can have a negative effect on body image, nutrition and dieting behaviors of young children and adolescents.

Tips for watching television

Both the American and Canadian pediatric societies have published suggestions for parents regarding the television that their children watch. These suggestions for parents include

1. Limit television viewing to a maximum of 1 to 2 hours per day
2. Emphasize alternative activities, including reading, athletics, hobbies and creative play
3. Participate in the selection of programs to be viewed
4. Watch TV with children and discuss it with them
5. Be a good media role model for children
6. Remove television sets from children's and adolescents' bedrooms
7. Avoid using the television as an "electronic babysitter"

The proper role of food

Food should not be used as a tool for reward, bribery or punishment. Parents will often use tactics to get kids to eat, to calm temper tantrums or to promote good behavior. Examples include, "Eat all your vegetables and then you may go and watch television," or "If you stop fighting with your sister, you may have a cookie." These feeding techniques can result in children who have a poor ability to regulate their caloric intake, and may contribute to overeating behavior and obesity.

Positive outlook

How you as a parent help to shape your children's attitudes toward eating and toward their body image could be the most important factor in preventing obesity and other eating disturbances.

Food is not a controlled substance

Parents should not try to control their child's food intake. Those who attempt to control their child's eating patterns are more likely to have children who are less capable of self-regulating their caloric intake. In other words, their children are less aware of using hunger to determine their eating habits — specifically, that they should eat when they are hungry and stop eating when they are full. Controlling a child's eating patterns includes forcing children to eat when they are told to, and to "eat what's on your plate."

Parents should provide healthy food choices, but must allow their children to assume control of their own intake. This can be difficult, because it is often tempting to place severe restrictions on a child's access to palatable foods that may be high in fat or sugar. While restrictions may seem to be an easy, straightforward way of decreasing the intake of these foods, it only focuses more attention on these "forbidden" foods, and can increase a child's desire to obtain and eat them. Ultimately, the strategy is self-defeating.

Promoting a positive body image

Parents who are concerned about their own body image or their child's weight need to be especially careful. It has been suggested that young girls, even as early as 5 years old, are more likely to develop a more negative self-perception of their weight when their parents are concerned about their own body image or their daughter's weight. One study found that parental concern about their child's weight — and the restriction of specific foods as a result — was associated with negative self-evaluations by young children.

Concerned parents often criticize their children (either directly or indirectly) or exert strict control over the types or quantities of foods to which their children have access. While their intent is well-meaning — that is, to encourage a behavior change, foster healthy eating habits or prevent an increase in weight gain — these attempts at control only send a message to children that their weight status is undesirable and that they are not capable of controlling their own eating habits.

Non-food-related tasks

Children's food preferences are influenced when foods are related to performing non-food-related tasks. For example, the child who is offered a cookie to stop fighting with his sister learns that a cookie must be a really good thing if he is rewarded with it. Likewise, children often learn to dislike certain foods that they are required to eat in order to obtain non-food-related rewards. For example, the child who is made to eat her vegetables before she can watch television learns that a vegetable must be a terrible thing to eat, if she must be bribed to do so. (This also reinforces the perceived value of television watching.)

Mothers and daughters

Between moms and dads, it is mothers who appear to play a particularly important role in determining whether or not their daughters will develop diet and other eating problems. This is especially true in the case of mothers who attempt to control their own weight or have a history of dieting. Some studies have suggested that daughters of "dieting mothers" have a comparable focus on dieting themselves. Parents must remember that their own dieting behavior influences their daughter's ideas and beliefs about dieting.

These messages, especially when the child is visibly overweight, can cause a child to have a poor body image and sense of self.

Research has shown that by 6 years of age, children have learned societal messages that say being overweight is undesirable. This can be especially detrimental to children who are already overweight, since these children are at an increased risk of having psychosocial problems that may persist into adulthood. Children need to be encouraged to have a positive body image and to be reassured about the range of healthy and acceptable body weights and shapes. Children also need to feel valued for their abilities and talents — not just their appearance — if they are to foster a positive self-image.

Breakfast

Here's a zesty variation on bananas that will start your child's day (and yours) with a bang. Serve alone, with a slice of toast on the side, or as an accompaniment to pancakes or toaster waffles.

Spiced Bananas

¼ cup	orange juice	60 mL
1 tsp	grated orange zest	5 mL
2 tbsp	cream cheese	30 mL
Pinch	ground cinnamon	Pinch
Pinch	ground ginger	Pinch
2 tbsp	liquid honey	30 mL
4	medium bananas, cut into slices	4

1. In a bowl, with an electric mixer, combine orange juice and zest, cream cheese, cinnamon and ginger; beat until smooth. Transfer mixture to a large nonstick skillet. Add honey and cook, stirring, over medium heat until mixture is warm and thoroughly blended.

2. Add bananas to skillet; cook, turning slices frequently, until bananas are softened and warm. Serve banana slices topped with some sauce.

NUTRITIONAL ANALYSIS (PER SERVING)

Energy	Protein	Carbohydrate	Fat	Fiber	Calcium	Iron	Sodium
177 kcal	2 g	40 g	3 g	4 g	10 mg	0.4 mg	23 mg

Homemade Fruit Yogurt

Delicious served by itself, this yogurt is also wonderful served over cottage cheese, or with pancakes or waffles. Youngsters love it as a dip for fresh fruit.

1 cup	raspberries or sliced strawberries or peaches	250 mL
1 tbsp	frozen orange juice concentrate	15 mL
1 cup	plain yogurt	250 mL
	Fresh fruit, such as mandarin orange sections, whole strawberries, banana chunks, apple or pear slices	

1. In a food processor or blender, purée fruit and orange juice concentrate until smooth. Transfer mixture to a microwave-safe container.
2. Microwave, covered, on High for 2 minutes or until warm. Cool before whisking in yogurt. Serve as a topping or sauce or as a dip with a variety of fruit.

NUTRITIONAL ANALYSIS (PER ½ CUP/125 ML)

Energy	Protein	Carbohydrate	Fat	Fiber	Calcium	Iron	Sodium
60 kcal	3 g	9 g	1 g	2 g	108 mg	0.2 mg	43 mg

**Makes 2 cups
(500 mL)**

This fast and delicious beverage is a breakfast favorite. It also makes a great snack.

Breakfast Fruit Smoothie

1 cup	2% milk	250 mL
½ cup	fresh or frozen strawberries or raspberries	125 mL
1 tsp	liquid honey	5 mL
½ cup	vanilla-flavored yogurt	125 mL
1 tbsp	wheat germ	15 mL

1. In a blender, process milk and fruit until very smooth. (If there are too many seeds, strain through a sieve, discard seeds and return mixture to blender.) Add honey, yogurt and wheat germ; process until smooth. Pour into glasses and serve.

NUTRITIONAL ANALYSIS (PER ½ CUP/125 ML)							
Energy	Protein	Carbohydrate	Fat	Fiber	Calcium	Iron	Sodium
79 kcal	4 g	11 g	2 g	1 g	129 mg	0.2 mg	43 mg

**Makes 1½ cups
(375 mL)**

Smoothies are what you get from blending just about any fruit or fruits with a dairy product such as milk or yogurt. This combination is one of our favorites.

Strawberry Banana Smoothie

¾ cup	sliced strawberries	175 mL
1	small banana, sliced	1
½ cup	plain yogurt	125 mL
¼ cup	orange juice	60 mL
½ tsp	vanilla extract	2 mL

1. In a blender, process strawberries, banana, yogurt, orange juice and vanilla until very smooth. Pour into glasses and serve.

NUTRITIONAL ANALYSIS (PER ½ CUP/125 ML)							
Energy	Protein	Carbohydrate	Fat	Fiber	Calcium	Iron	Sodium
80 kcal	3 g	16 g	0.8 g	2 g	77 mg	0.3 mg	29 mg

Try this easy and delicious dish using one or more of your child's favorite fruits. Add toast squares and you've got a healthy breakfast.

Food Safety Tip

To avoid spoilage, be sure to store perishable foods in the refrigerator (set no higher than 40°F/4°C) or in the freezer.

Creamy Breakfast Fruit Mix

¼ cup	cottage cheese	60 mL
2 tbsp	plain yogurt	30 mL
¼ cup	chopped fresh fruit (such as orange, pineapple, banana, apple, strawberry, kiwifruit, peach or pear)	60 mL
Pinch	brown sugar	Pinch
Pinch	ground cinnamon	Pinch

1. In a small bowl, stir together cottage cheese, yogurt and fruit. Sprinkle with brown sugar and cinnamon.

NUTRITIONAL ANALYSIS (PER SERVING)							
Energy	Protein	Carbohydrate	Fat	Fiber	Calcium	Iron	Sodium
83 kcal	8 g	8 g	2 g	1 g	111 mg	0.3 mg	208 mg

Let your kids build this easy breakfast treat with their favorite toppings.

Breakfast Pizza

2 tbsp	light cream cheese or peanut butter	30 mL
1	4-inch (10 cm) whole-grain pita	1
½	apple or banana, thinly sliced	½
1 tbsp	crisp rice cereal	15 mL
1 tbsp	chopped dried fruit, such as apricots, raisins and/or cranberries	15 mL
1 tbsp	chopped nuts or unsweetened shredded coconut	15 mL
1 tbsp	strawberry jam, melted	15 mL

1. Spread cream cheese on pita. Arrange apple over top. Sprinkle with cereal, dried fruit and nuts. Drizzle with strawberry jam. Cut into 4 to 6 wedges.

NUTRITIONAL ANALYSIS (PER SERVING)							
Energy	Protein	Carbohydrate	Fat	Fiber	Calcium	Iron	Sodium
295 kcal	9 g	39 g	13 g	5 g	58 mg	2 mg	244 mg

The berry sauce is a delicious change from maple syrup.

Variation

Multigrain Pancakes: Prepare batter as for waffles. Heat a large nonstick skillet over medium heat; brush lightly with oil or spray with vegetable spray. For each pancake, pour 1/4 cup (60 mL) batter into skillet and cook for 1 1/2 to 2 minutes or until bottom is brown and bubbles break on top but do not fill in. Turn and cook for about 1 minute or until bottom is golden brown. Repeat with remaining batter, greasing skillet and adjusting heat as necessary. Makes about 12 pancakes.

Multigrain Waffles with Warm Berry Sauce

• *Waffle maker, lightly brushed with oil or sprayed with vegetable spray, then preheated*

Warm Berry Sauce

1/3 cup	orange juice	75 mL
4 tsp	cornstarch	20 mL
3 cups	mixed frozen berries, thawed	750 mL
2 tbsp	liquid honey	30 mL

Waffles

1 cup	multigrain or whole wheat flour	250 mL
1 cup	all-purpose flour	250 mL
1 tbsp	granulated sugar	15 mL
2 tsp	baking powder	10 mL
1/2 tsp	baking soda	2 mL
1/4 tsp	salt	1 mL
2	eggs	2
2 cups	buttermilk	500 mL
2 tbsp	vegetable oil	30 mL

1. *Warm Berry Sauce:* In a small bowl, whisk together orange juice and cornstarch. In a saucepan, combine berries and any juices, orange juice mixture and honey. Bring to a boil over medium-high heat, stirring gently. Reduce heat to medium and cook, stirring gently, for 1 to 2 minutes or until thickened. Set aside and keep warm.
2. *Waffles:* In a large bowl, whisk together multigrain flour, all-purpose flour, sugar, baking powder, baking soda and salt.
3. In a separate bowl, whisk together eggs, buttermilk and oil; pour over flour mixture and stir just until combined.

If you prefer, you can, of course, serve the waffles plain or with a drizzle of maple syrup instead of the berry sauce.

4. Pour about $^1\!/_2$ cup (125 mL) batter into preheated waffle maker (or the amount that fits in your waffle maker), spreading to edges. Close lid and cook for 4 to 6 minutes or until crisp, golden and no longer steaming. Repeat with remaining batter, greasing waffle maker between waffles as necessary. Serve with berry sauce.

NUTRITIONAL ANALYSIS (PER 1 WAFFLE WITH 2 TBSP/30 ML SAUCE)

Energy	Protein	Carbohydrate	Fat	Fiber	Calcium	Iron	Sodium
250 kcal	9 g	38 g	7 g	3 g	145 mg	2 mg	407 mg

Makes 15 pancakes

Daina's dad used to make these for the kids on weekends. They were considered quite a treat!

Variation

For a delicious variation, add apple slices to this recipe. Peel 1 apple and cut into thin slices; add slices to batter at the end of step 1.

Dad's Pancakes

1	egg, lightly beaten	1
1 cup	2% milk, divided	250 mL
$^3\!/_4$ cup	all-purpose flour, divided	175 mL
$^1\!/_2$ tsp	salt	2 mL
1 tsp	granulated sugar	5 mL
2 tbsp	butter, divided	30 mL

1. In a large bowl, combine egg with $^1\!/_2$ cup (125 mL) of the milk, $^1\!/_2$ cup (125 mL) of the flour, salt and sugar; stir until batter is smooth and free of lumps. Stir in remaining milk and flour; mix until smooth.

2. In a nonstick skillet over medium-high heat, melt 2 tsp (10 mL) of the butter. For each 2-inch (5 cm) pancake, pour about 2 tbsp (25 mL) batter into skillet. (Vary amount according to size of pancake desired.) Cook on one side for about 2 minutes or until pancake starts to bubble. Turn pancake over and cook for another 1 minute, until browned. Repeat procedure for remaining batter, adding another 1 tsp (5 mL) butter for each batch.

NUTRITIONAL ANALYSIS (PER PANCAKE)

Energy	Protein	Carbohydrate	Fat	Fiber	Calcium	Iron	Sodium
43 kcal	2 g	6 g	1 g	0 g	22 mg	0.4 mg	94 mg

Making your own pancakes from scratch is easy, and you'll feel good about feeding them to your children, because you know exactly what ingredients went into them.

Kitchen Tip

Serve pancakes with maple syrup or our Tangy Fruit Sauce (see recipe, page 340).

Oatmeal Pancakes

1	egg	1
½ cup	2% milk	125 mL
2 tbsp	vegetable oil, divided	30 mL
¼ tsp	vanilla extract	1 mL
¾ cup	Homemade Oatmeal Pancake Mix (see recipe, below)	175 mL

1. In a bowl, whisk together egg, milk, half the oil and the vanilla. Stir in pancake mix. Let stand for 2 minutes.

2. In a nonstick skillet, heat the remaining oil over medium heat. Using a ¼-cup (60 mL) measure, pour batter into hot skillet; cook for 3 minutes or until bubbles break on surface and underside is golden brown. Turn pancakes with a spatula and cook just until bottom is slightly browned. Repeat with remaining batter.

Homemade Oatmeal Pancake Mix

1 cup	rolled oats	250 mL
1½ cups	whole wheat flour	375 mL
½ cup	skim milk powder	125 mL
2 tbsp	wheat germ	30 mL
2 tbsp	brown sugar	30 mL
4 tsp	baking powder	20 mL
½ tsp	baking soda	2 mL
½ tsp	salt	2 mL

1. In a food processor, combine oats, flour, milk powder, wheat germ, brown sugar, baking powder, baking soda and salt. Process until thoroughly mixed. Transfer to an airtight container and store in the refrigerator for up to 2 weeks or freeze for up to 3 months. Makes about 3 cups (750 mL).

NUTRITIONAL ANALYSIS (PER PANCAKE)							
Energy	Protein	Carbohydrate	Fat	Fiber	Calcium	Iron	Sodium
124 kcal	5 g	24 g	1 g	3 g	92 mg	1 mg	419 mg

Makes 16 pancakes

A nice change from traditional pancakes, these are wonderful topped with butter and maple syrup.

Kitchen Tips

For a slightly sweeter version of these pancakes, add 2 tsp (10 mL) granulated sugar to the batter at the end of step 2.

These pancakes freeze very well. Simply reheat frozen pancakes in your toaster oven.

Sweet Potato Pancakes

¾ cup	mashed cooked sweet potato (about ½ large)	175 mL
1 tbsp	butter or margarine, melted	15 mL
2	egg whites, lightly beaten	2
1½ cups	2% milk	375 mL
1 cup	all-purpose flour	250 mL
2 tsp	baking powder	10 mL
½ tsp	salt	2 mL
¼ tsp	ground cinnamon	1 mL

1. In a large bowl, combine sweet potato, margarine and egg whites. Stir in milk.
2. In another bowl, combine flour, baking powder, salt and cinnamon. Stir into the sweet potato mixture.
3. Heat a nonstick skillet sprayed with vegetable oil over medium-high heat. When pan is hot, pour in about 2 tbsp (30 mL) batter to make pancakes about 3 inches (7.5 cm) in diameter. Cook on one side for about 2 minutes or until pancake starts to bubble. Turn pancake over and cook for another 1 minute, until browned.

NUTRITIONAL ANALYSIS (PER PANCAKE)							
Energy	Protein	Carbohydrate	Fat	Fiber	Calcium	Iron	Sodium
67 kcal	2 g	10 g	2 g	1 g	42 mg	0.6 mg	134 mg

In our experience, a peanut butter and banana French toast sandwich is hard to beat!

Oven-Baked French Toast Sandwich

- 11- by 7-inch (2 L) baking pan, greased

8	slices white or whole wheat bread	8
⅓ cup	peanut butter	75 mL
2	bananas, sliced	2
3	eggs	3
⅓ cup	2% milk	75 mL
½ tsp	vanilla extract	2 mL
	Ground cinnamon	

1. Place 4 bread slices in prepared pan. Spread with peanut butter and top with a layer of sliced bananas. Cover with remaining slices of bread.

2. In a small bowl, whisk together eggs, milk and vanilla. Pour mixture evenly to cover each sandwich. Sprinkle lightly with cinnamon. Cover and refrigerate for 4 hours, or overnight if desired.

3. Preheat oven to 350°F (180°C). Bake sandwiches, uncovered, for 35 minutes or until golden brown and set in center. Cut each sandwich into smaller pieces and serve.

NUTRITIONAL ANALYSIS (PER SERVING)

Energy	Protein	Carbohydrate	Fat	Fiber	Calcium	Iron	Sodium
336 kcal	18 g	32 g	16 g	6 g	110 mg	2 mg	417 mg

Mexican Scrambled Eggs

1	10-inch (25 cm) whole wheat flour tortilla	1
1 tbsp	vegetable oil	15 mL
1	plum (Roma) tomato, diced	1
1	green onion, chopped	1
1 tbsp	minced jalapeño pepper (optional)	15 mL
6	eggs	6
2 tbsp	water	30 mL
¼ tsp	salt	1 mL
¼ tsp	freshly ground black pepper	1 mL
¼ cup	salsa	60 mL
¼ cup	shredded Cheddar cheese (optional)	60 mL

1. Cut tortilla into thirds and stack them. Cut into ¹/₂-inch (1 cm) strips.
2. Heat a large nonstick skillet over medium-high heat. Cook tortilla strips, stirring, for 4 to 6 minutes or until crisp and golden brown. Transfer to a plate.
3. In the same skillet, heat oil over medium heat. Sauté tomato, green onion and jalapeño pepper (if using) for about 3 minutes or until tender.
4. Meanwhile, in a large bowl, whisk together eggs, water, salt and pepper. Pour into skillet and sprinkle with tortilla strips. Cook, stirring, for about 3 minutes or until thickened and moist and no liquid remains.
5. Top each serving with a spoonful of salsa and a sprinkle of cheese (if using).

NUTRITIONAL ANALYSIS (PER SERVING)

Energy	Protein	Carbohydrate	Fat	Fiber	Calcium	Iron	Sodium
237 kcal	13 g	16 g	14 g	2 g	116 mg	2 mg	358 mg

Egg Fajitas

When time is short, this makes a fast and easy breakfast. It's great for lunch too!

4	eggs	4
¼ tsp	salt	1 mL
Pinch	freshly ground black pepper	Pinch
2 tsp	butter or margarine	10 mL
2	green onions, chopped	2
4	8-inch (20 cm) whole wheat flour tortillas	4
¼ cup	mild salsa	60 mL

1. In a small bowl, whisk together eggs, salt and pepper. Set aside.
2. In a nonstick skillet, melt butter over medium heat. Add green onions and cook for a few minutes or until softened. Add egg mixture and cook, without stirring, until almost set. Turn over to finish cooking. Remove to cutting board. Cut egg into strips.
3. Warm tortillas in microwave oven for 45 seconds on High or until heated through. Place several egg strips in center of each tortilla; top with 1 tbsp (15 mL) salsa. Roll up tortilla to enclose egg and salsa.

NUTRITIONAL ANALYSIS (PER SERVING)

Energy	Protein	Carbohydrate	Fat	Fiber	Calcium	Iron	Sodium
278 kcal	12 g	33 g	11 g	3 g	90 mg	2 mg	619 mg

Looking for a change from egg dishes at breakfast? Try this easy recipe next weekend.

Baked Vegetable Frittata

- *Preheat oven to 350°F (180°C)*
- *8-inch (2 L) square baking pan, greased*

½ cup	chopped cooked vegetables	125 mL
½ cup	dried bread cubes or seasoned croutons	125 mL
4	eggs	4
¼ cup	2% milk	60 mL
Pinch	salt	Pinch
Pinch	freshly ground black pepper	Pinch
½ cup	grated Cheddar or mozzarella cheese	125 mL
Pinch	dried basil	Pinch

1. In a bowl, combine vegetables and bread cubes. Sprinkle mixture evenly over bottom of prepared pan.

2. In a small bowl, whisk together eggs, milk, salt and pepper. Pour over vegetable mixture. Sprinkle with cheese and basil.

3. Bake in preheated oven for 20 minutes or until knife inserted in center comes out clean. Cut into 4 servings.

NUTRITIONAL ANALYSIS (PER SERVING)							
Energy	Protein	Carbohydrate	Fat	Fiber	Calcium	Iron	Sodium
122 kcal	10 g	6 g	6 g	1 g	145 mg	1 mg	346 mg

Eggs in Bread Baskets

A toasted bread basket makes a handy serving bowl for each egg. For breakfast, omit the shredded cheese and tomato. Add them for a tasty lunch.

Kitchen Tip

Save the bread crusts to make fresh bread crumbs.

- *Preheat oven to 400ºF (200ºC)*
- *4 greased custard or muffin cups*

4	slices whole wheat bread, crusts removed	4
1 tbsp	melted butter or margarine	15 mL
4	eggs	4
	Salt and freshly ground black pepper (optional)	
½ cup	shredded Cheddar cheese (optional)	125 mL
1	small tomato, diced (optional)	1

1. Roll each bread slice with a rolling pin or water glass to flatten. Lightly brush with melted butter. Press into prepared custard cups.

2. Break 1 egg into each bread cup. Season lightly with salt and pepper, if using.

3. Bake in preheated oven for about 15 minutes or until egg whites are set and edges of bread are toasted. If using cheese and tomato, sprinkle over egg during the last 5 minutes.

NUTRITIONAL ANALYSIS (PER SERVING)							
Energy	Protein	Carbohydrate	Fat	Fiber	Calcium	Iron	Sodium
234 kcal	13 g	16 g	13 g	4 g	281 mg	2 mg	306 mg

Variation

Asparagus or corn kernels make a nice change from broccoli.

Weekend Breakfast Quiche

* *Preheat oven to 375°F (190°C)*
* *10-inch (25 cm) quiche pan, greased*

1 cup	chopped broccoli	250 mL
1 cup	shredded Swiss cheese	250 mL
½ cup	finely chopped onion	125 mL
3	eggs	3
1 cup	2% milk	250 mL
½ cup	biscuit baking mix	125 mL
¼ tsp	ground nutmeg	1 mL
¼ tsp	salt	1 mL
Pinch	freshly ground black pepper	Pinch

1. Sprinkle broccoli, cheese and onion in bottom of prepared pan.

2. In a bowl, with an electric mixer, combine eggs, milk, baking mix and seasonings; beat at high speed for 1 minute. Pour over broccoli mixture in pan.

3. Bake in preheated oven for 45 minutes or until a knife inserted in center comes out clean. Transfer to a wire rack and allow to cool for 5 minutes before cutting into 6 wedges.

NUTRITIONAL ANALYSIS (PER SERVING)							
Energy	Protein	Carbohydrate	Fat	Fiber	Calcium	Iron	Sodium
165 kcal	10 g	13 g	8 g	1 g	214 mg	0.9 mg	377 mg

Cooked ham or chicken make good substitutes for the bacon.

Kitchen Tip

Serve this quiche with toast, bagel or English muffin.

Easy Quiche

- *4-cup (1 L) microwave-safe casserole, greased*

3	eggs	3
1 cup	2% milk	250 mL
¼ tsp	salt	1 mL
¼ tsp	paprika	1 mL
Pinch	ground nutmeg	Pinch
2	green onions, chopped	2
¾ cup	grated Swiss cheese	175 mL
¼ cup	grated Parmesan cheese	60 mL
3	strips bacon, chopped and cooked, fat drained	3

1. In a bowl, with an electric mixer, combine eggs, milk, salt, paprika and nutmeg; beat at high speed for 1 minute.
2. Place green onions, Swiss cheese, Parmesan cheese and bacon in bottom of prepared dish. Pour egg mixture over. Microwave, uncovered, on High for 5 minutes. Stir egg and microwave for another 6 minutes or until firm (not runny). Let stand for 5 minutes before serving.

NUTRITIONAL ANALYSIS (PER SERVING)

Energy	Protein	Carbohydrate	Fat	Fiber	Calcium	Iron	Sodium
128 kcal	8 g	3 g	10 g	0 g	155 mg	0.5 mg	237 mg

To save time in the morning, prepare this simple, tasty breakfast treat the night before. By morning, the berries will have thawed and the granola will have softened slightly. Make a bowl for each member of the family. It's also a great after-school snack.

Kitchen Tips

For the berries, try raspberries, blueberries, sliced strawberries or a combination.

This looks beautiful in clear bowls, so you can see the different layers.

Make-Ahead Breakfast Granola

¾ cup	frozen berries	175 mL
½ cup	plain or lightly sweetened yogurt	125 mL
2 tbsp	granola	30 mL

1. Place berries in a bowl, add yogurt and top with granola. Cover with plastic wrap and refrigerate overnight.

NUTRITIONAL ANALYSIS (PER SERVING)							
Energy	Protein	Carbohydrate	Fat	Fiber	Calcium	Iron	Sodium
155 kcal	7 g	26 g	3 g	4 g	218 mg	0.5 mg	90 mg

Homemade Microwave Granola

Commercially prepared granola is convenient, but may contain added ingredients you don't want. Here's a homemade version that's packed with nutritious goodness. And because it's cooked in the microwave, preparation is a snap.

Kitchen Tips

You can find wheat and rye flakes (and other grains used in this recipe) at health food stores, as well as some supermarkets.

Use whatever fruit you like best. Good choices include dried apricots, dates, apples or raisins.

• *4-cup (1 L) microwave-safe casserole, greased*

1 cup	large-flake rolled oats	250 mL
½ cup	wheat flakes (see tip, at left)	125 mL
½ cup	rye flakes	125 mL
¼ cup	unsweetened flaked coconut	60 mL
¼ cup	natural wheat bran	60 mL
Pinch	salt	Pinch
¼ cup	liquid honey	60 mL
2 tbsp	vegetable oil	30 mL
½ cup	chopped dried fruit, optional (see tip, at left)	125 mL

1. In prepared casserole, combine oats, wheat and rye flakes, coconut, bran and salt.

2. In a 1-cup (250 mL) measure, whisk together honey and oil. Pour over oat mixture; toss until well mixed.

3. Microwave on High for 6 minutes, stirring well every 2 minutes, until mixture is slightly brown. Stir in fruit, if using. Allow granola to cool before storing in a tightly covered container. Keeps for up to 1 month.

NUTRITIONAL ANALYSIS (PER ½ CUP/125 ML)							
Energy	Protein	Carbohydrate	Fat	Fiber	Calcium	Iron	Sodium
224 kcal	6 g	35 g	8 g	6 g	11 mg	1 mg	50 mg

Makes 24 squares

These unbaked squares are a snap to prepare in the microwave. Kids love them — and because they contain less sugar and fat than commercial granola treats, you'll love them too!

Granola Breakfast Squares

- *7- by 11-inch (2 L) baking pan, greased*

½ cup	corn syrup	125 mL
2 tbsp	brown sugar	30 mL
⅓ cup	peanut butter	75 mL
3 cups	Homemade Microwave Granola (see recipe, page 154)	750 mL
¼ cup	sunflower seeds	60 mL
½ tsp	ground cinnamon	2 mL
½ tsp	ground nutmeg	2 mL

1. In a large microwave-safe bowl, combine corn syrup and brown sugar. Microwave on High for 2 minutes or until mixture is boiling. Stir in peanut butter until smooth.

2. Quickly stir in granola, sunflower seeds, cinnamon and nutmeg. Press firmly into prepared pan. Cut into squares when cool. Transfer to an airtight container and store in the refrigerator.

NUTRITIONAL ANALYSIS (PER SQUARE)							
Energy	Protein	Carbohydrate	Fat	Fiber	Calcium	Iron	Sodium
110 kcal	3 g	16 g	5 g	2 g	7 mg	0.5 mg	46 mg

These nutritious, filling scones will delight kids and adults alike and make a nice change from the usual breakfast fare. They have a great texture, with soft bananas and raspberries combined with crunchy almonds. Best of all, they can be made the night before, for a quick start in the morning.

Kitchen Tip

To toast almonds, place in a small dry skillet and toast over medium heat, stirring constantly, for about 3 minutes or until fragrant.

Best Breakfast Berry Scones

- *Preheat oven to 325°F (160°C)*
- *Large baking sheet, greased*

2⅔ cups	all-purpose flour	650 mL
⅓ cup	quick-cooking rolled oats	75 mL
5 tsp	baking powder	30 mL
1 tsp	baking soda	5 mL
½ cup	butter, slightly softened	125 mL
½ cup	granola	125 mL
½ cup	whipping (35%) cream	125 mL
3 tbsp	packed brown sugar	45 mL
2 tbsp	liquid honey	30 mL
1	banana, sliced	1
1 cup	frozen raspberries, thawed	250 mL
¾ cup	slivered almonds, toasted (see tip, at left)	175 mL
2 tbsp	2% milk	30 mL
½ tsp	vanilla extract	2 mL

1. In a medium bowl, combine flour, oats, baking powder and baking soda. Cut in butter with two knives until mixture resembles coarse meal. Stir in granola.
2. In another bowl, combine cream, brown sugar and honey. Using a fork, gently stir into flour mixture. Stir in banana, raspberries and almonds until just combined. Do not overmix.
3. Use a spoon to scoop 5 to 6 tbsp (75 to 90 mL) batter onto baking sheet. Repeat to form 18 scones total, placing them about 2 inches (5 cm) apart. Combine milk and vanilla; brush over scones.
4. Bake in preheated oven for 20 to 25 minutes or until golden brown.

NUTRITIONAL ANALYSIS (PER SCONE)							
Energy	Protein	Carbohydrate	Fat	Fiber	Calcium	Iron	Sodium
205 kcal	4 g	25 g	10 g	2 g	53 mg	1 mg	196 mg

These great-looking muffins combine wonderful taste and texture.

Rolled Oat Muffins

- *Preheat oven to 375°F (190°C)*
- *12-cup muffin pan, greased or paper-lined*

1 cup	all-purpose flour	250 mL
1 cup	whole wheat flour	250 mL
1 cup	rolled oats	250 mL
½ cup	granulated sugar	125 mL
1 tbsp	baking powder	15 mL
1 tsp	ground cinnamon	5 mL
½ tsp	baking soda	2 mL
½ tsp	salt	2 mL
1½ cups	2% milk	375 mL
¼ cup	vegetable oil	60 mL
1	egg	1
¼ cup	molasses	60 mL

1. In a large bowl, combine all-purpose flour, whole wheat flour, rolled oats, sugar, baking powder, cinnamon, baking soda and salt.

2. In another bowl, combine milk, oil, egg and molasses. Add to dry ingredients; stir just until moistened.

3. Spoon batter into prepared muffin cups. Bake in preheated oven for 20 minutes or until muffins are firm to the touch.

NUTRITIONAL ANALYSIS (PER MUFFIN)							
Energy	Protein	Carbohydrate	Fat	Fiber	Calcium	Iron	Sodium
202 kcal	5 g	33 g	6 g	2 g	86 mg	2 mg	308 mg

Makes 24 muffins

Here's a great way to start the day. Serve with cheese and milk for a complete breakfast.

Variation

For a special treat, add 1 cup (250 mL) chocolate chips to this recipe. Fold in at the end of step 3.

Banana Oatmeal Muffins

- *Preheat oven to 375°F (190°C)*
- *Two 12-cup muffin pans, greased or paper-lined*

1 cup	rolled oats	250 mL
1 cup	2% milk	250 mL
2 cups	all-purpose flour	500 mL
½ cup	lightly packed brown sugar	125 mL
½ cup	granulated sugar	125 mL
1 tsp	baking soda	5 mL
1 tsp	salt	5 mL
½ tsp	ground cinnamon	2 mL
¼ tsp	ground nutmeg	1 mL
½ cup	butter or margarine, softened	125 mL
2	eggs, beaten	2
2 tsp	vanilla extract	10 mL
2 cups	mashed bananas	500 mL

1. In a bowl, combine oats and milk. Set aside to soak.
2. In another bowl, combine flour, brown sugar, granulated sugar, baking soda, salt, cinnamon and nutmeg.
3. Add butter, eggs, vanilla and bananas to oatmeal mixture; stir until thoroughly combined. Add mixture to dry ingredients; stir just until moistened.
4. Spoon batter into prepared muffin cups, filling about three-quarters full. Bake in preheated oven for 20 minutes or until muffins are firm to the touch.

NUTRITIONAL ANALYSIS (PER MUFFIN)							
Energy	Protein	Carbohydrate	Fat	Fiber	Calcium	Iron	Sodium
138 kcal	3 g	22 g	5 g	1 g	20 mg	0.8 mg	186 mg

The combination of orange juice and bananas makes these muffins incredibly moist and flavorful.

Kitchen Tip

For added fiber, use natural bran instead of cornmeal.

Orange Banana Muffins

- *Preheat oven to 400°F (200°C)*
- *12-cup muffin pan, greased or paper-lined*

1 cup	whole wheat flour	250 mL
1 cup	all-purpose flour	250 mL
¼ cup	cornmeal	60 mL
1 tsp	baking soda	5 mL
1 tsp	baking powder	5 mL
Pinch	salt	Pinch
1 cup	mashed bananas	250 mL
½ cup	frozen orange juice concentrate, thawed	125 mL
¼ cup	packed brown sugar	60 mL
¼ cup	vegetable oil	60 mL
¼ cup	2% milk	60 mL
1	egg	1

1. In a large bowl, combine whole wheat flour, all-purpose flour, cornmeal, baking soda, baking powder and salt.

2. In another bowl, stir together bananas, orange juice concentrate, brown sugar, oil, milk and egg. Add mixture to dry ingredients; stir just until mixed.

3. Spoon batter into prepared muffin cups. Bake in preheated oven for 20 to 25 minutes or until muffins are firm to the touch.

NUTRITIONAL ANALYSIS (PER MUFFIN)							
Energy	Protein	Carbohydrate	Fat	Fiber	Calcium	Iron	Sodium
183 kcal	4 g	31 g	6 g	2 g	38 mg	1 mg	220 mg

Along with a glass of milk, these muffins make for a great quick breakfast on the run or an energy-filled snack on the way to a soccer or hockey practice.

Apple Muffins

- *Preheat oven to 400°F (200°C)*
- *Two 12-cup muffin pans, greased or paper-lined*

2½ cups	all-purpose flour	625 mL
2 cups	quick-cooking rolled oats	500 mL
1 cup	lightly packed brown sugar	250 mL
2 tsp	baking soda	10 mL
2 tsp	ground cinnamon	10 mL
3 cups	coarsely chopped apples	750 mL
1½ cups	plain yogurt	375 mL
1 cup	vegetable oil	250 mL
4	eggs	4

1. In a large bowl, combine flour, oats, brown sugar, baking soda and cinnamon; mix well.

2. In another bowl, combine apples, yogurt, oil and eggs; mix well. Add to dry ingredients, stirring just until moistened. (Do not overmix.)

3. Spoon batter into prepared muffin cups and bake for 18 minutes or until muffins are firm to the touch.

NUTRITIONAL ANALYSIS (PER MUFFIN)

Energy	Protein	Carbohydrate	Fat	Fiber	Calcium	Iron	Sodium
214 kcal	4 g	26 g	11 g	2 g	39 mg	1 mg	126 mg

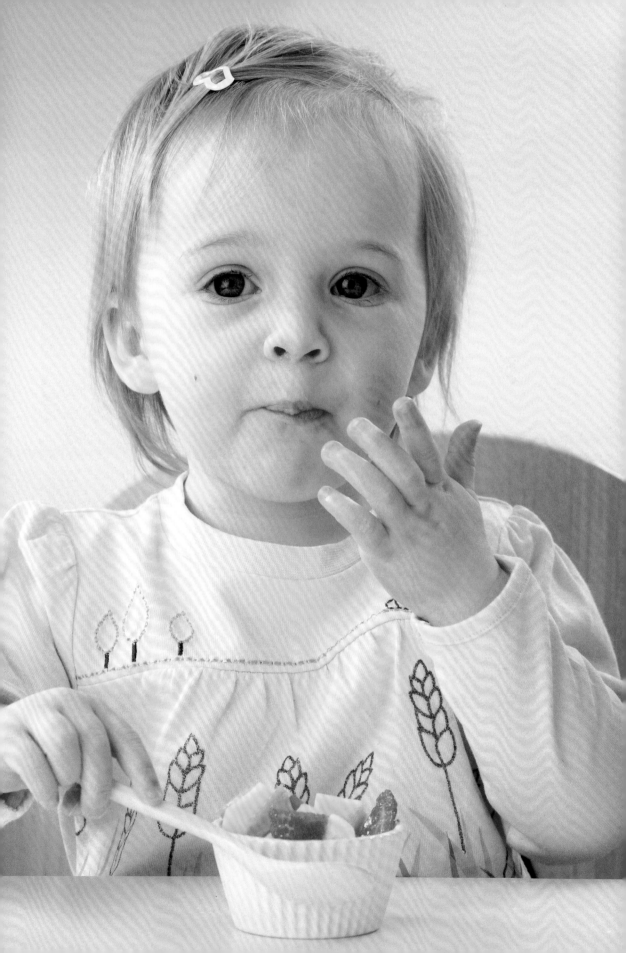

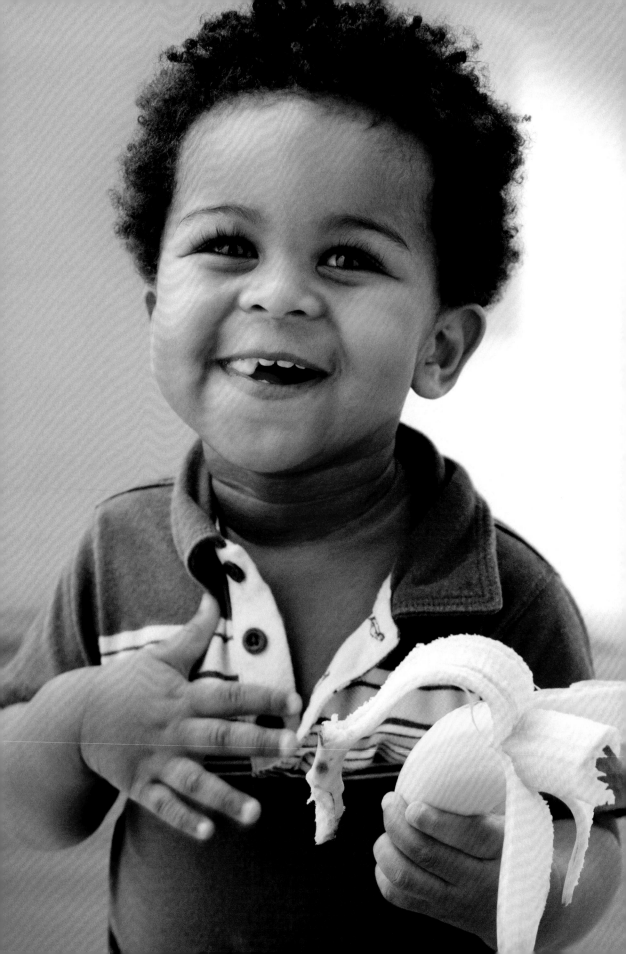

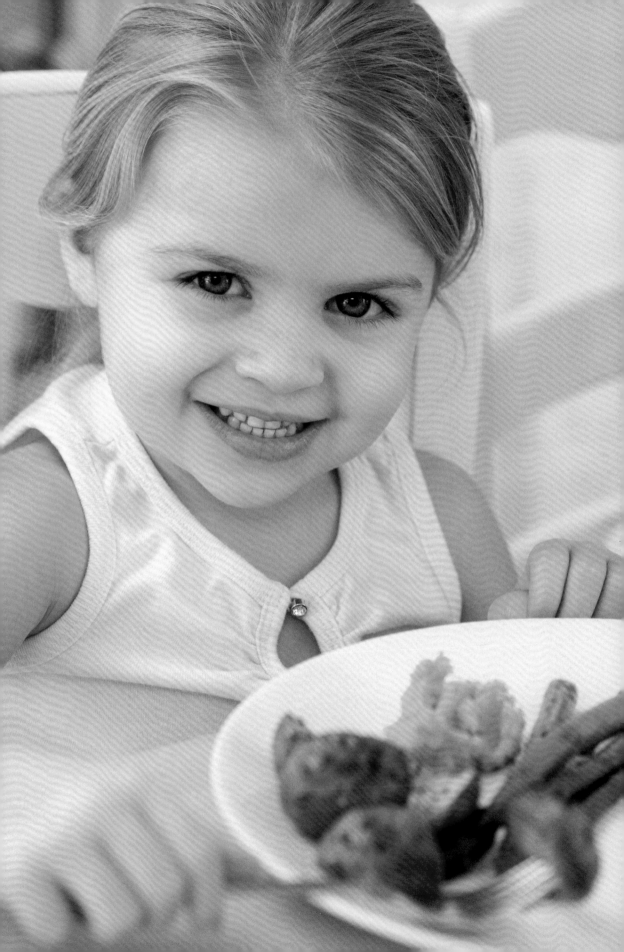

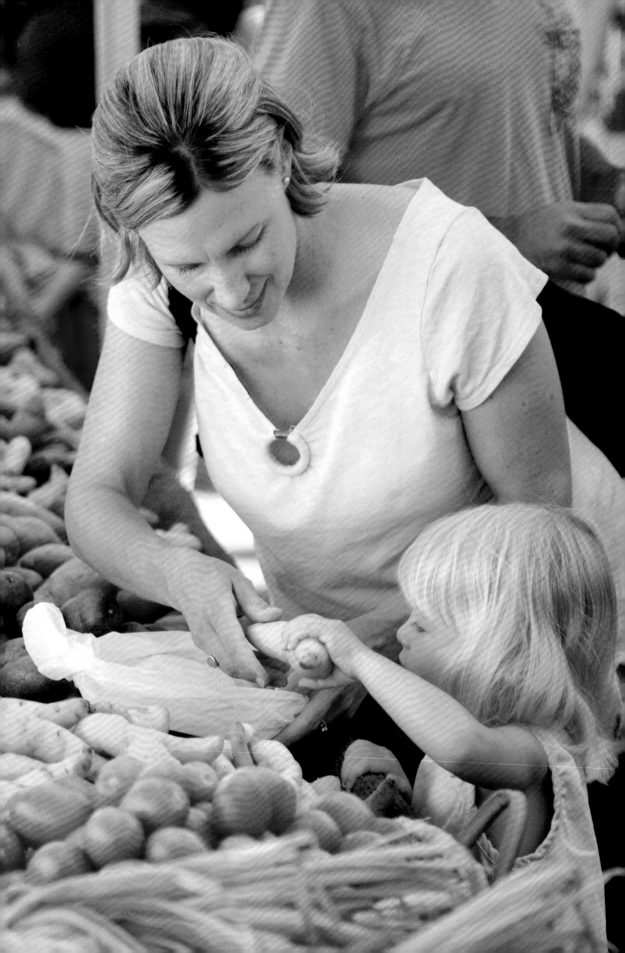

Makes 12 muffins

Wonderful and moist, these nutritious muffins have great flavor. They're sure to be a hit with the entire family.

Apple and Cheese Whole Wheat Muffins

- *Preheat oven to 375°F (190°C)*
- *12-cup muffin pan, greased or paper-lined*

1¼ cups	all-purpose flour	300 mL
1 cup	whole wheat flour	250 mL
1 cup	lightly packed brown sugar	250 mL
1 tsp	baking soda	5 mL
½ tsp	ground cinnamon	2 mL
½ tsp	ground nutmeg	2 mL
1	egg	1
1 cup	plain yogurt	250 mL
⅓ cup	vegetable oil	75 mL
2 cups	diced peeled apples	500 mL
½ cup	shredded old Cheddar cheese	125 mL

1. In a large bowl, combine all-purpose flour, whole wheat flour, brown sugar, baking soda, cinnamon and nutmeg.

2. In another bowl, combine egg, yogurt, oil, apple and cheese. Add to dry ingredients; stir just until moistened.

3. Spoon batter into prepared muffin cups. Bake in preheated oven for 20 minutes or until muffins are firm to the touch.

NUTRITIONAL ANALYSIS (PER MUFFIN)							
Energy	Protein	Carbohydrate	Fat	Fiber	Calcium	Iron	Sodium
238 kcal	5 g	37 g	8 g	2 g	77 mg	1 mg	154 mg

Not too sweet and really quick to prepare, these muffins are an excellent on-the-go breakfast or snack choice. They also freeze well.

Kitchen Tip

Oat bran and natural wheat bran can both be found in the hot cereal aisle of well-stocked supermarkets.

Blueberry Bran Muffins

- *Preheat oven to 400°F (200°C)*
- *12-cup muffin pan, lightly greased*

¾ cup	oat bran	175 mL
½ cup	quick-cooking rolled oats	125 mL
½ cup	natural wheat bran	125 mL
½ cup	whole wheat flour	125 mL
½ cup	all-purpose flour	125 mL
½ cup	lightly packed brown sugar	125 mL
1 tbsp	baking powder	15 mL
½ tsp	baking soda	2 mL
½ tsp	ground cinnamon	2 mL
Pinch	salt	Pinch
2	eggs	2
½ cup	skim milk	125 mL
⅓ cup	butter, melted	75 mL
1 cup	blueberries	250 mL

1. In a large bowl, combine oat bran, oats, wheat bran, whole wheat flour, all-purpose flour, brown sugar, baking powder, baking soda, cinnamon and salt.

2. In another bowl, whisk together eggs, milk and butter. Add to flour mixture and stir with a wooden spoon until just combined. Fold in blueberries.

3. Spoon batter into prepared muffin cups. Bake in preheated oven for 20 minutes or until a toothpick inserted in the center comes out clean.

NUTRITIONAL ANALYSIS (PER MUFFIN)							
Energy	Protein	Carbohydrate	Fat	Fiber	Calcium	Iron	Sodium
171 kcal	5 g	28 g	7 g	4 g	51 mg	1.4 mg	267 mg

*Moist and delicious,
these muffins have a mild
crunchiness thanks to the
poppy seeds, which also
provide some calcium.
They're great for breakfast,
with cheese or yogurt, or
as a school snack with
some fruit.*

Kitchen Tips

Enjoy warm out of the oven
or let cool and store in an
airtight container at room
temperature for up 1 week.

These freeze well, so you
may want to make an extra
batch. Store in an airtight
container in the freezer for
up to 3 months.

Poppy Seed Muffins

- *Preheat oven to 400°F (200°C)*
- *12-cup muffin pan, lightly greased or paper-lined*

2 cups	all-purpose flour	500 mL
1/2 cup	poppy seeds	125 mL
1 tbsp	baking powder	15 mL
1 tsp	baking soda	5 mL
1/4 tsp	salt	1 mL
3/4 cup	granulated sugar	175 mL
2	eggs	2
1/2 cup	butter, melted	125 mL
3/4 cup	sour cream or plain yogurt	175 mL
1/4 cup	orange juice	60 mL
2 tbsp	lemon juice	30 mL
1/2 tsp	almond extract or vanilla extract	2 mL

1. In a large bowl, combine flour, poppy seeds, baking powder, baking soda and salt. Set aside.

2. In another bowl, whisk together sugar, eggs and butter. Stir in yogurt, orange juice, lemon juice and almond extract. Add to dry ingredients; stir just until moistened.

3. Spoon batter into prepared muffin cups. Bake in preheated oven for 15 to 20 minutes or until tops are golden brown.

NUTRITIONAL ANALYSIS (PER MUFFIN)							
Energy	Protein	Carbohydrate	Fat	Fiber	Calcium	Iron	Sodium
254 kcal	5 g	32 g	12 g	1 g	132 mg	2 mg	170 mg

Corn Muffins

Kitchen Tip

These muffins are best served warm from the oven. Serve with fruit jam or preserves.

* Preheat oven to 350°F (180°C)
* 12-cup muffin pan, greased or paper-lined

1½ cups	all-purpose flour	375 mL
⅔ cup	granulated sugar	175 mL
½ cup	cornmeal	125 mL
1 tbsp	baking powder	15 mL
½ tsp	salt	2 mL
1¼ cups	2% milk	300 mL
2	eggs, slightly beaten	2
⅓ cup	vegetable oil	75 mL
¼ cup	butter or margarine, melted	60 mL

1. In a large bowl, combine flour, sugar, cornmeal, baking powder and salt.
2. In another bowl, whisk together milk, eggs, oil and melted butter. Add to dry ingredients; stir just until moistened.
3. Spoon batter into prepared muffin cups, filling about three-quarters full. Bake in preheated oven for 18 to 20 minutes or until muffins are firm to the touch.

NUTRITIONAL ANALYSIS (PER MUFFIN)

Energy	Protein	Carbohydrate	Fat	Fiber	Calcium	Iron	Sodium
218 kcal	4 g	27 g	12 g	1 g	78 mg	1 mg	354 mg

Lunch

Carrot-Potato Soup

The creamy texture of this soup comes from the starch in the potatoes. It's delicious — and healthy too!

Kitchen Tips

If you have it (or have the time to make it), use homemade stock, so you can control the amount of added salt. Otherwise, purchase reduced-sodium ready-to-use broth.

Kids generally prefer their soup warm. But this recipe also makes a great summertime starter for adults when served cold.

1 tbsp	olive oil	15 mL
1/3 cup	chopped onion	75 mL
3	green onions, chopped	3
2 cups	finely chopped carrots	500 mL
2 cups	diced potatoes	500 mL
2 tsp	grated gingerroot (optional)	10 mL
3 cups	reduced-sodium chicken stock	750 mL
1/4 tsp	curry powder	1 mL
1/4 tsp	ground cinnamon	1 mL
1/4 tsp	ground nutmeg	1 mL
Pinch	freshly ground black pepper	Pinch
1	bay leaf	1
	Sour cream (optional)	

1. In a large saucepan, heat oil over medium heat. Add green onions and sauté for 3 minutes. Add carrots and potatoes; cook for 2 minutes.
2. Add ginger, if using, along with stock, curry, cinnamon, nutmeg, pepper and bay leaf. Bring to a boil. Reduce heat and simmer, covered, for about 45 minutes or until vegetables are very tender. Remove and discard bay leaf. Allow soup to cool slightly.
3. Transfer soup to a blender or food processor; purée until smooth. Return mixture to saucepan and heat to serving temperature. Ladle soup into bowls and, if desired, garnish with a small dollop of sour cream.

NUTRITIONAL ANALYSIS (PER 1/2 CUP/125 ML)							
Energy	Protein	Carbohydrate	Fat	Fiber	Calcium	Iron	Sodium
61 kcal	2 g	9 g	2 g	2 g	21 mg	0.6 mg	42 mg

Sweet and oh-so-simple, this soup is a great source of beta carotene.

Kitchen Tips

If using ready-to-use chicken broth, look for the reduced-sodium variety.

Garnish the soup with a little plain yogurt or sour cream before serving.

Sweet Potato Soup

1 tbsp	vegetable oil	15 mL
1	small onion, chopped	1
6 cups	chicken stock	1.5 L
2	large sweet potatoes, peeled and chopped	2
½ tsp	ground nutmeg	2 mL
¼ tsp	freshly ground black pepper	1 mL

1. In a large saucepan, warm oil over medium-high heat. Add onions and sauté for 2 to 3 minutes or until onions are soft and translucent. Add chicken stock, sweet potatoes, nutmeg and pepper. Cover and bring to a boil; reduce heat and simmer for 25 minutes or until potatoes are tender.

2. Remove soup from heat and, in batches, purée soup in a blender or food processor until smooth. Return soup to saucepan and heat to serving temperature.

NUTRITIONAL ANALYSIS (PER ½ CUP/125 ML)							
Energy	Protein	Carbohydrate	Fat	Fiber	Calcium	Iron	Sodium
47 kcal	2 g	7 g	1 g	1 g	13 mg	0.2 mg	311 mg

Aztec Squash Soup

Aztec soup glows with the golden colors of squash and corn. It can be served as is or garnished with shredded cheese, crisp tortilla pieces, diced avocado and/or pumpkin seeds to suit each taste.

Kitchen Tip

Purée the soup if your children prefer a smoother, thicker consistency. You can use an immersion blender right in the pot, or transfer the soup in batches to a blender or food processor.

2 tbsp	butter or margarine, divided	30 mL
1	onion, diced (about ¾ cup/175 mL)	1
2	cloves garlic, minced	2
6 cups	reduced-sodium vegetable stock	1.5 L
3 cups	diced butternut squash	750 mL
2 cups	frozen corn kernels	500 mL
1	avocado, diced (optional)	1
2 cups	shredded Monterey Jack cheese	500 mL
½ cup	toasted pumpkin seeds (optional)	125 mL
	Crisp corn tortillas, broken into pieces	

1. In a large pot, melt butter over medium heat. Sauté onion and garlic for 5 minutes or until softened. Add stock and squash; bring to a boil. Reduce heat and simmer for 10 minutes or until squash is tender. Add corn and simmer for 5 minutes.
2. Ladle soup into bowls and offer avocado (if using), cheese, pumpkin seeds (if using) and tortilla pieces at the table.

NUTRITIONAL ANALYSIS (PER ½ CUP/125 ML)							
Energy	Protein	Carbohydrate	Fat	Fiber	Calcium	Iron	Sodium
212 kcal	8 g	16 g	13 g	3 g	175 mg	1.3 mg	253 mg

Makes 4 cups (1 L)

Here's another wonderfully creamy soup that uses milk (not cream) and can be made with all kinds of different vegetables.

Kitchen Tips

Add whatever seasonings you like, depending on the vegetables used. See our Seasoning Guide, at right, for suggestions.

This soup freezes well.

Creamy Vegetable Soup

3 tbsp	butter or margarine	45 mL
3 tbsp	all-purpose flour	45 mL
2 cups	reduced-sodium vegetable or chicken stock	500 mL
2 cups	chopped cooked vegetables	500 mL
1 cup	2% milk	250 mL

1. In a large saucepan, melt butter over medium heat. Add flour and cook, stirring, for 2 minutes or until bubbly. Gradually whisk in stock; cook until smooth and thickened.

2. Add cooked vegetables. Remove from heat and transfer soup to food processor or blender. Purée until smooth. Return to saucepan. Slowly stir in milk and heat to serving temperature.

NUTRITIONAL ANALYSIS (PER ½ CUP/125 ML)							
Energy	Protein	Carbohydrate	Fat	Fiber	Calcium	Iron	Sodium
104 kcal	4 g	8 g	6 g	1 g	50 mg	0.6 mg	156 mg

Vegetable Soup Seasoning Guide

VEGETABLE	SEASONING
Asparagus	Ground nutmeg or white pepper
Broccoli	Lemon zest or juice
Carrot	Ground nutmeg, ginger, curry
Cauliflower	Ground nutmeg or white pepper
Cream-style corn	Cayenne pepper
Green bean	Dried tarragon or basil
Green pea	Dried mint or parsley; lemon zest
Mushroom	Ground white pepper, cayenne
Spinach	Lemon zest or ground nutmeg
Tomato	Dried thyme or basil

This tasty, healthy soup is a wonderful way to eat a variety of vegetables. Serve it with fresh whole-grain bread or whole-grain pitas.

Kitchen Tip

You can also serve these tasty roasted vegetables on their own, alongside chicken or fish. Simply prepare the recipe through step 2.

Variations

For a creamy version, add about 2 tbsp (25 mL) milk or cream to each serving of soup.

To make the soup heartier, add 1 to 2 tbsp (15 to 30 mL) cooked rice, quinoa or other grain to each serving of soup.

Roasted Vegetable Soup

- *Preheat oven to 400°F (200°C)*
- *Large rimmed baking sheet, lined with foil*

5	carrots, sliced	5
2	zucchini, sliced	2
1	large tomato, cut into quarters	1
1	large red onion, sliced	1
1	red bell pepper, cut into strips	1
1	orange or yellow bell pepper, cut into strips	1
2 tbsp	olive oil	30 mL
½ tsp	sea salt	2 mL
½ tsp	freshly ground black pepper	2 mL
3½ cups	reduced-sodium vegetable stock	875 mL

1. In a large bowl, combine carrots, zucchini, tomato, red onion, red pepper and orange pepper. Add oil, salt and pepper; toss to coat.

2. Spread vegetables in a single layer on prepared baking sheet. Roast in preheated oven for 35 to 40 minutes, stirring every 10 minutes, until vegetables are lightly browned.

3. Working in batches, transfer vegetables to a food processor and purée until smooth. Transfer to a medium saucepan, add stock and bring to a simmer over medium-low heat. Simmer for about 20 minutes to blend the flavors.

NUTRITIONAL ANALYSIS (PER ½ CUP/125 ML)							
Energy	Protein	Carbohydrate	Fat	Fiber	Calcium	Iron	Sodium
92 kcal	2 g	13 g	4 g	4 g	44 mg	0.8 mg	137 mg

Tuscan Bean Soup

Known in its native Italy as ribolitta, this thick bean soup is the ideal comfort food to fend off the winter blues.

Kitchen Tips

The traditional texture of this soup is quite chunky. If your children prefer a smoother soup (as some seem to do), purée their portion and keep the remainder as is for adults.

You can use 1 tbsp (15 mL) dried rosemary in place of the fresh.

1 cup	dried cannellini or white kidney beans	250 mL
2 tbsp	olive oil	30 mL
1	small onion, finely chopped	1
1	large stalk celery, finely chopped	1
1	sprig fresh rosemary leaves, chopped	1
1	large carrot, finely chopped	1
2	cloves garlic, finely chopped	2
4 cups	reduced-sodium chicken stock	1 L
2 tbsp	tomato paste	30 mL
2	leeks, white part only, chopped	2
2	zucchini, chopped	2
½ cup	chopped fresh basil	125 mL
	Salt and freshly ground black pepper	
	Toasted bread slices	
	Grated Parmesan cheese	

1. In a large saucepan, add enough cold water to cover beans. Cover and bring to a boil; reduce heat and cook for 5 minutes. Remove from heat and allow to stand for 1 hour. Drain and discard liquid. Return drained beans to saucepan and add 4 cups (1 L) cold water. Bring to a boil; reduce heat and cook for 1 hour or until beans are tender. Drain.
2. Meanwhile, in a large nonstick skillet, heat oil over medium heat. Add onion, celery, rosemary, carrot and garlic; cook for 10 minutes.
3. Add vegetable mixture to cooked drained beans. Stir in chicken stock and tomato paste; cook, uncovered, over medium heat for 10 minutes. Add leeks and zucchini; cover and cook for 15 minutes or until all vegetables are tender. Add basil and season to taste with salt and pepper.
4. Place toasted bread in each soup bowl. Ladle soup over and sprinkle with Parmesan.

NUTRITIONAL ANALYSIS (PER ½ CUP/125 ML)							
Energy	Protein	Carbohydrate	Fat	Fiber	Calcium	Iron	Sodium
50 kcal	2 g	6 g	2 g	1 g	25 mg	0.8 mg	44 mg

*Here's a simple and
delicious way to use up
leftover cooked ham.*

Variation

For a more colorful soup, try
adding ½ to 1 cup (125 to
250 mL) tomato juice.

Easy Bean Soup with Ham

1 lb	Great Northern beans	500 g
8 cups	cold water (used in step 2)	2 L
1	medium onion, chopped	1
3	carrots, chopped	3
3	stalks celery, diced	3
2 cups	chopped cooked ham	500 mL
1	bay leaf	1
	Salt and freshly ground black pepper to taste	

1. In a large saucepan, add sufficient cold water to cover beans. Cover and bring to a boil; reduce heat and cook for 5 minutes. Remove from heat and allow to stand for 1 hour. Drain and discard liquid. Return drained beans to saucepan and add 4 cups (1 L) cold water. Bring to a boil; reduce heat and cook for 1 hour or until beans are tender. Drain.

2. In a large stockpot, stir together beans, 8 cups (2 L) cold water, onion, carrots, celery, ham and bay leaf. Season to taste with salt and pepper. Bring to a boil; reduce heat, cover and simmer for 1½ hours or until beans are soft. Remove and discard bay leaf before serving.

NUTRITIONAL ANALYSIS (PER ½ CUP/125 ML)							
Energy	Protein	Carbohydrate	Fat	Fiber	Calcium	Iron	Sodium
55 kcal	5 g	5 g	2 g	2 g	22 mg	0.6 mg	21 mg

Here's a good opportunity for you and your kids to try some vegetables that you may not have very often — kohlrabi and parsnips, which add a sweet flavor to this soup.

Kitchen Tip

Kohlrabi can be found at most supermarkets.

Serve this hearty soup over cooked rice or noodles.

Hungarian Chicken Soup

4	bone-in chicken thighs, with skin, rinsed under cold running water	4
5 cups	water	1.25 L
1 tsp	salt	5 mL
¼ tsp	freshly ground black pepper	1 mL
2	carrots, peeled and sliced	2
2	parsnips, peeled and sliced	2
1	kohlrabi, peeled and chopped	1
3	sprigs fresh parsley, chopped	3

1. In a large saucepan, combine chicken and water. Add salt and pepper. Bring to a boil; reduce heat and simmer, skimming off any froth from the surface, for $1\frac{1}{2}$ hours or until chicken falls off the bone.

2. Remove bones from broth and add vegetables. Simmer for another 45 minutes or until the vegetables are tender. Transfer soup to a serving bowl and garnish with parsley.

NUTRITIONAL ANALYSIS (PER ½ CUP/125 ML)							
Energy	Protein	Carbohydrate	Fat	Fiber	Calcium	Iron	Sodium
46 kcal	4 g	4 g	1 g	1 g	14 mg	0.3 mg	214 mg

These tasty little sandwiches will appeal to children, as they are just the right size for smaller mouths.

Mini Grilled Ham 'n' Cheese Sandwiches

6	slices whole wheat bread	6
	Mustard	
6	slices Cheddar or mozzarella cheese	6
3	slices deli or cooked ham, beef or turkey	3
2	eggs	2
¼ cup	evaporated milk	60 mL
Pinch	freshly ground black pepper	Pinch
	Canola oil	
	Salsa (optional)	

1. Spread 3 of the bread slices lightly with mustard. Top each with 1 slice of cheese, 1 slice of meat and another slice of cheese. Cover with the remaining bread slices and press sandwiches together lightly. Cut off crusts, then cut each sandwich into 4 triangles.

2. In a small bowl, whisk together eggs, milk and pepper. Dip sandwich pieces in egg mixture.

3. In a nonstick skillet, heat a small amount of oil over medium-high heat. Cook sandwich pieces in batches for about 3 minutes per side or until lightly browned on both sides and cheese is melted, adding oil to the skillet and adjusting heat between batches as necessary. Serve with salsa (if using).

NUTRITIONAL ANALYSIS (PER SANDWICH WEDGE)

Energy	Protein	Carbohydrate	Fat	Fiber	Calcium	Iron	Sodium
130 kcal	8 g	8 g	7 g	2 g	194 mg	0.7 mg	243 mg

Super Salmon Sandwiches

Salmon is one of the world's favorite sandwich fillings — and we think this version is one of the best. See if you agree.

KITCHEN TIP

Mashing the bones with the salmon (instead of discarding them) provides as much extra calcium as is contained in a small glass of milk.

We like the taste and texture of English muffins, but any bread will work with this filling.

If you have any filling left over, just cover and refrigerate for up to 2 days.

Variation

Oven-Toasted Cheese: Broil each muffin half on a baking sheet until toasted; spread with salmon filling. Top each half with a slice of cheese, return to broiler and broil until cheese melts.

1	can (7½ oz/213 g) salmon, undrained	1
¼ cup	mayonnaise	60 mL
2 tbsp	finely chopped onion	30 mL
2 tsp	lemon juice	10 mL
¼ tsp	salt	1 mL
Pinch	freshly ground black pepper	Pinch
4	whole wheat English muffins split and toasted (see tip, at left)	4

1. In a small bowl, flake salmon. Remove and discard skin, but mash bones with salmon. Stir in mayonnaise, onion, lemon juice, salt and pepper.

2. Spread filling on one half of each toasted muffin and top with other half. Cut each assembled sandwich into 2 pieces and serve.

NUTRITIONAL ANALYSIS (PER HALF SANDWICH)							
Energy	Protein	Carbohydrate	Fat	Fiber	Calcium	Iron	Sodium
158 kcal	9 g	14 g	8 g	2 g	104 mg	1 mg	274 mg

The relish gives these sandwiches zip. Panini buns are slightly smaller than sub buns and are perfect for lunch.

Homemade Subs with Tomato Pepper Relish

Tomato Pepper Relish

½ cup	finely chopped tomato	125 mL
¼ cup	finely chopped green bell pepper	60 mL
1	green onion, finely chopped	1
1	small clove garlic, minced	1
1 tsp	olive oil	5 mL
1 tsp	red or white wine vinegar	5 mL
Pinch	salt	Pinch
Pinch	freshly ground black pepper	Pinch
4	whole wheat panini buns	4
4	leaves lettuce	4
4	slices Cheddar or Havarti cheese (optional)	4
6 oz	deli roast beef, smoked turkey or ham, sliced	175 g

1. *Tomato Pepper Relish:* In a small bowl, combine tomato, green pepper, green onion, garlic, oil, vinegar, salt and pepper; let stand for 10 minutes.

2. Cut buns in half lengthwise. Spoon relish on bottom halves. Place a lettuce leaf on each. Top with cheese (if using) and roast beef. Cover with top halves. Cut in half, if desired.

NUTRITIONAL ANALYSIS (PER SERVING)							
Energy	Protein	Carbohydrate	Fat	Fiber	Calcium	Iron	Sodium
330 kcal	24 g	32 g	12 g	3 g	231 mg	2 mg	827 mg

Stromboli is an enclosed sandwich made of pizza dough filled with a variety of fillings. It is similar to a calzone or a panzerotto. Serve with tomato pasta sauce for dipping.

Kitchen Tip

Bake the stromboli in the bottom third of the oven.

Mushroom and Broccoli Stromboli

- *Preheat oven to 400°F (200°C)*
- *Baking sheet, lined with parchment paper or greased*

1 cup	broccoli florets	250 mL
2 tbsp	olive oil, divided	30 mL
2 cups	sliced mushrooms	500 mL
1	clove garlic, minced	1
½	red or yellow bell pepper, chopped	½
½ tsp	dried basil	2 mL
Pinch	salt	Pinch
Pinch	freshly ground black pepper	Pinch
1 lb	whole wheat pizza dough	500 g
⅔ cup	tomato pasta sauce	150 mL
1 cup	shredded part-skim mozzarella	250 mL
½ cup	chopped pepperoni (optional)	125 mL

1. In a small saucepan of boiling water, cook broccoli for 1 minute. Drain and rinse under cold water.
2. In a nonstick skillet, heat half the oil over medium heat. Sauté mushrooms, garlic, red pepper, basil, salt and pepper for 5 to 8 minutes or until vegetables are tender. Add broccoli and set aside.
3. Divide dough into 4 pieces. On a floured work surface, roll or stretch each piece of dough into an 8- by 6-inch (20 by 15 cm) oval.
4. Spread pasta sauce over each oval, leaving a 1-inch (2.5 cm) border. Sprinkle with mushroom mixture, cheese and pepperoni (if using). Fold short ends over filling, overlapping to enclose it, leaving the sides open. Pinch seam to seal.
5. Place on prepared baking sheet and brush dough with remaining oil. Bake in preheated oven for about 20 minutes or until dough is puffed and golden.

NUTRITIONAL ANALYSIS (PER SERVING)							
Energy	Protein	Carbohydrate	Fat	Fiber	Calcium	Iron	Sodium
387 kcal	16 g	50 g	12 g	4 g	183 mg	4 mg	696 mg

This lunch can be made in the proverbial "blink of an eye" — or close to it! Keep the necessary ingredients on hand and you'll always be ready with an instant meal.

Kitchen Tip

For added convenience, look for pre-shredded cheese in the dairy case of your supermarkets. Typically, these are available in a number of varieties, including Cheddar, mozzarella, Monterey Jack — or a combination of cheeses.

Hasty Pita Lunch

- Preheat broiler

2	7-inch (18 cm) whole wheat pitas	2
3/4 cup	shredded Cheddar cheese (see tip, at left)	175 mL
1	green onion, finely chopped	1
1	medium tomato, diced	1
1/4 tsp	dried basil	1 mL
1/4 tsp	dried oregano	1 mL

1. With kitchen scissors, cut around edge of each pita to separate it into 2 rounds. Place cut side up on baking sheet and broil for 2 minutes or until lightly golden.

2. Divide cheese between rounds, being careful to spread evenly to their edges. Sprinkle with green onion and tomato, then with basil and oregano. Return to oven and broil for 3 minutes or until cheese starts to melt.

NUTRITIONAL ANALYSIS (PER PITA HALF)

Energy	Protein	Carbohydrate	Fat	Fiber	Calcium	Iron	Sodium
189 kcal	9 g	21 g	9 g	2 g	210 mg	1 mg	231 mg

Make these the night before and wrap them tightly in plastic wrap for lunch to go.

Kitchen Tip

You can substitute whole-grain pitas for the tortillas, or simply make sandwiches using whole-grain buns.

Tuna Veggie Wraps

1	can (6 oz/170 g) water-packed tuna, drained	1
2 tbsp	light mayonnaise	30 mL
1 tbsp	light sour cream or plain yogurt	15 mL
1 tbsp	dill pickle relish	15 mL
Pinch	freshly ground black pepper	Pinch
2	leaves leaf lettuce	2
2	10-inch (25 cm) whole wheat flour tortillas	2
1/3 cup	sliced English cucumber	75 mL
1/2	carrot, grated	1/2
1/2	avocado, thinly sliced (optional)	1/2

1. In a bowl, combine tuna, mayonnaise, sour cream, relish and pepper.

2. Place a lettuce leaf on each tortilla. Top with tuna mixture, cucumber, carrot and avocado (if using). Fold up bottom of tortilla. Fold in sides and roll up.

NUTRITIONAL ANALYSIS (PER SERVING)

Energy	Protein	Carbohydrate	Fat	Fiber	Calcium	Iron	Sodium
263 kcal	24 g	20 g	9 g	4 g	55 mg	2 mg	573 mg

Makes 12 wraps

Mexican dishes are zesty but simple — often requiring only everyday ingredients you already have in your refrigerator. These wraps are a great way to use up leftover turkey.

Kitchen Tip

If desired, spread additional salsa over cheese before baking.

Tex-Mex Turkey Wraps

- *Preheat oven to 350°F (180°C)*
- *Large baking pan*

1 tbsp	vegetable oil	15 mL
2	small onions, finely chopped	2
2	cloves garlic, minced	2
4 cups	chopped cooked turkey	1 L
2 cups	medium or mild salsa	500 mL
1 tsp	chili powder	5 mL
12	10-inch (25 cm) whole wheat flour tortillas	12
2 cups	shredded Cheddar cheese, divided	500 mL

1. In a nonstick skillet, heat oil over medium-high heat. Add onions and garlic; sauté for 5 minutes or until softened but not browned. Stir in turkey, salsa and chili powder; cook until warmed through.

2. Place tortillas on a flat surface. Divide turkey mixture between tortillas, spreading evenly over each. Divide $1\frac{1}{2}$ cups (375 mL) of the cheese over the tortillas. Roll tortillas and place in a single layer on baking pan. Top with remaining cheese and bake in preheated oven until cheese is melted.

NUTRITIONAL ANALYSIS (PER WRAP)							
Energy	Protein	Carbohydrate	Fat	Fiber	Calcium	Iron	Sodium
369 kcal	25 g	35 g	13 g	3 g	209 mg	2 mg	643 mg

Lettuce Wraps

Boston lettuce has a softer
texture than other lettuces,
which makes it easier to roll.
You can serve the filling in
lettuce cups rather than rolls
or use small flour tortillas.

4 tsp	vegetable oil	20 mL
1 tbsp	rice vinegar	15 mL
1 tsp	reduced-sodium soy sauce	5 mL
1 tsp	sesame oil (optional)	5 mL
½ tsp	minced gingerroot (or pinch ground ginger)	2 mL
½ tsp	liquid honey	2 mL
	Salt and freshly ground black pepper	
1 cup	chopped cooked chicken or whole small cooked shrimp	250 mL
1 cup	halved or quartered cherry tomatoes	250 mL
½ cup	chopped English cucumber	125 mL
1	carrot, grated	1
1	green onion, sliced	1
8	leaves Boston lettuce	8

1. In a large bowl, whisk together vegetable oil, vinegar, soy sauce, sesame oil (if using), ginger and honey. Season to taste with salt and pepper. Add chicken, tomatoes, cucumber, carrot and green onion; toss to coat.
2. Spoon chicken mixture in the center of each lettuce leaf, dividing evenly. Fold in sides of lettuce leaves and roll up from the bottom.

NUTRITIONAL ANALYSIS (PER WRAP)							
Energy	Protein	Carbohydrate	Fat	Fiber	Calcium	Iron	Sodium
106 kcal	6 g	3 g	8 g	1 g	15 mg	0.5 mg	43 mg

Focaccia is a type of Italian flatbread that is widely available in grocery stores today. It makes an ideal base for various toppings, and an easy pizza lunch or snack.

Focaccia Pizza Squares

- *Preheat oven to 425°F (220°C)*
- *Large baking pan*

1	focaccia or Italian-style flatbread (about 14 oz/400 g)	1
1	can (7½ oz/213 mL) tomato sauce	1
½ tsp	dried basil	2 mL
½ tsp	dried oregano	2 mL
½ cup	finely minced ham	125 mL
¼ cup	diced green or red bell pepper	60 mL
1 cup	shredded Cheddar cheese	250 mL

1. Place flatbread on baking pan. In a bowl, combine tomato sauce, basil and oregano. Spread sauce mixture evenly over bread. Sprinkle with ham, green pepper and cheese.

2. Bake in preheated oven for 15 minutes or until crust is golden and cheese has melted. Remove from oven and cut into 36 small pieces.

NUTRITIONAL ANALYSIS (PER SQUARE)

Energy	Protein	Carbohydrate	Fat	Fiber	Calcium	Iron	Sodium
48 kcal	2 g	6 g	2 g	0 g	24 mg	0.5 mg	115 mg

Makes 12 muffins

These tasty muffins are ideal to have tucked away in the freezer for those days when you need lunch (or breakfast) in a hurry. Served with a glass of milk, they also make an ideal snack.

Cheese Pizza Muffins

- *Preheat oven to 375°F (190°C)*
- *12-cup muffin pan, greased or paper-lined*

1½ cups	all-purpose flour	375 mL
1 cup	whole wheat flour	250 mL
2 tbsp	granulated sugar	30 mL
2 tsp	baking powder	10 mL
1 tsp	dried basil	5 mL
½ tsp	dried oregano	2 mL
½ tsp	baking soda	2 mL
½ tsp	salt	2 mL
2 cups	shredded Cheddar cheese	500 mL
1	egg	1
1½ cups	buttermilk	375 mL
⅓ cup	vegetable oil	75 mL

1. In a bowl, combine all-purpose flour, whole wheat flour, sugar, baking powder, basil, oregano, baking soda, salt and cheese.
2. In another bowl, whisk together egg, buttermilk and oil. Add to dry ingredients. Stir just until moistened.
3. Spoon batter into prepared muffin pan. Bake in preheated oven for 25 minutes or until muffins are firm to the touch. Cool 10 minutes before removing from pan to wire rack to cool completely.

NUTRITIONAL ANALYSIS (PER MUFFIN)							
Energy	Protein	Carbohydrate	Fat	Fiber	Calcium	Iron	Sodium
245 kcal	9 g	23 g	13 g	2 g	197 mg	1 mg	364 mg

For a change of pace from the usual sandwiches, serve this roasted red pepper hummus with whole wheat mini pitas or any other kind of flatbread.

Roasted Red Pepper Hummus

3 tbsp	tahini	45 mL
2 tbsp	cold water (approx.)	30 mL
1	can (19 oz/540 mL) chickpeas (or 2 cups/500 mL), drained and rinsed	1
1	clove garlic, coarsely chopped	1
1	roasted red bell pepper	1
	Juice of 1 lemon	

1. In a small bowl, combine tahini and cold water, stirring until tahini turns white.

2. In a food processor, process chickpeas and tahini mixture until just combined. Add garlic, roasted red pepper and lemon juice; purée until desired consistency is reached, adding more cold water if necessary.

NUTRITIONAL ANALYSIS (PER 2 TBSP/30 ML)

Energy	Protein	Carbohydrate	Fat	Fiber	Calcium	Iron	Sodium
65 kcal	3 g	8 g	3 g	2 g	22 mg	0.8 mg	131 mg

Another speedy lunchtime treat, antijitos (pronounced an-te-hee-toes) are a favorite with kids and adults alike.

Kitchen Tip

Antijitos make great appetizers for entertaining. For grown-ups who prefer a little extra spice, add 1 tsp (5 mL) chopped jalapeño peppers to each tortilla before rolling.

Antijitos

2	10-inch (25 cm) whole wheat flour tortillas	2
1/4 cup	spreadable cream cheese	60 mL
1/4 cup	salsa	60 mL

1. On each tortilla, thinly spread 2 tbsp (30 mL) each cream cheese and salsa. Roll each tortilla up tightly and cut the roll into 1 1/2-inch (4 cm) slices. Serve cold or bake in a preheated 350°F (180°C) oven for 5 minutes or until warmed through.

NUTRITIONAL ANALYSIS (PER "BITE")

Energy	Protein	Carbohydrate	Fat	Fiber	Calcium	Iron	Sodium
199 kcal	5 g	23 g	10 g	2 g	59 mg	0.6 mg	365 mg

Lunchtime Burritos

1 cup	shredded cooked chicken, turkey or beef	250 mL
¾ cup	shredded Monterey Jack cheese	175 mL
⅓ cup	salsa (store-bought or see recipe, page 187)	75 mL
¼ cup	low-fat sour cream or plain yogurt	60 mL
4	8-inch (20 cm) whole wheat flour tortillas	4
1	green onion, chopped	1
⅓ cup	chopped red bell pepper	75 mL
½ cup	chopped romaine lettuce	125 mL
1	avocado, thinly sliced (optional)	1

1. In a bowl, combine chicken, cheese, salsa and sour cream. Divide mixture evenly among tortillas, spreading to within 1 inch (2.5 cm) of edges.

2. Evenly sprinkle green onion, red pepper and lettuce over chicken mixture. Top each with thin slices of avocado (if using). Fold in sides of tortillas and roll up from the bottom.

NUTRITIONAL ANALYSIS (PER SERVING)

Energy	Protein	Carbohydrate	Fat	Fiber	Calcium	Iron	Sodium
409 kcal	23 g	35 g	20 g	6 g	245 mg	2 mg	552 mg

Kitchen Tips

These burritos are excellent when topped with 1 to 2 tsp (5 to 10 mL) sour cream.

If your children are not accustomed to spicy food, you may wish to use only 1 tbsp (15 mL) chili powder.

Black Bean Burritos

2 tbsp	vegetable oil	30 mL
1	clove garlic, minced	1
½	red onion, chopped	½
1	green pepper, chopped	1
1	red bell pepper, chopped	1
1 cup	canned black beans, rinsed and drained	250 mL
3	carrots, shredded	3
½ cup	chopped broccoli	125 mL
2 tbsp	chili powder (see tip, at left)	30 mL
1 tbsp	ground cumin	15 mL
¼ cup	red wine vinegar	60 mL
¼ cup	water	60 mL
1 tbsp	brown sugar	15 mL
8	8-inch (20 cm) whole wheat flour tortillas	8

1. In a large saucepan, heat oil over medium-high heat. Add garlic, onion and peppers; sauté for about 5 minutes or until softened. Stir in beans, carrots, broccoli, chili powder, cumin, vinegar, water and brown sugar. Increase heat to high and cook for 5 minutes or until vegetables are tender.
2. In microwave, heat tortillas, 2 at a time, on High for 20 to 30 seconds.
3. Place ½ cup (125 mL) bean mixture into middle of each tortilla and fold all sides over to enclose.

NUTRITIONAL ANALYSIS (PER SERVING)							
Energy	Protein	Carbohydrate	Fat	Fiber	Calcium	Iron	Sodium
282 kcal	9 g	43 g	9 g	7 g	97 mg	2 mg	481 mg

Makes 12 wedges

We are sure these Tex-Mex quesadillas will become a favorite lunch meal. You can use bottled salsa or make your own.

Cheese and Bean Quesadillas

¾ cup	nonfat refried beans	175 mL
½ cup	frozen corn kernels, thawed	125 mL
⅓ cup	salsa (store-bought or see recipe, below)	75 mL
4	8-inch (20 cm) whole wheat flour tortillas	4
1 cup	shredded Cheddar cheese	250 mL
2 tsp	vegetable oil, divided	10 mL
	Additional salsa	

1. In a nonstick skillet, heat beans, corn and salsa over medium heat, stirring constantly, until hot.
2. Arrange 2 tortillas on a cutting board and divide bean mixture between them. Sprinkle with cheese and top with remaining tortillas; press firmly to seal.
3. In clean skillet, heat half the oil over medium-high heat. Place one filled tortilla in skillet and cook for about 2 minutes per side, until tortilla is light brown on both sides and cheese is melted. Transfer to cutting board. Repeat with second tortilla, adding the remaining oil between batches.
4. When cool enough to handle, cut tortillas into wedges. Serve with additional salsa.

Fresh Salsa

1	large tomato, chopped,	1
1	avocado, chopped	1
	Juice of 1 lime	
½ to 1 tsp	chili powder (optional)	2 to 5 mL

1. In a bowl, combine tomato, avocado, lime juice and chili powder (if using). Use right away or cover and refrigerate for up to 2 days.

Makes about 1 cup (250 mL)

Use this salsa in place of commercial varieties as a dip, in recipes or as a condiment.

NUTRITIONAL ANALYSIS (PER 2 WEDGES)							
Energy	Protein	Carbohydrate	Fat	Fiber	Calcium	Iron	Sodium
255 kcal	11 g	28 g	11 g	4 g	186 mg	1 mg	547 mg

The all-time favorite with kids of all ages is easy to make from scratch!

Homemade Mac 'n' Cheese

2 cups	elbow macaroni	500 mL
2 cups	2% milk	500 mL
2 tbsp	all-purpose flour	30 mL
Pinch	salt	Pinch
Pinch	freshly ground black pepper	Pinch
2 tbsp	butter or margarine	30 mL
2 cups	coarsely shredded Cheddar cheese	500 mL

1. In a large saucepan, cook macaroni in boiling water according to package instructions until tender but firm. Drain and set aside.

2. In the same saucepan, whisk together milk, flour, salt and pepper. Bring to a gentle boil over medium heat. Cook, stirring often, for 2 minutes or until thickened and smooth. Remove from heat.

3. Stir in butter and cheese until cheese is melted. Stir in macaroni.

NUTRITIONAL ANALYSIS (PER SERVING)							
Energy	Protein	Carbohydrate	Fat	Fiber	Calcium	Iron	Sodium
563 kcal	26 g	52 g	28 g	1 g	551 mg	2 mg	531 mg

Kids love the flavor of tomato and cheese — and this classic dish has plenty of both!

Cheese and Tomato Macaroni

2 cups	elbow macaroni	500 mL
1 tbsp	butter or margarine	15 mL
3 tbsp	all-purpose flour	45 mL
2 cups	2% milk, warmed to room temperature	500 mL
1½ cups	shredded Cheddar cheese	375 mL
1	can (19 oz/398 mL) tomatoes, drained	1
½ tsp	salt	2 mL
Pinch	freshly ground black pepper	Pinch

1. In a large saucepan, cook pasta in boiling water according to package instructions or until tender but firm. Drain.
2. In a second large saucepan, melt butter over medium heat. Add flour and cook, stirring, until it starts to bubble. Gradually add milk, whisking constantly, and cook until thickened. Add shredded cheese; stir until melted. Stir in drained tomatoes, salt and pepper.
3. Pour sauce over macaroni and toss to coat.

NUTRITIONAL ANALYSIS (PER SERVING)							
Energy	Protein	Carbohydrate	Fat	Fiber	Calcium	Iron	Sodium
257 kcal	12 g	29 g	10 g	1 g	234 mg	1 mg	437 mg

*For children and parents
who love the flavor of
peanuts (and are not
allergic to them), here's a
great combination of pasta,
vegetables and sauce.*

Kitchen Tip

To reduce the amount of
sodium in this recipe, choose
reduced-sodium soy sauce
and peanut butter.

Pasta with Vegetables and Asian Peanut Sauce

2 cups	short pasta (such as fusilli)	500 mL
½	red bell pepper, cut into thin strips	½
1	large carrot, peeled and cut into thin strips	1
1	clove garlic	1
½ cup	cilantro leaves (optional)	125 mL
½ cup	creamy peanut butter	125 mL
¼ cup	soy sauce	60 mL
1 tbsp	lemon juice	15 mL
2 tsp	sesame oil	10 mL
1 cup	diced cucumber	250 mL
1	green onion, sliced	1
Pinch	salt	Pinch
Pinch	freshly ground black pepper	Pinch

1. In a large saucepan, cook pasta in boiling water according to package instructions or until tender but firm. A few minutes before the end of cooking time, add red pepper and carrot. Drain well and return to saucepan.

2. Meanwhile, in a food processor, process garlic and cilantro with on/off turns until chopped. Transfer to a bowl. Stir in peanut butter, soy sauce, lemon juice and sesame oil.

3. When pasta and vegetables are cooked and drained, add peanut sauce. Toss to coat. Stir in cucumber and green onions, and season with salt and pepper.

NUTRITIONAL ANALYSIS (PER SERVING)							
Energy	Protein	Carbohydrate	Fat	Fiber	Calcium	Iron	Sodium
449 kcal	17 g	55 g	20 g	4 g	34 mg	2 mg	1555 mg

Perogies

*This authentic East European
dish makes great use of
leftover mashed potatoes.*

Kitchen Tip

Cook perogies in boiling
water or, for a change,
pan-fry with a little butter
and sliced onion.

Perogies freeze extremely
well. Place assembled
(uncooked) perogies on a
baking sheet and freeze.
Once frozen, transfer
perogies to freezer bags
and store in freezer. Cook
perogies from frozen, adding
about 3 minutes to boiling
time.

2 cups	all-purpose flour	500 mL
1 tsp	salt	5 mL
1	egg, beaten	1
²⁄₃ cup	cold water	150 mL
1 cup	mashed potatoes	250 mL
½ cup	shredded Cheddar cheese	125 mL
	Salt and freshly ground pepper to taste	
	Plain yogurt or sour cream	

1. In a large bowl, combine flour, salt, egg and water. Mix together to form dough. Cover bowl and set aside.
2. In another bowl, combine mashed potatoes, cheese, salt and pepper.
3. *Assembly:* On a lightly floured surface, roll out dough. Cut circles out of dough using a 3-inch (7.5 cm) round cookie cutter or drinking glass. Place about 1 tsp (5 mL) potato mixture in center of each circle and fold over, pinching edges to seal.
4. In a large pot of boiling water, cook perogies 8 to 12 at a time for 4 to 5 minutes or until they float. Serve with yogurt or sour cream.

NUTRITIONAL ANALYSIS (PER 3 PEROGIES)							
Energy	Protein	Carbohydrate	Fat	Fiber	Calcium	Iron	Sodium
120 kcal	5 g	19 g	3 g	1 g	48 mg	1 mg	304 mg

If you're going to try just one
lentil recipe, this is the one
to make. Your kids and the
rest of the family will love
the flavor of these patties.
They're also great as a
snack, since they don't need
to be reheated.

Kitchen Tips

Serve plain or with dip
(ranch-style is good), or try
plum sauce.

These patties take a bit of
time to prepare, so you may
want to make them ahead
and freeze until needed.
When ready to serve, just
thaw in the microwave.

Lentil Patties

1 cup	red lentils	250 mL
2 tsp	olive oil	10 mL
2	small onions, chopped	2
2	large tomatoes, chopped	2
1	small apple, peeled and chopped	1
2¼ cups	bread crumbs, divided	550 mL
1 tsp	dried sage	5 mL
Pinch	salt	Pinch
Pinch	freshly ground black pepper	Pinch
1	egg, lightly beaten	1
4 tbsp	olive oil, divided	60 mL

1. Rinse lentils and transfer to a saucepan. Add 3 cups
(750 mL) water. Bring to a boil; cook for about
30 minutes or until soft. Drain and set aside.

2. In a skillet, heat 2 tsp (10 mL) olive oil over
medium-high heat. Add onions, tomatoes and apples;
cook for about 10 minutes or until soft. Transfer
mixture to saucepan containing lentils, along with
¼ cup (50 mL) of the bread crumbs, sage, salt and
pepper. Add egg and mix well.

3. Wipe skillet clean and heat 1 tbsp (15 mL) of the olive
oil over medium-high heat. Using your hands, form
lentil mixture into patties. Roll each patty in remaining
bread crumbs and cook for about 5 minutes per side
or until crisp. Cook remaining patties, adding oil as
required, 1 tbsp (15 mL) at a time.

NUTRITIONAL ANALYSIS (PER PATTY)							
Energy	Protein	Carbohydrate	Fat	Fiber	Calcium	Iron	Sodium
88 kcal	4 g	12 g	2 g	3 g	20 mg	1 mg	85 mg

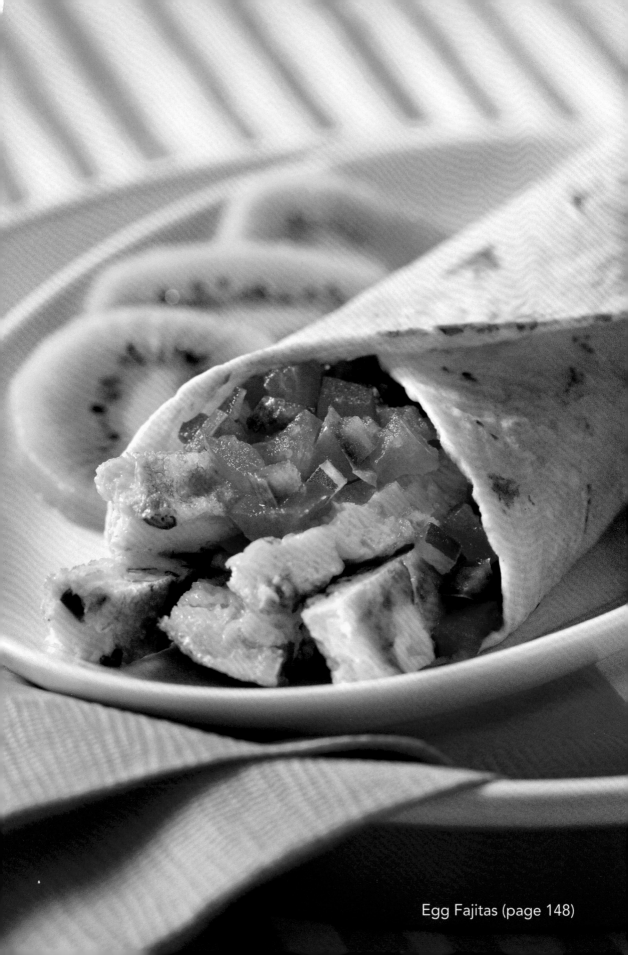

Egg Fajitas (page 148)

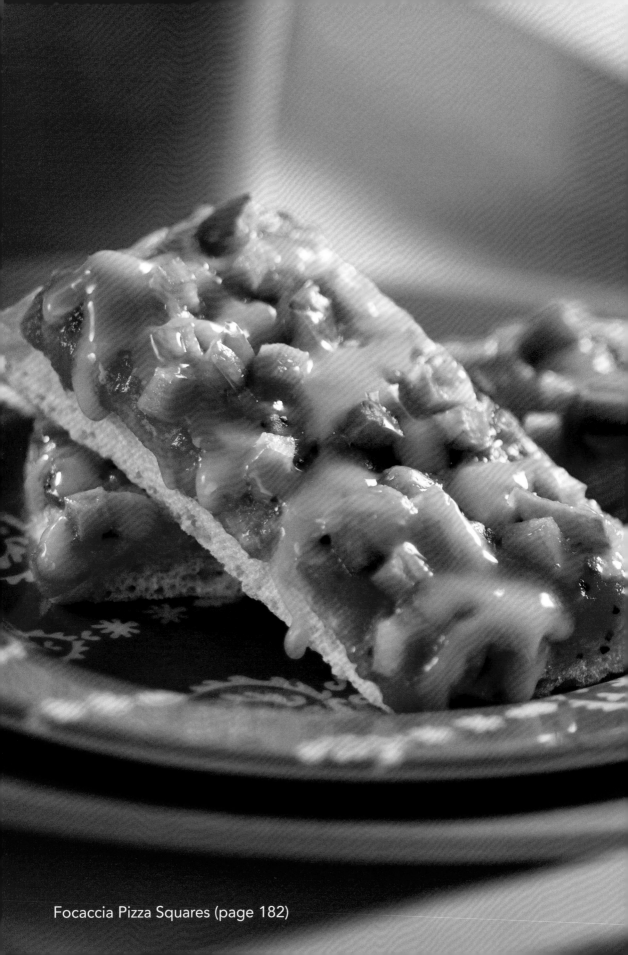

Focaccia Pizza Squares (page 182)

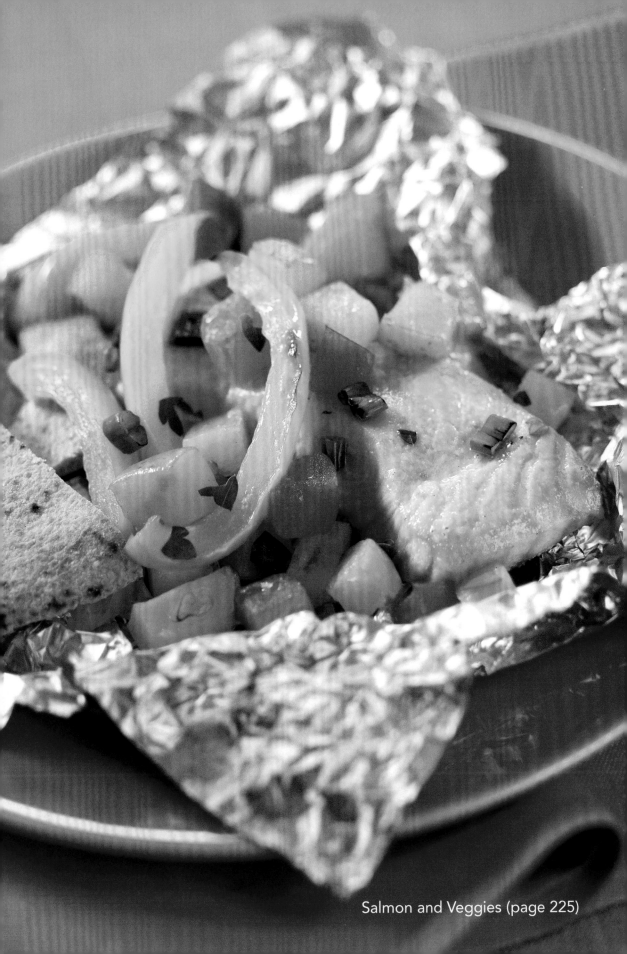

Salmon and Veggies (page 225)

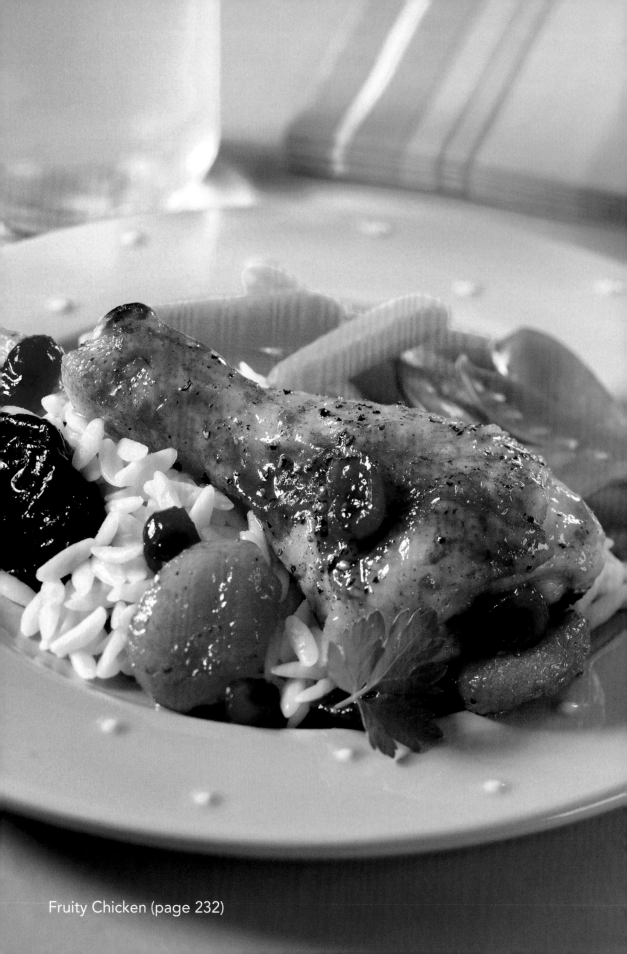

Fruity Chicken (page 232)

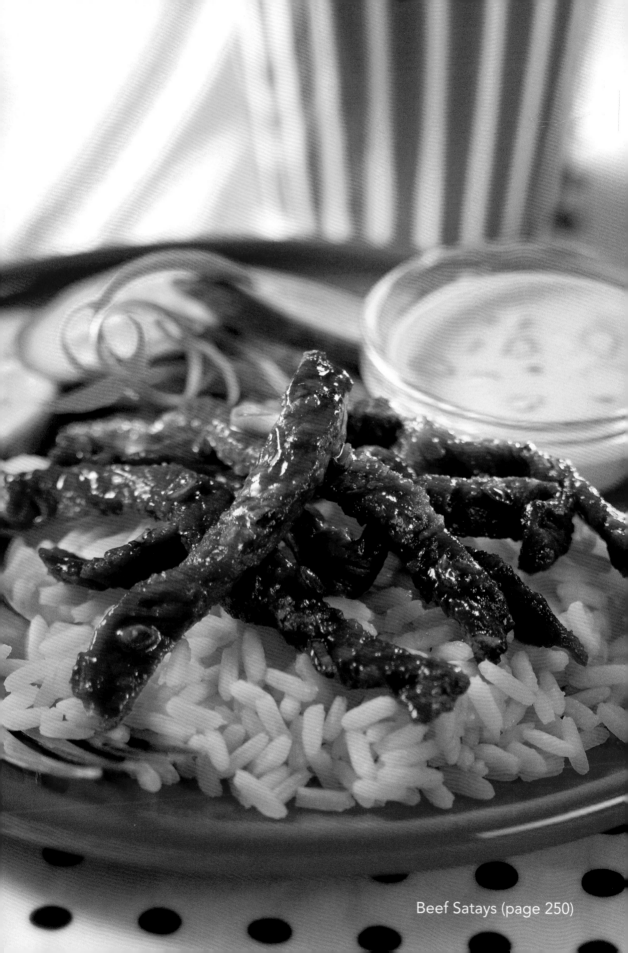

Beef Satays (page 250)

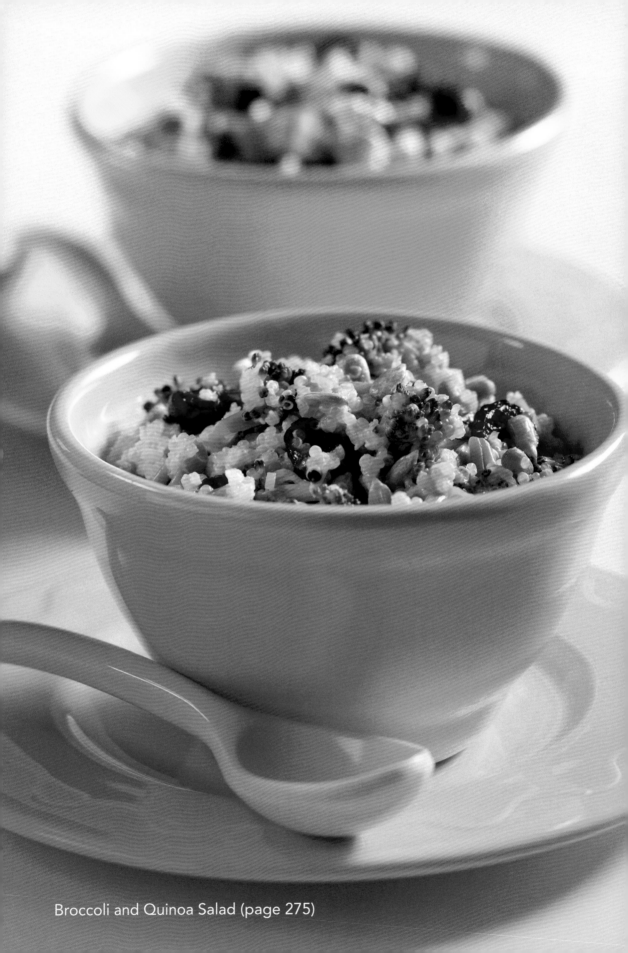
Broccoli and Quinoa Salad (page 275)

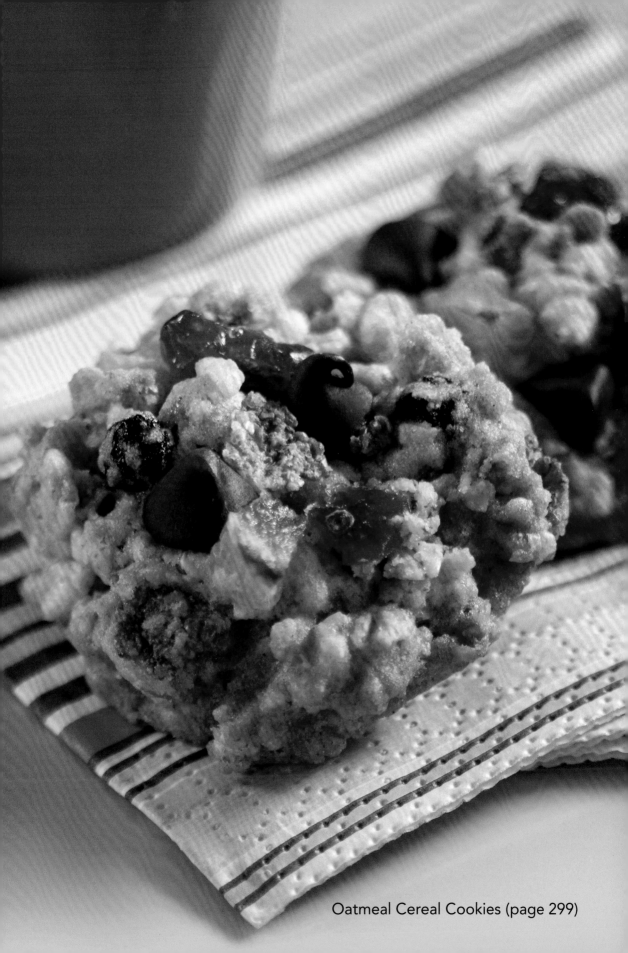

Oatmeal Cereal Cookies (page 299)

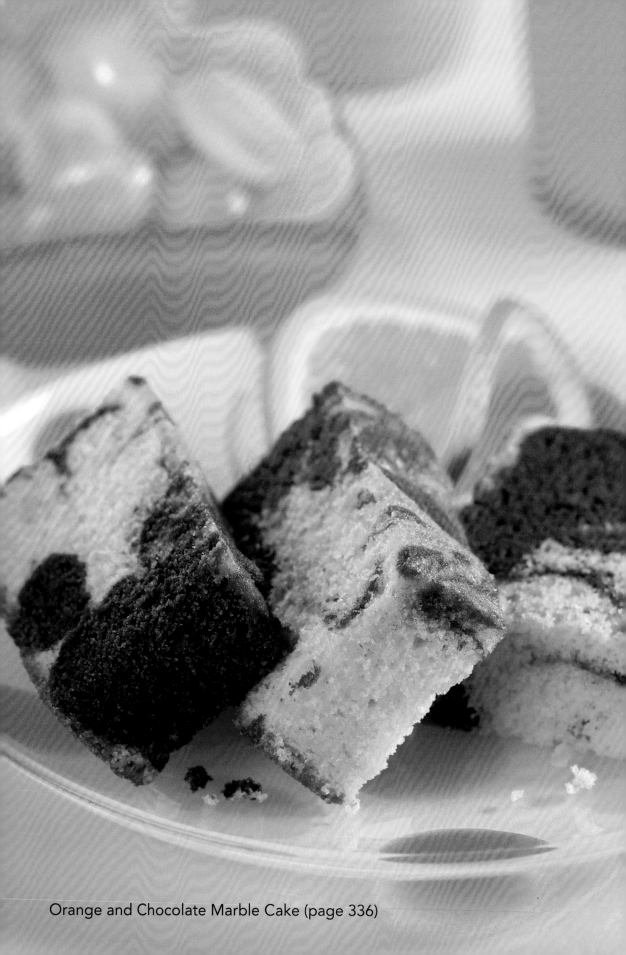

Orange and Chocolate Marble Cake (page 336)

Makes 4 servings

Here's an amazingly easy and tasty way to add eggs to your child's meals.

Eggs Baked in Cheese

- *Preheat oven to 350°F (180°C)*
- *8-inch (2 L) baking pan, greased*

⅔ cup	shredded Cheddar cheese	150 mL
4	eggs	4
½ cup	whole milk or light (5%) cream	125 mL
¼ tsp	salt	1 mL
Pinch	freshly ground black pepper	Pinch
Pinch	paprika	Pinch
	Finely chopped fresh parsley (optional)	

1. Sprinkle cheese over bottom of prepared pan. Break eggs over cheese.

2. In a bowl, whisk together milk, salt and pepper. Pour over eggs. Sprinkle lightly with paprika.

3. Bake in preheated oven for 20 minutes or until eggs are just set. Sprinkle with parsley, if desired.

NUTRITIONAL ANALYSIS (PER SERVING)							
Energy	Protein	Carbohydrate	Fat	Fiber	Calcium	Iron	Sodium
158 kcal	11 g	2 g	12 g	0 g	194 mg	1 mg	336 mg

These scrambled eggs with a Mexican twist will soon become a family favorite.

Kitchen Tip

When you're warming the tortillas in the microwave, check them after 30 seconds. If they're not warm enough, microwave them for another 30 seconds.

Huevos Rancheros

4	eggs	4
1 tbsp	butter or margarine	15 mL
4	10-inch (25 cm) whole wheat flour tortillas	4
½ cup	salsa (store-bought or see recipe, page 187)	125 mL

1. In a bowl, whisk eggs until fluffy. In a nonstick skillet, melt butter over medium heat. Add eggs to skillet and cook, stirring frequently, for 5 minutes or until firm.
2. Wrap tortillas in paper towels and microwave on High for 30 to 60 seconds or until warm.
3. Divide egg mixture among tortillas and top with salsa. Fold in sides of tortillas and roll up from the bottom. Serve warm.

NUTRITIONAL ANALYSIS (PER SERVING)

Energy	Protein	Carbohydrate	Fat	Fiber	Calcium	Iron	Sodium
283 kcal	12 g	32 g	12 g	3 g	84 mg	2 mg	480 mg

This is a great alternative to traditional quiche Lorraine. The salmon is tender and flavorful, and is a great way to incorporate fish in your family's diet. Feel free to experiment with ingredients (see Variations, below).

Variations

Cheddar Cheese and Ham: Use Cheddar cheese and replace salmon with diced cooked ham. Replace nutmeg with a pinch of dry mustard or Dijon mustard.

Savory Leek: Replace green onion with 1 leek (white and light green parts only), sliced, washed and blanched for 5 minutes.

Salmon Quiche

• *Preheat oven to 400°F (200°C)*

1	9-inch (23 cm) frozen pastry shell, thawed	1
4	eggs	4
1½ cups	whole milk	375 mL
½ tsp	salt	2 mL
Pinch	ground nutmeg	Pinch
Pinch	freshly ground black pepper	Pinch
1 cup	shredded Swiss or Cheddar cheese	250 mL
½ cup	canned boneless skinless salmon	125 mL
2	green onions, finely chopped	2

1. Prick bottom of pastry shell with a fork; partially bake in preheated oven for 8 minutes. Remove from oven; reduce heat to 350°F (180°C).
2. In a small bowl, lightly beat eggs. Stir in milk, salt, nutmeg and pepper.
3. Spread cheese, salmon and green onions in pastry shell. Pour in egg mixture. Bake for 35 minutes or until knife inserted in center comes out clean. Remove from oven and let stand for 10 minutes before cutting into 6 pieces.

NUTRITIONAL ANALYSIS (PER SERVING)							
Energy	Protein	Carbohydrate	Fat	Fiber	Calcium	Iron	Sodium
310 kcal	16 g	16 g	20	1 g	231 mg	2 mg	434 mg

*A favorite weekend
breakfast or lunch recipe,
strata can be made ahead
when life is busy and you are
having overnight guests.*

Make-Ahead Ham 'n' Egg Strata

- *9-inch (23 cm) casserole dish, lightly greased*

2 cups	chopped broccoli	500 mL
4 cups	cubed whole wheat bread	1 L
1 cup	diced ham	250 mL
1 cup	shredded mozzarella cheese, divided	250 mL
4	eggs	4
1½ cups	2% milk	375 mL
Pinch	salt	Pinch
Pinch	freshly ground black pepper	Pinch
2	tomatoes, chopped	2

1. In a small saucepan of boiling water, cook broccoli for 1 minute. Drain and rinse under running water to cool.
2. Arrange bread in prepared casserole dish. Top with broccoli, ham and half the cheese.
3. In a large bowl, whisk together eggs, milk, salt and pepper. Pour over bread mixture. Sprinkle with remaining cheese. Cover and refrigerate overnight.
4. Preheat oven to 350°F (180°C). Uncover pan and top strata with tomatoes. Bake for 40 minutes or until edges are golden and tester inserted in center comes out clean.

NUTRITIONAL ANALYSIS (PER SERVING)

Energy	Protein	Carbohydrate	Fat	Fiber	Calcium	Iron	Sodium
236 kcal	20 g	19 g	9 g	5 g	348 mg	2 mg	390 mg

*This is actually a
soufflé — we just
thought "puff" sounds
less intimidating! There's
no reason to be worried
about making this dish.
It's easy enough for
anyone to prepare.*

Salmon Puff

- *Preheat oven to 375°F (190°C)*
- *4-cup (1 L) casserole, greased*

1	can (7½ oz/213 g) salmon	1
½ cup	2% milk	125 mL
1	slice white bread, crust removed	1
3	eggs, separated	3
½ tsp	salt	2 mL
¼ tsp	freshly ground black pepper	1 mL
	Toast triangles as accompaniment	

1. Drain liquid from salmon into a small saucepan. Transfer salmon to a bowl; flake salmon with a fork and set aside. Add milk to saucepan and warm gently over low heat.

2. In another bowl, cover bread slice with milk mixture. Allow to sit in a warm location until soft, then break apart with a fork. Add flaked salmon, egg yolks, salt and pepper; stir until smooth.

3. In a bowl, with an electric mixer, beat egg whites until stiff. Fold into salmon mixture. Gently transfer mixture into prepared casserole or 3 individual dishes. Bake in preheated oven for about 20 minutes or until puffed and golden. Serve with toast triangles.

NUTRITIONAL ANALYSIS (PER SERVING)							
Energy	Protein	Carbohydrate	Fat	Fiber	Calcium	Iron	Sodium
196 kcal	21 g	4 g	11 g	0 g	191 mg	1 mg	798 mg

Zucchini Pudding

Kitchen Tip

To make individual puddings, bake in a lightly greased 12-cup muffin tin.

- *Preheat oven to 350°F (180°C)*
- *8-cup (2 L) casserole, lightly greased*

3 cups	grated zucchini, rinsed and drained (about 2 medium zucchini)	750 mL
½	medium onion, chopped	½
4	eggs	4
½ cup	vegetable oil	125 mL
¼ tsp	freshly ground pepper	1 mL
Pinch	salt	Pinch
2 tsp	chopped fresh parsley	10 mL
1 cup	dry bread crumbs	250 mL

1. Squeeze zucchini to remove any excess moisture. Set aside
2. In a bowl, combine onion and eggs. Add zucchini and oil; mix well. Add pepper, salt, parsley and bread crumbs. Stir until well mixed. Transfer to casserole and bake for 45 minutes or until firm.

NUTRITIONAL ANALYSIS (PER SERVING)							
Energy	Protein	Carbohydrate	Fat	Fiber	Calcium	Iron	Sodium
217 kcal	5 g	13 g	17 g	1 g	41 mg	1 mg	182 mg

Kids love french fries, and here we serve them up using both potatoes and sweet potatoes. Serve plain or with ketchup.

Kitchen Tip

These french fries cook with only a small amount of oil. Canola or sunflower oil are good choices.

Safety Tip

Make sure the frying pan is placed on the back burner while cooking. And, as always when cooking with young children around, never leave the pan unattended — not even for a minute.

Maria's Colorful French Fries

- *Preheat oven to 350°F (180°C)*
- *Rimmed baking sheet*

2	white (or Yukon gold) potatoes, peeled and cut into 2- by ½-inch (5 by 1 cm) pieces	2
½	large sweet potato, peeled and cut into 2- by ½-inch (5 by 1 cm) pieces	½
2 tbsp	vegetable oil (see tip, at left)	30 mL
½ tsp	salt (optional)	2 mL

1. In a bowl, toss potatoes and sweet potatoes with oil and salt (if using). Spread out in a single layer on baking sheet. Bake in preheated oven for 45 minutes or until lightly browned.

NUTRITIONAL ANALYSIS (PER SERVING)							
Energy	Protein	Carbohydrate	Fat	Fiber	Calcium	Iron	Sodium
51 kcal	0.6 g	7 g	2 g	1 g	5 mg	0.1 mg	101 mg

Zucchini Sticks

Kitchen Tip

Serve with sour cream or a creamy dressing.

- *Preheat oven to 400°F (200°C)*
- *Baking sheet, lightly greased*

¾ cup	dry bread crumbs	175 mL
¼ cup	grated Parmesan cheese	60 mL
½ tsp	garlic powder	2 mL
½ tsp	dried sage	2 mL
¼ tsp	salt	1 mL
¼ tsp	freshly ground black pepper	1 mL
2	eggs	2
3	medium zucchini, cut into 3- by ½-inch (7.5 by 1 cm) sticks	3
¼ cup	vegetable oil	60 mL

1. In a bowl, combine bread crumbs, Parmesan, garlic powder, sage, salt and pepper; mix well.

2. In another bowl, beat eggs lightly.

3. Dip zucchini sticks in eggs, then in the bread crumb mixture; transfer to prepared baking sheet. Drizzle sticks with oil and bake for 20 minutes or until lightly browned, turning sticks over once halfway through baking time.

NUTRITIONAL ANALYSIS (PER STICK)

Energy	Protein	Carbohydrate	Fat	Fiber	Calcium	Iron	Sodium
19 kcal	0.6 g	1 g	1 g	0 g	8 mg	0.1 mg	27 mg

This is a great way to introduce tofu to your children. The sesame seeds add crunch and a light flavor. Serve with reduced-sodium hoisin sauce or soy sauce.

Tofu in Sesame Crust

¼ cup	dry whole wheat bread crumbs	60 mL
3 tbsp	sesame seeds	45 mL
2	eggs	2
¼ cup	2% milk	60 mL
Pinch	sea salt	Pinch
Pinch	freshly ground black pepper	Pinch
1 tbsp	vegetable oil, divided	15 mL
12 oz	firm tofu, drained and cut crosswise into 15 slices	350 g

1. On a plate, combine bread crumbs and sesame seeds. In a small bowl, whisk together eggs, milk, salt and pepper. Dip tofu slices in egg mixture, then in sesame seed mixture, coating evenly and shaking off excess. Discard excess egg and seed mixtures.
2. In a large nonstick skillet, heat half the oil over medium heat. Spread half the tofu slices evenly in the pan and cook for 2 to 2½ minutes per side or until lightly browned on both sides. Transfer to a plate and keep warm. Repeat with remaining tofu slices, adding remaining oil to the skillet and adjusting heat between batches as necessary.

NUTRITIONAL ANALYSIS (PER SERVING)

Energy	Protein	Carbohydrate	Fat	Fiber	Calcium	Iron	Sodium
170 kcal	11 g	7 g	11 g	1 g	182 mg	2 mg	103 mg

Tasty Tofu

Kitchen Tips

For young children who don't like the strong taste of garlic, omit this ingredient from step 2. If you wish, once the child has been served, you can season the remaining sauce with garlic powder.

Serve this dish on its own or over rice. For added flavor and texture, try adding snow peas at the end of cooking.

1 tbsp	vegetable oil	15 mL
12 oz	extra-firm tofu, patted dry and cut into 1/2-inch (1 cm) cubes	350 g
1	clove garlic, minced (see tip, at left)	1
1 tsp	ground ginger	5 mL
1/3 cup	teriyaki sauce	75 mL
2 tbsp	brown sugar	30 mL
2 tsp	molasses	10 mL
1 tbsp	sesame oil	15 mL
1	green onion, chopped	1

1. In a saucepan, heat oil over medium-high heat. Add tofu and sauté for 10 minutes or until browned on all sides. (Cubes should be crispy.) Transfer to a bowl and set aside.
2. Add the garlic and ginger to pan; cook, stirring, for about 15 seconds. Add teriyaki sauce, brown sugar, molasses, sesame oil and onions. Bring to a boil, stirring occasionally. Add tofu and cook for 3 minutes, tossing cubes gently until thoroughly glazed and sauce is syrupy in texture.

NUTRITIONAL ANALYSIS (PER SERVING)							
Energy	Protein	Carbohydrate	Fat	Fiber	Calcium	Iron	Sodium
97 kcal	5 g	7 g	6 g	1 g	89 mg	0.9 mg	408 mg

Tofu with Hoisin Sauce

2 tbsp	reduced-sodium hoisin sauce	30 mL
1 tbsp	reduced-sodium soy sauce	15 mL
1 tbsp	orange juice	15 mL
1 tbsp	balsamic vinegar	15 mL
12 oz	firm tofu, cut into 12 slices	350 g
1 tbsp	vegetable oil, divided	15 mL

1. In a medium bowl, combine hoisin sauce and soy sauce. Stir in orange juice and balsamic vinegar. Add tofu slices a few at a time, stirring to coat.

2. In a large nonstick skillet, heat half the oil over low heat. Working in batches, spread tofu slices evenly in pan and cook for $1\frac{1}{2}$ to 2 minutes per side or until lightly browned on both sides, adding oil to the skillet and adjusting heat between batches as necessary.

NUTRITIONAL ANALYSIS (PER SERVING)							
Energy	Protein	Carbohydrate	Fat	Fiber	Calcium	Iron	Sodium
40 kcal	3 g	1 g	3 g	0 g	56 mg	0.4 mg	98 mg

Variations

For flavor variety, sprinkle with reduced-sodium soy sauce or teriyaki sauce.

Try different vegetables, such as zucchini, corn or spinach. Diced cooked chicken or beef can also replace the tofu.

Rice and Tofu

2 tbsp	butter, divided	30 mL
2 cups	cooked rice	500 mL
1	egg, lightly beaten	1
4 oz	firm tofu, drained and cubed	125 g
1/3	medium onion, diced	1/3
1/2 cup	cooked diced carrots	125 mL
1/2 cup	cooked green peas	125 mL

1. In a saucepan, melt 1 tbsp (15 mL) butter over medium-high heat. Add rice and cook, stirring, for 3 minutes or until cooked through. Transfer to a bowl and set aside.

2. Using same pan, melt 1 tsp (5 mL) butter. Add egg and scramble until cooked. Transfer to another bowl and set aside.

3. Wipe pan clean, and melt another 1 tsp (5 mL) butter. Add tofu and cook, stirring, for 2 minutes or until lightly browned. Transfer to another bowl and set aside.

4. Wipe pan clean, and melt remaining 1 tsp (5 mL) butter. Add onion and cook for 2 minutes or until softened. Add reserved rice, egg and tofu. Stir in carrots and peas. Cook mixture until heated through. Serve immediately.

NUTRITIONAL ANALYSIS (PER SERVING)							
Energy	Protein	Carbohydrate	Fat	Fiber	Calcium	Iron	Sodium
120 kcal	4 g	17 g	4 g	1 g	38 mg	1 mg	34 mg

Dinner

Beans, corn and Mexican seasonings give this soup its authentic flavors. It works well as a vegetarian dish or with meat added.

Kitchen Tip

If your children are not accustomed to spicy food, you may wish to use only 1 tsp (5 mL) chili powder.

Sopa de Mexico

½ cup	dried pinto or kidney beans	125 mL
2 tsp	vegetable oil	10 mL
½ cup	chopped onion	125 mL
2	cloves garlic, crushed	2
2 tsp	chili powder	10 mL
½ tsp	ground cumin	2 mL
½ tsp	ground oregano	2 mL
Pinch	freshly ground black pepper	Pinch
3 cups	reduced-sodium beef or vegetable stock	750 mL
1	large carrot, peeled and sliced	1
1 cup	frozen corn kernels	250 mL

Garnishes: Sour cream, corn tortilla chips, shredded cheese, chopped avocado, tomato, green onions and cilantro

1. In a saucepan, combine beans with 1½ cups (375 mL) cold water. Cover and bring to a boil; reduce heat and cook for 5 minutes. Remove from heat and let stand for 1 hour. Drain and discard liquid. Transfer to a bowl and set aside.

2. In same pan, heat oil over medium-high heat. Add onion and garlic; sauté for 5 minutes or until softened. Stir in chili powder, cumin, oregano and pepper. Add stock and reserved beans. Cover and bring to a boil; reduce heat and simmer, stirring occasionally, for 1½ hours or until beans are tender.

3. Add carrots and corn; cook for 10 minutes or until vegetables are tender. Serve with a variety of garnishes at the table. You may need to assist younger children with their choices.

NUTRITIONAL ANALYSIS (PER ½ CUP/125 ML)

Energy	Protein	Carbohydrate	Fat	Fiber	Calcium	Iron	Sodium
54 kcal	3 g	9 g	1 g	3 g	22 mg	1 mg	54 mg

Here's an easy way to make a comforting thick chowder for dinner.

Chicken Corn Chowder

2	boneless skinless chicken breasts	2
2 cups	water	500 mL
½ tsp	salt	2 mL
Pinch	freshly ground black pepper	Pinch
1	stalk celery, finely chopped	1
½	small onion, finely chopped	½
1	large potato, peeled and cubed	1
1	large carrot, peeled and sliced	1
1	can (14 oz/341 mL) creamed corn	1
1 cup	2% milk	250 mL

1. In a large saucepan, bring chicken, water, salt and pepper to a boil. Reduce heat, cover and cook for about 20 minutes or until chicken is no longer pink. Remove chicken from cooking liquid and, when cool enough to handle, cut into cubes. Set aside.

2. Add celery, onion, potato, and carrot to cooking liquid. Bring to a boil, reduce heat and simmer for 10 minutes or until vegetables are tender. Add corn, milk and reserved chicken. Reheat to serving temperature.

NUTRITIONAL ANALYSIS (PER ½ CUP/125 ML)							
Energy	Protein	Carbohydrate	Fat	Fiber	Calcium	Iron	Sodium
85 kcal	6 g	13 g	1 g	1 g	34 mg	0.3 mg	209 mg

Warm, gooey and great-tasting — what more could a child want from a meal? Fondues can be a little messy, but they're great fun for the whole family.

Kitchen Tips

For a grown-up version, replace chicken stock with white wine. Vegetarians can substitute vegetable stock.

Cheese fondue thickens as it cools, which makes it less likely to drip, and therefore easier for a child to eat. If you wish a thinner consistency, however, just whisk in a little more milk or stock.

Instead of (or in addition to) bread cubes, dippers can include blanched vegetables or apple slices.

You can prepare fondues in the microwave. Set power to Medium and stir frequently, making sure the container is microwave-safe, of course!

Family Cheese Fondue

2 tbsp	butter or margarine	30 mL
2 tbsp	all-purpose flour	30 mL
⅔ cup	chicken stock (see tip, at left)	150 mL
1 lb	shredded Swiss or Cheddar cheese	500 g
½ tsp	ground nutmeg	2 mL
Pinch	salt	Pinch
Pinch	freshly ground black pepper	Pinch
3 cups	cubed French bread	750 mL

1. In a saucepan or fondue pot, melt butter over medium heat. Whisk in flour and cook for 1 minute or until bubbly. Gradually whisk in stock, stirring constantly until smooth and thickened.

2. Reduce heat to low. Add cheese and cook, stirring constantly, for 3 minutes or until cheese is melted. Stir in nutmeg, salt and pepper. Remove from heat.

3. Spoon fondue into individual small bowls and serve with bread cubes for dipping. Be sure that the child's portion has cooled to a safe temperature before serving.

NUTRITIONAL ANALYSIS (PER ¼ CUP/60 ML)							
Energy	Protein	Carbohydrate	Fat	Fiber	Calcium	Iron	Sodium
409 kcal	25 g	16 g	27 g	1 g	668 mg	0.9 mg	348 mg

Makes 8 wedges

Keep several prebaked pizza crusts in the freezer so crusts are always handy for last-minute dinner preparation.

Cheesy Chicken Pizza

- *Preheat oven to 425°F (220°C)*
- *Large baking pan or pizza pan*

1	10-inch (25 cm) whole wheat prebaked pizza crust	1
½ cup	tomato sauce	125 mL
1	cooked boneless skinless chicken breast, diced	1
1	green onion, minced	1
1 cup	shredded Monterey Jack or mozzarella cheese	250 mL

1. Place pizza crust on pan. Spread tomato sauce evenly over crust and top with chicken, green onion and cheese.

2. Bake in preheated oven for about 10 minutes or until cheese has melted and crust is brown. Cut into 8 wedges and serve.

NUTRITIONAL ANALYSIS (PER WEDGE)

Energy	Protein	Carbohydrate	Fat	Fiber	Calcium	Iron	Sodium
81 kcal	8 g	8 g	2 g	1 g	100 mg	0.4 mg	270 mg

Summertime is definitely the time to make this fresh tomato sauce. However, if local fresh tomatoes are not available, you can use canned tomatoes to make it at any time of year.

Kitchen Tip

To easily peel tomatoes, use a sharp knife to cut a star in the stem end. Plunge each tomato into a saucepan of boiling water just until skin starts to pull away from flesh. Remove to ice cold water to stop further cooking. Peel off skin.

Tomato Vegetable Pasta Sauce

- Preheat oven to 375°F (180°C)
- 2 large baking sheets, lined with parchment paper

2	red bell peppers	2
1	large onion, chopped	1
3	cloves garlic, minced	3
3 tbsp	olive or canola oil, divided	45 mL
1	eggplant, cut into small cubes	1
6	large ripe plum (Roma) tomatoes, peeled and diced	6
2 tbsp	tomato paste	30 mL
1 tsp	dried oregano	5 mL
1 tsp	dried basil	5 mL
Pinch	salt	Pinch
Pinch	freshly ground black pepper	Pinch

1. Place peppers on a prepared baking sheet. Roast in preheated oven for 40 minutes, turning once, until tender. Remove from baking sheet, place in a paper or plastic bag and let cool.

2. Meanwhile, in a large bowl, toss onion and garlic with 1 tbsp (15 mL) of the oil. Spread out in a single layer on baking sheet. Roast for about 30 minutes or until softened.

3. In the same bowl, toss eggplant with remaining oil. Spread out in a single layer on the other baking sheet. Place in the oven with the onion and garlic; roast for 25 minutes or until edges start to brown.

4. Peel and seed roasted peppers. Purée one of the peppers in a food processor until smooth. Cut the second pepper into small pieces.

Kitchen Tip

You can replace the fresh tomatoes with a 28-oz (796 mL) can of diced tomatoes, with juice.

5. In a medium saucepan, combine puréed pepper, roasted onion and garlic, tomatoes, 1 cup (250 mL) water and tomato paste; bring to a boil over medium-high heat. Reduce heat and simmer, stirring frequently, for 20 minutes. Stir in eggplant and chopped pepper; simmer, stirring occasionally, for about 20 minutes or until sauce thickens.

NUTRITIONAL ANALYSIS (PER ½ CUP/250 ML)

Energy	Protein	Carbohydrate	Fat	Fiber	Calcium	Iron	Sodium
110 kcal	2 g	14 g	5 g	4 g	38 mg	1 mg	287 mg

Makes 4 servings

Variations

Try adding sautéed vegetables or grilled chicken — or whatever you have available in your refrigerator.

For a richer version of this dish, use half-and-half (10%) cream instead of milk.

Speedy Fettuccine Alfredo

8 oz	fettuccine	250 g
3 tbsp	butter	45 mL
¾ cup	grated Parmesan cheese	175 mL
⅔ cup	whole milk	150 mL
	Salt and freshly ground black pepper	

1. In a large saucepan, cook pasta in boiling water according to package instructions until tender but firm. Drain.

2. In another saucepan, melt butter over medium heat. Add Parmesan and milk; bring to a boil, stirring constantly. Reduce heat and simmer for 10 minutes or until sauce has thickened slightly. Season to taste with salt and pepper. Pour sauce over pasta and toss to coat.

NUTRITIONAL ANALYSIS (PER SERVING)

Energy	Protein	Carbohydrate	Fat	Fiber	Calcium	Iron	Sodium
392 kcal	16 g	49 g	15 g	2 g	224 mg	2 mg	309 mg

Kitchen Tip

For a burst of tomato flavor, serve this dish drizzled with cream of tomato soup.

Mushroom Zucchini Pasta

8 oz	rotini or other short pasta	250 g
2 tbsp	butter or margarine, divided	30 mL
2	cloves garlic, minced, divided	2
6 oz	mushrooms, sliced	175 g
2 tsp	lemon juice	10 mL
6 oz	zucchini, unpeeled, diced	175 g
1 tbsp	minced fresh parsley, divided	15 mL
1/2 tsp	crushed dried basil	2 mL
Pinch	salt and freshly ground black pepper	Pinch

1. In a large saucepan, cook pasta in boiling water according to package instructions or until tender but firm. Drain.

2. In a large skillet, melt 1 tbsp (15 mL) butter over medium heat. Add one-half of the minced garlic and cook for 3 minutes. Add mushrooms and lemon juice; toss well. Stir in zucchini, 2 tsp (10 mL) of the parsley, basil, salt and pepper. Cover and cook, stirring often, for 3 to 5 minutes or until the vegetables are tender-crisp.

3. In a large bowl, place remaining butter, garlic and parsley. Add hot pasta and toss well. Add vegetables and toss again.

NUTRITIONAL ANALYSIS (PER SERVING)							
Energy	Protein	Carbohydrate	Fat	Fiber	Calcium	Iron	Sodium
298 kcal	11 g	50 g	7 g	3 g	28 mg	3 mg	51 mg

Kids love pasta of all types, including the rice-shaped orzo used in this dish. It makes an ideal accompaniment to the bounty of summer vegetables.

Kitchen Tip

If you are using frozen corn, there's no need to thaw it first; just add it directly to the hot orzo.

Summer Vegetable Orzo

2 cups	orzo	500 mL
2 cups	snow peas or sugar-snap peas, trimmed and halved	500 mL
1/4 cup	olive oil, divided	60 mL
1 cup	corn kernels, fresh or frozen (see tip, at left)	250 mL
1 1/2 cups	diced tomatoes	375 mL
1 cup	diced seedless cucumber	250 mL
1/2 cup	finely chopped red onion	125 mL
1/4 cup	chopped fresh mint (optional)	60 mL
1 tsp	grated lemon zest	5 mL
1/4 cup	lemon juice	60 mL
1/2 tsp	salt	2 mL
1/2 tsp	freshly ground black pepper	2 mL

1. In a large saucepan of boiling water, cook orzo for 6 minutes. Add snow peas and cook for 2 minutes or until peas and orzo are just tender. Drain well.
2. In a large bowl, combine orzo, peas and 1 tbsp (15 mL) olive oil. Stir in corn, tomato, cucumber, onion, mint (if using) and lemon zest.
3. In a small bowl, whisk together remaining oil, lemon juice, salt and pepper. Add to orzo mixture and toss to coat. Serve warm or allow to cool.

NUTRITIONAL ANALYSIS (PER SERVING)							
Energy	Protein	Carbohydrate	Fat	Fiber	Calcium	Iron	Sodium
189 kcal	5 g	27 g	7 g	2 g	41 mg	2 mg	235 mg

Kitchen Tip

Lasagna is a great meal to make ahead and freeze.

Spinach and Mushroom Lasagna Roll-Ups

- *Preheat oven to 375°F (190°C)*
- *13- by 9-inch (3 L) glass baking dish, greased*

Tomato Sauce

1 tbsp	olive oil	15 mL
1	onion, chopped	1
2	cloves garlic, minced	2
3 cups	sliced mushrooms	750 mL
1 tsp	dried oregano	5 mL
¼ tsp	salt	1 mL
¼ tsp	freshly ground black pepper	1 mL
1	can (28 oz/796 mL) crushed tomatoes	1
8	lasagna noodles	8
1	package (10 oz/300 g) frozen chopped spinach, thawed	1
1 cup	2% cottage cheese	250 mL
2 tbsp	grated Parmesan cheese	30 mL
Pinch	salt	Pinch
Pinch	freshly ground black pepper	Pinch
¾ cup	shredded part-skim mozzarella cheese	175 mL

1. *Tomato Sauce:* In a large saucepan, heat oil over medium heat. Sauté onion, garlic, mushrooms, oregano, salt and pepper for about 8 minutes or until vegetables are softened. Add tomatoes and bring to a boil. Reduce heat and simmer, stirring occasionally, for 10 minutes or until thickened.
2. Meanwhile, in a large saucepan, cook lasagna noodles in boiling water according to package instructions until tender but firm. Drain and rinse under running water to cool. Pat dry and set aside.
3. In a sieve, drain spinach, pressing with a spoon to remove as much moisture as possible. In a bowl, combine spinach, cottage cheese, Parmesan, salt and pepper.

Kitchen Tip

Consider doubling this recipe. Eat half for dinner tonight and freeze the rest for a quick and easy meal some other time.

4. Spread half the tomato sauce in prepared baking dish. Arrange noodles on work surface. Spread spinach mixture over noodles and roll up. Place seam side down on top of sauce. Pour remaining sauce over top. Sprinkle with mozzarella. Cover with foil and bake in preheated oven for 30 minutes or until sauce is bubbly.

NUTRITIONAL ANALYSIS (PER ROLL-UP)

Energy	Protein	Carbohydrate	Fat	Fiber	Calcium	Iron	Sodium
218 kcal	14 g	30 g	5 g	5 g	207 mg	3 mg	493 mg

Makes 8 servings

This version of an old favorite makes a fast and easy skillet dinner.

Macaroni and Beef with Cheese

8 oz	ground beef	250 g
1	small onion, finely chopped	1
1	can (14 oz/398 mL) tomatoes, with juice	1
1/3 cup	elbow macaroni	75 mL
1/2 cup	shredded Cheddar cheese	125 mL
1/4 tsp	dried basil	1 mL
1/4 tsp	dried oregano	1 mL
1/4 tsp	chili powder	1 mL

1. In a large nonstick skillet over medium heat, combine beef and onion; cook, stirring frequently to break up meat, for 5 minutes or until browned. Drain fat. Add tomatoes and macaroni. Bring to a boil, cover and cook for 10 minutes or until macaroni is tender. (If mixture becomes too thick, add a little water.)

2. Remove skillet from heat. Stir in cheese, basil, oregano and chili powder. Cover and allow to sit for 5 minutes or until cheese has melted.

NUTRITIONAL ANALYSIS (PER SERVING)

Energy	Protein	Carbohydrate	Fat	Fiber	Calcium	Iron	Sodium
98 kcal	9 g	7 g	4 g	1 g	63 mg	1 mg	185 mg

Not nearly as high in fat as it sounds, this dish gets its creamy taste from evaporated milk.

Creamy Salmon Fettuccine

12 oz	fettuccine	375 g
1 tbsp	butter or margarine	15 mL
1	small onion, finely chopped	1
1 tbsp	all-purpose flour	15 mL
1	can (14 oz/385 mL) 2% evaporated milk	1
1	can (7½ oz/213 g) salmon	1
1 tbsp	lemon juice	15 mL
1 tsp	grated lemon zest	5 mL
	Chopped fresh parsley	

1. In a large saucepan, cook pasta in boiling water according to package instructions or until tender but firm. Drain.

2. In another saucepan, melt butter over medium heat. Add onion and cook for 5 minutes or until soft. Stir in flour and cook for 1 minute. Gradually whisk in milk. Cook, stirring constantly, for 5 minutes or until sauce has thickened.

3. Drain salmon. Remove and discard skin, but mash bones (for extra calcium). Flake salmon with a fork and add to sauce; cook just until heated through. Stir in lemon juice and zest. Pour sauce over cooked pasta and toss to coat. Serve with chopped parsley.

NUTRITIONAL ANALYSIS (PER SERVING)							
Energy	Protein	Carbohydrate	Fat	Fiber	Calcium	Iron	Sodium
552 kcal	31 g	85 g	10 g	3 g	399 mg	4 mg	370 mg

Pizza Spaghetti

You can add your family's favorite pizza toppings to this tasty pasta.

½ cup	chopped pepperoni	125 mL
2	strips bacon, chopped (optional)	2
1	onion, chopped	1
1	clove garlic, minced	1
1	zucchini, diced	1
½	yellow or red bell pepper, chopped	½
1 cup	sliced mushrooms	250 mL
1 tsp	dried basil	5 mL
1 tsp	dried oregano	5 mL
¼ tsp	freshly ground black pepper	1 mL
1	can (28 oz/796 mL) tomatoes, puréed	1
12 oz	whole wheat spaghetti	375 g
2 tbsp	grated Parmesan cheese (optional)	30 mL

1. In a large nonstick skillet, sauté pepperoni and bacon (if using) over medium-high heat for about 4 minutes or until browned. Drain off fat.
2. Add onion, garlic, zucchini, yellow peppers, mushrooms, basil, oregano and pepper to skillet. Sauté for 5 to 8 minutes or until vegetables are tender.
3. Add tomatoes and bring to a boil. Reduce heat and simmer, stirring occasionally, for about 20 minutes or until thickened.
4. Meanwhile, in a large saucepan, cook spaghetti in boiling water according to package instructions until tender but firm. Drain and return to saucepan.
5. Add sauce to spaghetti and toss to coat. Serve sprinkled with cheese (if using).

NUTRITIONAL ANALYSIS (PER SERVING)

Energy	Protein	Carbohydrate	Fat	Fiber	Calcium	Iron	Sodium
309 kcal	14 g	52 g	7 g	9 g	54 mg	3 mg	279 mg

These are a nutritious
change from beef tacos.
Set out all of the toppings in
bowls so everyone can help
themselves.

Fish Tacos

- *Preheat broiler*
- *Baking sheet, lined with foil and greased*

1 lb	skinless white fish fillets, such as sole or cod	500 g
2 tsp	vegetable oil	10 mL
1 tsp	chili powder	5 mL
1/4 tsp	dried oregano	1 mL
Pinch	salt	Pinch
Pinch	freshly ground black pepper	Pinch
2	lime wedges	2
8	6-inch (15 cm) flour or corn tortillas, warmed	8
1	plum (Roma) tomato, chopped	1
1/2	avocado, diced	1/2
2 tbsp	chopped fresh cilantro (optional)	30 mL
1/2 cup	salsa	125 mL
1/4 cup	light sour cream or plain yogurt	60 mL

1. Arrange fish fillets on prepared baking sheet. Brush with oil. Sprinkle with chili powder, oregano, salt and pepper. Broil for about 5 minutes or until fish flakes easily with a fork. Squeeze lime wedges over fish.

2. Break fish into chunks and divide among tortillas. Top with tomato, avocado, cilantro (if using), salsa and sour cream. Fold in sides of tortillas and roll up from the bottom.

NUTRITIONAL ANALYSIS (PER TACO)							
Energy	Protein	Carbohydrate	Fat	Fiber	Calcium	Iron	Sodium
196 kcal	13 g	20 g	7 g	2 g	48 mg	1 mg	359 mg

Makes 4 servings

Our families love this combination of baked fish on a bed of spinach with a light creamy cheese sauce and crispy topping.

Kitchen Tip

Don't try making the sauce with regular cheese; the processed type provides a much smoother result.

Fish Fillets Florentine

- *Preheat oven to 400°F (200°C)*
- *8-inch (2 L) square baking pan, greased*

1	package (10 oz/300 g) frozen chopped spinach, thawed	1
1 tbsp	butter or margarine	15 mL
1	small onion, finely chopped	1
1 lb	fish fillets, such as sole or cod	500 g
⅔ cup	2% milk	150 mL
½ cup	processed Cheddar cheese (see tip, at left)	125 mL
2 tbsp	dry bread crumbs	30 mL
2 tbsp	grated Parmesan cheese	30 mL

1. In a sieve, drain spinach, pressing with a spoon to remove as much moisture as possible.

2. In a small skillet, melt butter over medium heat. Add onion and cook for 5 minutes or until translucent. Add spinach and cook, stirring frequently, for 5 minutes or until moisture has evaporated. Transfer mixture to prepared pan, spreading evenly. Place fish on top of spinach.

3. In a saucepan over medium heat, stir together milk and processed cheese until smooth and melted. Pour sauce over fish; top with bread crumbs and Parmesan cheese.

4. Bake in preheated oven for 10 minutes or until fish is almost opaque. Turn on broiler and place pan 3 inches (7.5 cm) under heat; broil for 3 minutes or until crumbs are golden and fish flakes easily with a fork.

NUTRITIONAL ANALYSIS (PER SERVING)							
Energy	Protein	Carbohydrate	Fat	Fiber	Calcium	Iron	Sodium
250 kcal	32 g	10 g	9 g	2 g	351 mg	2 mg	566 mg

Here's a special fish recipe that kids enjoy, but is elegant enough to serve to dinner guests. The combination of textures and colors makes a very attractive entrée.

Kitchen Tips

Choose a firm white fish such as sole, haddock or whitefish.

If serving adults, you can replace chicken stock with white wine.

Safety Tip

For small children, remove toothpicks before serving.

Rolled Fish Fillets with Salmon Filling

- *Preheat oven to 350°F (180°C)*
- *8-cup (2 L) baking dish, greased*

4	fish fillets (about 1 lb/500 g) (see tip, at left)	4
	Salt and freshly ground black pepper	
1	can (7½ oz/213 g) salmon, drained	1
¼ cup	finely chopped celery	60 mL
2 tbsp	finely chopped fresh parsley	30 mL
2 tbsp	tomato sauce or ketchup	30 mL
½ cup	reduced-sodium chicken stock (see tip, at left)	125 mL
2 tbsp	butter or margarine	30 mL
2 tbsp	all-purpose flour	30 mL
¼ cup	2% milk or light (5%) cream	60 mL

1. Pat fish dry with paper towels; sprinkle lightly with salt and pepper.

2. Place salmon in a bowl. Remove and discard skin; mash salmon and bones with a fork. Add celery, parsley and tomato sauce; stir until combined. Divide mixture evenly over fillets; roll and fasten with toothpicks. Transfer to prepared baking dish.

3. Pour stock over fish. Cover and bake in preheated oven for 20 minutes or until fish flakes easily with a fork. With a slotted spoon, transfer fish to a warm serving plate, leaving juices in dish.

4. Pour fish juices into a small saucepan. Whisk in butter and flour; cook over medium heat, stirring constantly, until sauce thickens. Stir in cream and heat until warmed through. Pour sauce over rolled fish and serve.

NUTRITIONAL ANALYSIS (PER SERVING)							
Energy	Protein	Carbohydrate	Fat	Fiber	Calcium	Iron	Sodium
270 kcal	37 g	6 g	10 g	0 g	197 mg	1 mg	459 mg

Serve this Japanese-inspired dish with brown rice and steamed broccoli and carrots.

Kitchen Tip

Miso, a Japanese fermented soybean paste, has the consistency of peanut butter. Look for white miso, which is the mildest and is perfect in soups, salad dressings and fish marinades.

Miso-Glazed Haddock

- *Preheat oven to 400°F (200°C)*
- *Baking sheet, lined with foil and greased*

2 tbsp	miso	30 mL
1 tbsp	rice vinegar	15 mL
1 tbsp	finely chopped green onions	15 mL
2 tsp	granulated sugar	10 mL
1 tsp	minced gingerroot	5 mL
1 tsp	sesame oil	5 mL
1 lb	skinless haddock fillets	500 g

1. In a small bowl, whisk together miso, vinegar, green onions, sugar, ginger and oil.

2. Place fish on prepared baking sheet. Spread miso mixture over both sides of fish. Let stand for 10 minutes.

3. Roast in preheated oven for 10 to 12 minutes or until fish flakes easily with a fork. If desired, broil until browned.

NUTRITIONAL ANALYSIS (PER SERVING)							
Energy	Protein	Carbohydrate	Fat	Fiber	Calcium	Iron	Sodium
131 kcal	22 g	4 g	3 g	1 g	42 mg	1 mg	398 mg

A fresh cilantro sauce is a perfect match for the light taste of halibut. Serve with cooked spinach on the side.

Delicious Halibut in Fresh Cilantro Sauce

- *Preheat oven to 400°F (200°C)*
- *Stoneware or glass baking dish*

4	skinless halibut fillets (each 4 oz/125 g)	4
	Juice of 1 lime	
Pinch	sea salt	Pinch
Pinch	freshly ground black pepper	Pinch
1 tbsp	olive oil	15 mL
4	cloves garlic, minced	4
½ cup	chopped fresh cilantro	125 mL
5 tsp	butter	25 mL

1. Place halibut fillets in baking dish. Squeeze lime juice over halibut and sprinkle with salt and pepper. Roast in preheated oven for about 10 minutes or until fish flakes easily with a fork. Transfer to a plate and keep warm.
2. In a small saucepan, heat oil over medium-high heat. Sauté garlic for 1 minute. Add cilantro and butter; sauté for about 1 minute or until butter is melted. Drizzle sauce over fish.

NUTRITIONAL ANALYSIS (PER SERVING)							
Energy	Protein	Carbohydrate	Fat	Fiber	Calcium	Iron	Sodium
214 kcal	26 g	4 g	11 g	1 g	77 mg	1 mg	130 mg

A can of salmon and a
microwave oven are the
main requirements for this
quick and easy recipe. The
light lemon sauce adds a
nice highlight to the salmon.

Kitchen Tip

The child's cup cooks
faster than the 2 larger
adult portions, so you will
need to remove it from the
microwave before the full 3
minutes of cooking time.

Individual Salmon Cups

- *3 ovenproof custard cups*

1	can (7½ oz/213 g) salmon, drained	1
½ cup	finely chopped carrots	125 mL
½ cup	fresh bread crumbs	125 mL
1	egg	1
¼ tsp	dried thyme	1 mL
¼ tsp	salt	1 mL

Sauce

½ cup	2% milk	125 mL
1 tbsp	all-purpose flour	15 mL
1 tbsp	butter or margarine, melted	15 mL
2 tsp	lemon juice	10 mL
Pinch	freshly ground black pepper	Pinch

1. In a bowl, remove skin from salmon, flake salmon and mash bones. Add carrots, bread crumbs, egg, thyme and salt; mix well.

2. Spoon mixture into 3 custard cups, dividing mixture to make the child's portion smaller than those of the 2 adults. Arrange cups in a circle in microwave and cook on High for 3 minutes, slightly less for child's portion (see tip, at left) or until almost set. Let stand for 2 minutes before serving.

3. *Sauce:* In a small microwave-safe bowl or glass measure, whisk together milk, flour, butter, lemon juice and pepper. Microwave on High for 1 minute. Stir, then cook for another 45 seconds or until mixture comes to a boil and thickens. Spoon a small amount of sauce over each salmon cup.

NUTRITIONAL ANALYSIS (PER CHILD SERVING)							
Energy	Protein	Carbohydrate	Fat	Fiber	Calcium	Iron	Sodium
162 kcal	12 g	12 g	8 g	1 g	124 mg	1 mg	435 mg

Fish is a wonderful addition to a family's meal plan, and poaching is an excellent way to maintain the moisture that makes fish so enjoyable. This dish is served with a refreshing Lemon Yogurt Sauce.

Kitchen Tip

Although salmon fillets are usually boneless, it's a good idea to check for bones before serving.

Poached Salmon with Lemon Yogurt Sauce

Lemon Yogurt Sauce

1 cup	low-fat plain yogurt	250 mL
1 tsp	grated lemon zest	5 mL
1 tbsp	fresh lemon juice	15 mL
⅓ cup	fresh orange juice	75 mL
4	skinless salmon fillets (each about 4 oz/125 g)	4
1	large orange, cut into sections	1

1. *Lemon Yogurt Sauce:* Whisk together yogurt, lemon zest and lemon juice. Cover and refrigerate for up to 3 hours.

2. In a large skillet, bring orange juice and ⅓ cup (75 mL) water to a boil. Add salmon; reduce heat to low, cover and simmer for 8 minutes or until salmon flakes easily with a fork.

3. Using a slotted spatula, transfer salmon to a large plate. Surround with orange sections and serve with Lemon Yogurt Sauce on the side.

NUTRITIONAL ANALYSIS (PER SERVING)							
Energy	Protein	Carbohydrate	Fat	Fiber	Calcium	Iron	Sodium
240 kcal	28 g	10 g	9 g	1 g	131 mg	1 mg	99 mg

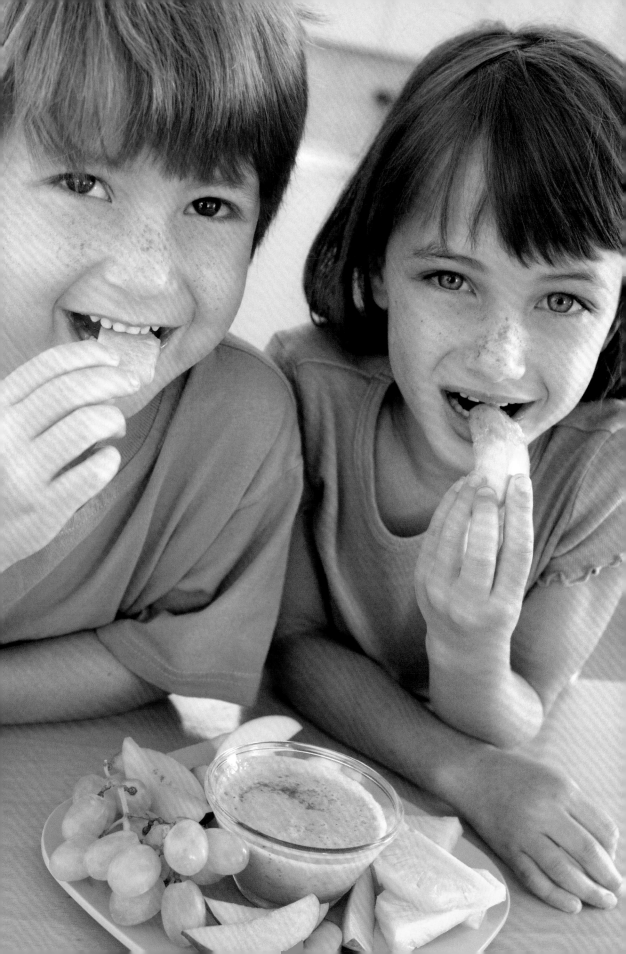

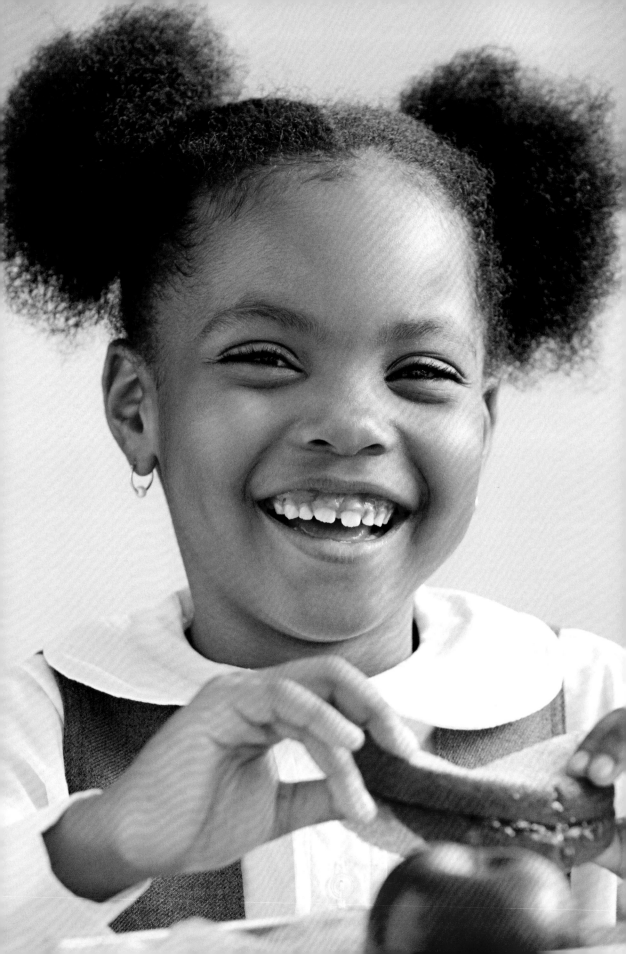

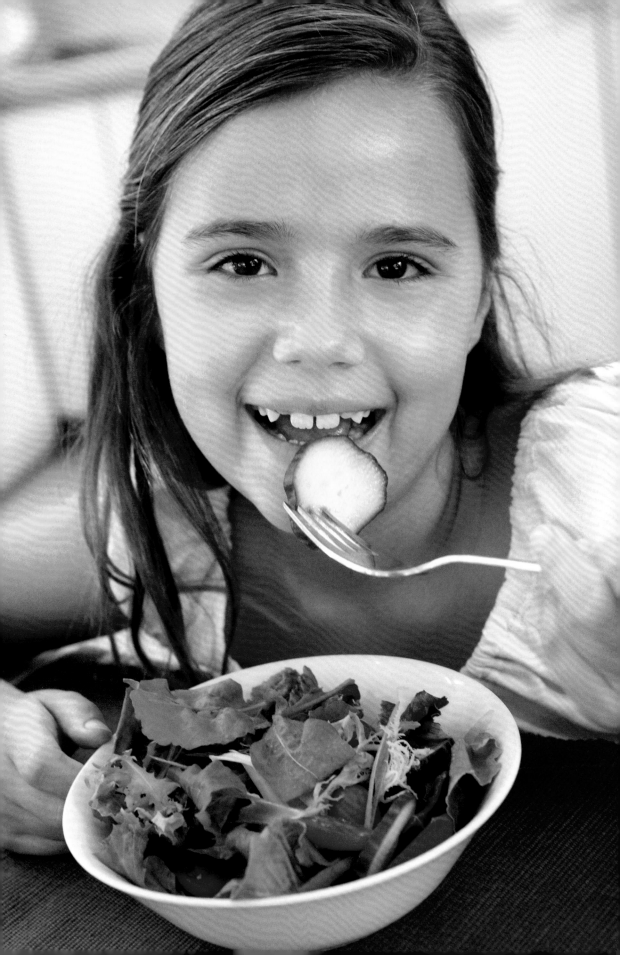

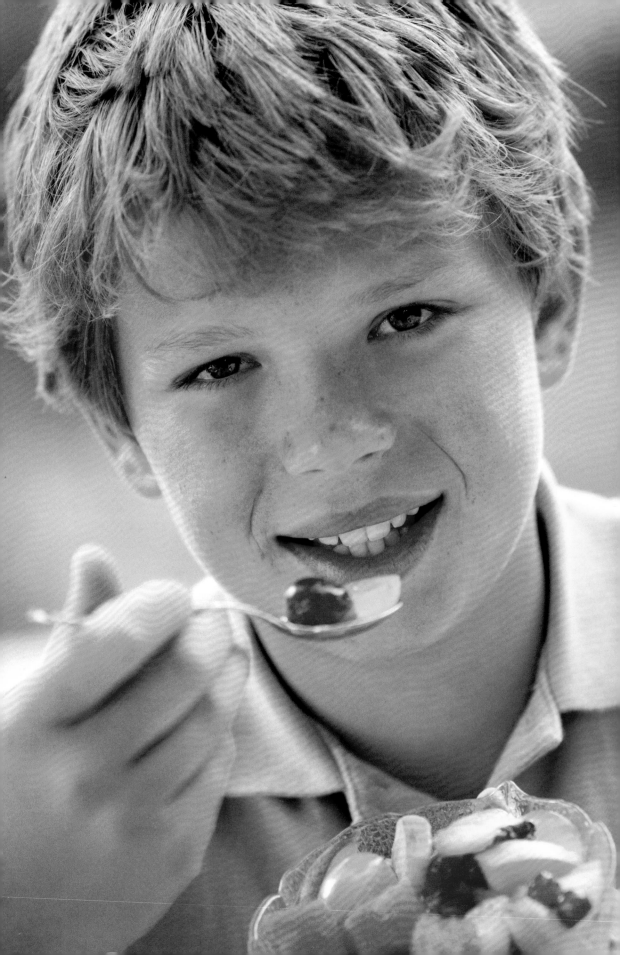

Here's a colorful, kid-sized recipe that's packed with nutrition.

Kitchen Tip

Serve this dish with whole grain pita bread to scoop up vegetables.

Salmon and Veggies

- *Preheat oven to 425°F (220°C)*
- *Baking sheet*

½	medium potato, diced	½
½ tsp	olive oil	2 mL
4 oz	salmon fillet	125 g
1	green onion, chopped	1
1	slice tomato, diced	1
3 or 4	strips yellow or red bell pepper, diced	3 or 4
½ tsp	lemon juice	2 mL
½ tsp	chopped fresh parsley	2 mL
Pinch	salt	Pinch

1. In a pot of boiling water, cook potato for about 5 minutes. Drain.

2. Tear off a square of aluminum foil and place on baking sheet. Brush center of foil with olive oil. Place fish fillet on oiled area. Top fish with potato, green onion, tomato and pepper strips. Drizzle with lemon juice and sprinkle with parsley and salt.

3. Fold edges of foil up to enclose fish tightly. Bake in preheated oven for 15 minutes or until fish flakes easily with a fork.

NUTRITIONAL ANALYSIS (PER SERVING)							
Energy	Protein	Carbohydrate	Fat	Fiber	Calcium	Iron	Sodium
224 kcal	17 g	28 g	6 g	4 g	56 mg	2 mg	186 mg

Kids love eating fish when it's prepared as simply and easily as it is here.

Kitchen Tips

This recipe is also delicious using trout instead of salmon.

If you wish, you can make this recipe with frozen fish. Just increase cooking time to 30 minutes.

Baked Salmon

- *Preheat oven to 425°F (220°C)*
- *Baking sheet*

1 lb	salmon fillet	500 g
2 tbsp	olive oil	30 mL
3 tbsp	honey garlic sauce	60 mL

1. Cover baking sheet with a length of foil. Place salmon on foil and drizzle with oil and honey garlic sauce. Wrap foil around fish and bake in preheated oven for 10 minutes per 1 inch (2.5 cm) thickness or until fish flakes easily with a fork.

NUTRITIONAL ANALYSIS (PER SERVING)

Energy	Protein	Carbohydrate	Fat	Fiber	Calcium	Iron	Sodium
239 kcal	23 g	4 g	14 g	0 g	14 mg	0.9 mg	193 mg

For speed, simplicity, flavor and lasting kid appeal, this recipe is an absolute must!

Kitchen Tip

For a complete meal, serve with green beans or broccoli and a slice of fresh bread.

Lemon Yogurt Sole

- *Preheat broiler*
- *Baking sheet, lined with foil*

2 tbsp	light mayonnaise	30 mL
2 tbsp	plain yogurt	30 mL
1 tsp	all-purpose flour	5 mL
1 tsp	lemon juice	5 mL
½ tsp	dried thyme	2 mL
14 oz	frozen sole fillets, thawed and thoroughly patted dry	400 g

1. In a bowl, combine mayonnaise, yogurt, flour, lemon juice and thyme; mix well.

2. Arrange sole fillets in a single layer on baking sheet. Spread mayonnaise-yogurt over fish. Broil for about 8 minutes or until fish flakes easily with a fork.

NUTRITIONAL ANALYSIS (PER SERVING)

Energy	Protein	Carbohydrate	Fat	Fiber	Calcium	Iron	Sodium
124 kcal	20 g	2 g	4 g	0 g	34 mg	0.6 mg	146 mg

Makes 4 servings

Commercially prepared fish sticks can't compare with these. Kids love to dip them.

Kitchen Tip

Serve with rice or potatoes.

Ranch-style dressing makes a great dip for these sticks.

Savory Sole Fingers

1 cup	dry bread crumbs	250 mL
½ cup	grated Parmesan cheese	125 mL
14 oz	frozen sole fillets, thawed, thoroughly patted dry and cut into strips	400 g
3 tbsp	olive oil, divided	45 mL
2 tbsp	butter or margarine, divided	30 mL

1. In a bowl, combine bread crumbs and Parmesan; stir to mix well. Dredge fish strips in crumbs to coat completely and transfer to a plate.

2. In a skillet, heat half of the oil and half of the butter over medium heat. In batches, add fish and cook for 5 minutes on one side; turn over and cook for another 2 minutes or until lightly browned.

NUTRITIONAL ANALYSIS (PER SERVING)							
Energy	Protein	Carbohydrate	Fat	Fiber	Calcium	Iron	Sodium
384 kcal	26 g	20 g	22 g	1 g	170 mg	2 mg	496 mg

Makes 4 servings

A fresh tomato salsa tastes like summer on this trout.

Broiled Trout with Fresh Salsa

- *Preheat broiler*
- *Baking sheet, lined with foil and greased*

Salsa

1 cup	chopped cherry or plum (Roma) tomatoes	250 mL
¼ cup	finely chopped yellow or green bell pepper	60 mL
1	clove garlic, minced	1
1 tbsp	chopped fresh cilantro or parsley	15 mL
1 tbsp	lime juice	15 mL
Pinch	salt	Pinch
Pinch	freshly ground black pepper	Pinch
1 lb	rainbow trout fillets	500 g
1 tbsp	olive oil	15 mL
¼ tsp	salt	1 mL
¼ tsp	freshly ground black pepper	1 mL

1. *Salsa:* In a small bowl, combine tomatoes, yellow pepper, garlic, cilantro, lime juice, salt and pepper. Set aside.
2. Arrange trout fillets, skin side down, on prepared baking sheet. Brush flesh side with oil and sprinkle with salt and pepper.
3. Broil for 6 to 8 minutes or until fish flakes easily with a fork. Serve topped with fresh salsa.

NUTRITIONAL ANALYSIS (PER SERVING)							
Energy	Protein	Carbohydrate	Fat	Fiber	Calcium	Iron	Sodium
200 kcal	24 g	3 g	10 g	1 g	84 mg	0.5 mg	260 mg

Trout is mild in flavor and high in omega-3 fatty acids. Serve it with lemon wedges to squeeze over top.

Lemon Dill Trout

- *Preheat broiler*
- *Baking sheet, lined with foil and greased*

2 tbsp	minced onion	30 mL
½ tsp	grated lemon zest	2 mL
1 tbsp	fresh lemon juice	15 mL
2 tsp	chopped fresh dill (or ½ tsp/2 mL dried dillweed)	10 mL
2 tsp	olive oil	10 mL
Pinch	salt	Pinch
Pinch	freshly ground black pepper	Pinch
1 lb	rainbow trout fillets	500 g

1. In a small bowl, combine onion, lemon zest, lemon juice, dill, oil, salt and pepper.

2. Arrange trout fillets, skin side down, on prepared baking sheet. Spread onion mixture over trout.

3. Broil for 6 to 8 minutes or until fish flakes easily with a fork.

NUTRITIONAL ANALYSIS (PER SERVING)

Energy	Protein	Carbohydrate	Fat	Fiber	Calcium	Iron	Sodium
197 kcal	26 g	1 g	9 g	0 g	86 mg	0.4 mg	117 mg

Tuna Burgers

Kitchen Tip

Serve these patties with a
fresh whole wheat roll and
sliced tomatoes.

1	carrot, finely chopped	1
1	small onion, finely chopped	1
3 tbsp	green peas	45 mL
2	cans (each 6 oz/170 g) tuna, drained	2
2	eggs	2
3 tbsp	light mayonnaise	45 mL
1½ cups	dry bread crumbs	375 mL
Pinch	salt	Pinch
Pinch	freshly ground black pepper	Pinch
3 tbsp	vegetable oil	45 mL

1. In a food processor combine carrot, onion, peas, tuna, eggs, mayonnaise, bread crumbs, salt and pepper. Process until mixture is well blended and binds together. Using your hands, form into small (2½-inch/7 cm) patties.

2. In a skillet, heat oil over medium-high heat. Add patties in batches and cook for about 10 minutes on each side or until golden.

NUTRITIONAL ANALYSIS (PER PATTY)

Energy	Protein	Carbohydrate	Fat	Fiber	Calcium	Iron	Sodium
64 kcal	5 g	5 g	3 g	0 g	13 mg	0.6 mg	121 mg

Makes 4 servings

This easy-to-prepare chicken dinner is a go-to meal in the Saab household. Joanne can prepare it after work without blinking an eye, and her kids just gobble it up.

Roasted Chicken and Vegetables

- *Preheat oven to 350°F (180°C)*
- *Rimmed baking sheet*

8	bone-in chicken thighs or drumsticks (or 4 breasts), trimmed of excess fat	8
12	red-skinned baby potatoes, quartered	12
2	carrots, cut into 2-inch (5 cm) pieces	2
2	parsnips, cut into 2-inch (5 cm) pieces	2
1	clove garlic, minced	1
2 tbsp	vegetable oil	30 mL
1 tsp	salt	5 mL
½ tsp	freshly ground black pepper	5 mL
1 tsp	paprika	5 mL

1. Place chicken, potatoes, carrots and parsnips in a large bowl. Add garlic, oil, salt and pepper; toss to coat chicken and vegetables. Spread out in a single layer in baking sheet and sprinkle with paprika.

2. Roast in preheated oven for about 1 hour or until juices run clear when chicken is pierced with a fork and vegetables are tender.

NUTRITIONAL ANALYSIS (PER SERVING)							
Energy	Protein	Carbohydrate	Fat	Fiber	Calcium	Iron	Sodium
438 kcal	33 g	54 g	11 g	8 g	80 mg	3.3 mg	877 mg

Makes 4 to 6 servings

Kids love the flavor and sweetness of dried fruit — and it's a good source of iron, too!

Fruity Chicken

- *Preheat oven to 400°F (200°C)*
- *Roasting pan with lid*

1	whole chicken (about 5 lbs/2.5 kg)	1
1 tsp	paprika	5 mL
½ tsp	salt	2 mL
¼ tsp	freshly ground black pepper	1 mL
½	package (9 oz/275 g) pitted prunes	½
½	package (9 oz/275 g) dried apricots	½
½ cup	dried cranberries	125 mL
2 tbsp	honey	30 mL
½ cup	orange juice	125 mL
½ cup	water	125 mL

1. Season chicken with paprika, salt and pepper.
2. In a bowl, toss together prunes, apricots and cranberries until well mixed. Stuff chicken cavity with fruit and place in roasting pan. (Place any extra fruit around chicken in pan.)
3. In a small bowl, whisk together honey, juice and water. Drizzle over chicken.
4. Bake uncovered for 1 hour, then remove from oven, cover and bake for another 30 minutes or until chicken is no longer pink and juices run clear when pierced with a fork.

NUTRITIONAL ANALYSIS (PER SERVING)							
Energy	Protein	Carbohydrate	Fat	Fiber	Calcium	Iron	Sodium
502 kcal	26 g	76 g	11 g	8 g	64 mg	2.2 mg	538 mg

Makes 6 servings

This dish is so quick and easy, the kids can help to prepare it!

Kitchen Tip

Serve plain or with plum sauce for dipping.

Crispy Chicken

- *Preheat oven to 375°F (190°C)*
- *Baking sheet, lightly greased*

½ cup	plain low-fat yogurt	125 mL
½ tsp	dried tarragon (optional)	2 mL
¼ tsp	salt	1 mL
¼ tsp	freshly ground black pepper	1 mL
1½ cups	finely crushed corn flakes cereal	375 mL
¼ cup	grated Parmesan cheese	60 mL
12	boneless skinless chicken thighs (about 28 oz/800 g total), rinsed and patted dry	12

1. In a bowl, combine yogurt, tarragon, salt and pepper; stir to mix well. In another bowl, combine corn flakes and Parmesan.

2. Roll chicken in yogurt mixture to coat, then roll in crumb mixture. Place on prepared baking sheet and bake in preheated oven for 45 to 50 minutes or until chicken is no longer pink and juices run clear when pierced with a fork.

NUTRITIONAL ANALYSIS (PER SERVING)							
Energy	Protein	Carbohydrate	Fat	Fiber	Calcium	Iron	Sodium
210 kcal	26 g	10 g	12 g	0 g	72 mg	3 mg	564 mg

In this traditional Greek
recipe, yogurt makes the
chicken incredibly tender!
Serve with a side of rice pilaf
or roasted potatoes.

Kitchen Tip

If you don't have any
homemade chicken
stock, use ready-to-use
chicken broth, preferably a
reduced-sodium variety.

Yogurt Chicken

- Preheat oven to 350°F (180°C)
- 8-inch (2 L) square baking dish, ungreased

8	chicken pieces (drumsticks, thighs, breasts), rinsed and patted dry	8
2 cups	plain yogurt	500 mL
1	egg, beaten	1
1 tbsp	all-purpose flour	15 mL
1 tsp	salt	5 mL
½ tsp	freshly ground black pepper	2 mL
½ tsp	ground nutmeg	2mL
2 tbsp	butter	30 mL
2	cloves garlic, minced	2
1 cup	chicken stock	250 mL

1. Place chicken in baking dish and add sufficient cold water to cover by 1 inch (2.5 cm). Bake in preheated oven for 45 minutes.

2. Meanwhile, in a bowl, combine yogurt, egg, flour, salt, pepper and nutmeg. Set aside.

3. In a saucepan, melt butter over medium-high heat. Add garlic and sauté for 5 minutes or until just golden. (Be careful not to burn.) Add stock and bring to a boil. Gradually add reserved yogurt mixture, stirring continuously. Return to a boil and remove from heat. Pour over baked chicken. Reduce oven temperature to to 300°F (150°C). Cover chicken and bake for another 30 minutes or until no longer pink and juices run clear when pierced with a fork.

NUTRITIONAL ANALYSIS (PER SERVING)							
Energy	Protein	Carbohydrate	Fat	Fiber	Calcium	Iron	Sodium
294 kcal	41 g	7 g	10 g	0 g	159 mg	1 mg	579 mg

Fajita-Style Chicken

1 tbsp	cider vinegar	15 mL
1 tsp	Worcestershire sauce	5 mL
1 tsp	chili powder	5 mL
1	clove garlic, crushed	1
1 tbsp	canola oil	15 mL
2	boneless skinless chicken breasts (or 4 thighs), cut into strips	2
1 tbsp	canola oil	15 mL
1	onion, thinly sliced	1
½	green or red bell pepper, thinly sliced	½

1. In a shallow dish, combine vinegar, Worcestershire sauce, chili powder and garlic. Add chicken and turn to coat. Cover and refrigerate for 2 hours to blend the flavors.
2. In a nonstick skillet, heat oil over medium heat. Remove chicken from marinade, discarding marinade. Sauté chicken for 5 minutes or until browned. Add onion and green pepper; sauté for 5 minutes or until chicken is no longer pink inside and juices run clear.

NUTRITIONAL ANALYSIS (PER SERVING)

Energy	Protein	Carbohydrate	Fat	Fiber	Calcium	Iron	Sodium
122 kcal	14 g	4 g	5 g	1 g	17 mg	0.7 mg	43 mg

The tangy sauce in this recipe really perks up the mild flavors of chicken to make it something special. It also helps to keep the chicken wonderfully moist.

Kitchen Tips

When draining canned mushrooms, save the liquid to add flavor to soup or when cooking rice or other vegetables.

Serve with orzo or any shell pasta to soak up all the wonderful sauce.

Tomato Herbed Chicken

2 tbsp	vegetable oil	30 mL
4	boneless skinless chicken breasts	4
1 tbsp	all-purpose flour	15 mL
1	small onion, finely chopped	1
1	stalk celery, sliced	1
½	green pepper, chopped	½
1 tsp	dried oregano	5 mL
¼ tsp	dried thyme	1 mL
¼ tsp	salt	1 mL
1	can (19 oz/540 mL) tomatoes, crushed, with juice	1
1	can (10 oz/284 mL) sliced mushrooms, drained (see tip, at left)	1
	Cooked pasta (see tip, at left)	

1. In a skillet, heat oil over medium heat. Sprinkle chicken with flour and add to skillet. Cook, turning, until brown on all sides. Transfer chicken to a plate and set aside.

2. Add onion, celery and green pepper to skillet; sauté for 5 minutes or until softened. Add oregano, thyme, salt, tomatoes and mushrooms. Bring to a boil. Reduce heat and simmer, uncovered, for 10 minutes or until liquid is reduced and thickened. Add reserved chicken; cover and simmer for 20 minutes or until chicken is cooked and no longer pink.

3. Serve chicken and sauce over cooked pasta.

NUTRITIONAL ANALYSIS (PER SERVING)							
Energy	Protein	Carbohydrate	Fat	Fiber	Calcium	Iron	Sodium
285 kcal	19 g	5 g	11 g	0 g	89 mg	4 mg	614 mg

Daina's children can't get enough of these chicken fingers when Eva, their part-time caretaker, makes a batch. They are much better than store-bought, because you control the amount of salt added and the source of the chicken. Serve as is or with plum sauce or another favorite dipping sauce.

Kitchen Tip

Leftovers can be stored in an airtight container in the refrigerator for up to 2 days. Slice and add to a salad, use to make a chicken sandwich or chop and add to a pita wrap.

Eva's Simple Chicken Fingers

½ cup	dry whole wheat bread crumbs	125 mL
Pinch	salt	Pinch
2	eggs	2
3	boneless skinless chicken breasts, cut into 1-inch (2.5 cm) strips	3
3 tbsp	vegetable oil (approx.), divided	45 mL

1. On a plate, combine bread crumbs and salt. In a bowl, lightly beat eggs. Dip chicken strips in eggs, then in bread crumbs, coating evenly and shaking off excess. Discard excess eggs and bread crumbs.

2. In a large skillet, heat 1 tbsp (15 mL) oil over medium-high heat. Spread 6 to 8 chicken strips evenly in the pan and cook for 4 to 5 minutes per side or until lightly browned on both sides and no longer pink inside. Transfer to a plate and keep warm. Continue cooking chicken in batches, adding oil to the skillet and adjusting heat between batches as necessary.

NUTRITIONAL ANALYSIS (PER SERVING)							
Energy	Protein	Carbohydrate	Fat	Fiber	Calcium	Iron	Sodium
212 kcal	25 g	6 g	9 g	1 g	37 mg	1 mg	195 mg

Bruschetta Chicken

Cherry or plum (Roma) tomatoes have the best flavor all year round and make a tasty topping for the chicken.

Variation

This chicken is also perfect on the grill when the sun is shining. Cook for about 8 minutes per side over medium-high heat with the lid down. Spoon the topping on during the last few minutes.

• *Rimmed baking sheet, greased*

2 tbsp	red wine vinegar	30 mL
1 tbsp	olive oil	15 mL
1	clove garlic, minced	1
½ tsp	dried basil	2 mL
¼ tsp	salt	1 mL
¼ tsp	freshly ground black pepper	1 mL
4	boneless skinless chicken breasts	4

Tomato Topping

1 cup	chopped cherry or plum (Roma) tomatoes	250 mL
1	clove garlic, minced	1
2 tbsp	chopped fresh basil (or 1 tsp/5 mL dried)	30 mL
1 tsp	red wine vinegar	5 mL
Pinch	salt	Pinch
Pinch	freshly ground black pepper	Pinch

1. In a small bowl, whisk together vinegar, oil, garlic, basil, salt and pepper.

2. Place chicken in a shallow dish. Pour marinade over chicken. Cover and refrigerate, turning chicken occasionally, for 4 to 8 hours to blend the flavors.

3. *Topping:* In a small bowl, combine tomatoes, garlic, basil, vinegar, salt and pepper. Set aside.

4. Preheat oven to 400°F (200°C). Remove chicken from marinade, discarding marinade, and place on prepared baking sheet. Bake for 20 minutes. Spoon tomato topping over chicken. Bake for about 5 minutes or until chicken is no longer pink inside.

NUTRITIONAL ANALYSIS (PER SERVING)							
Energy	Protein	Carbohydrate	Fat	Fiber	Calcium	Iron	Sodium
185 kcal	27 g	2 g	7 g	1 g	32 mg	1 mg	357 mg

Here's a deliciously tangy chicken dish that requires just a few minutes of preparation time. Dinner's ready in half an hour!

Kitchen Tip

Instead of roasting in the oven, chicken can be grilled on a preheated barbecue. Cook for about 8 minutes per side over medium-high heat with barbecue lid down.

Lemon Mustard Chicken

• *Shallow baking dish*

2 tbsp	Dijon mustard	30 mL
1 tbsp	lemon juice	15 mL
1 tbsp	vegetable oil	15 mL
2	green onions, chopped	2
4	boneless skinless chicken breasts	4

1. In a small bowl, whisk together mustard, lemon juice, oil and green onions. Pour marinade into a sealable plastic bag and add chicken, making sure it is thoroughly coated. Seal bag and refrigerate for at least 2 hours or up to 8 hours.

2. Preheat oven to 375°F (190°C). Remove chicken from lemon mixture and transfer to a shallow baking dish. Bake for 30 minutes or until chicken is no longer pink and juices run clear when pierced with a fork.

NUTRITIONAL ANALYSIS (PER SERVING)							
Energy	Protein	Carbohydrate	Fat	Fiber	Calcium	Iron	Sodium
175 kcal	27 g	0.9 g	7 g	0 g	19 mg	1 mg	162 mg

This moist and delicious chicken dish combines everyday ingredients to create North African flavors that are unusual — but still enjoyable for children.

Kitchen Tip

Instead of roasting in the oven, chicken can be grilled on a preheated barbecue. Cook for about 8 minutes per side over medium-high heat with barbecue lid down.

Food Safety Tip

To minimize the risk of bacterial contamination, be sure that you thoroughly wash hands, utensils, cutting boards and all work surfaces before, during and after handling raw meat — especially poultry.

Moroccan Chicken Breasts

- *Preheat oven to 400°F (200°C)*
- *Baking sheet, greased*

½ cup	plain yogurt	125 mL
2 tbsp	orange juice	30 mL
2	cloves garlic, crushed	2
1 tsp	grated orange zest	5 mL
½ tsp	salt	2 mL
½ tsp	ground cinnamon	2 mL
½ tsp	ground cumin	2 mL
¼ tsp	ground cloves	1 mL
¼ tsp	ground ginger	1 mL
4	boneless skinless chicken breasts	4
⅔ cup	dried whole wheat bread crumbs	150 mL

1. In a small bowl, stir together yogurt, orange juice, garlic, zest, salt, cinnamon, cumin, cloves and ginger.

2. Place chicken in a shallow dish. Pour yogurt mixture over and turn chicken to coat. Cover and refrigerate for at least 4 hours, turning chicken occasionally.

3. Remove chicken from marinade and dredge in bread crumbs until thoroughly coated. Place on prepared baking sheet and bake in preheated oven for 20 minutes or until chicken is no longer pink and juices run clear when pierced with a fork.

NUTRITIONAL ANALYSIS (PER SERVING)							
Energy	Protein	Carbohydrate	Fat	Fiber	Calcium	Iron	Sodium
239 kcal	30 g	18 g	4 g	2 g	124 mg	2 mg	599 mg

Chicken thighs are slightly higher in fat than chicken breasts, but they stay moist and juicy on the grill.

Kitchen Tip

If you don't have a barbecue, or the weather is not cooperating, you can broil these kabobs on a greased foil-lined baking sheet instead. The timing is the same.

Marinated Chicken Kabobs

- *Four 12-inch (30 cm) metal or bamboo skewers*

2 tbsp	reduced-sodium soy sauce	30 mL
1 tbsp	lime juice	15 mL
1 tbsp	vegetable oil	15 mL
2 tsp	liquid honey	10 mL
1	green onion, finely chopped	1
1	clove garlic, minced	1
Pinch	freshly ground black pepper	Pinch
1 lb	boneless skinless chicken thighs, cut into 1½ inch (4 cm) cubes	500 g

1. In a large bowl, whisk together soy sauce, lime juice, oil, honey, green onion, garlic and pepper. Add chicken and stir to coat. Cover and refrigerate, stirring occasionally, for 4 to 8 hours to blend the flavors.

2. If using bamboo skewers, soak in water for at least 30 minutes. Grease barbecue grill and preheat to medium-high.

3. Thread chicken onto skewers. Place skewers on grill, close the lid and grill, turning once, for 10 to 12 minutes or until juices run clear when chicken is pierced.

NUTRITIONAL ANALYSIS (PER SERVING)							
Energy	Protein	Carbohydrate	Fat	Fiber	Calcium	Iron	Sodium
176 kcal	21 g	4 g	12 g	0 g	6 mg	0.2 mg	552 mg

Here's a great way to introduce kids to Thai cuisine. Serve with Thai or jasmine rice.

Kitchen Tip

Add steamed green beans on the side or mix in with the chicken near the end of the cooking time.

Best Chicken Curry

1 tbsp	olive oil	15 mL
2	large boneless skinless chicken breasts, cut into 2-inch (5 cm) pieces	2
1	can (14 oz/398 mL) unsweetened coconut milk	1
1 tbsp	packed brown sugar	15 mL
1 tbsp	fish sauce	15 mL
1 tbsp	red Thai curry paste	15 mL

1. In a skillet, heat oil over medium heat. Cook chicken pieces, stirring occasionally, for 3 to 4 minutes or until lightly browned on all sides.

2. In a bowl, combine coconut milk, brown sugar, fish sauce and curry paste. Pour over chicken, reduce heat and simmer for 15 to 20 minutes or until chicken is no longer pink inside.

NUTRITIONAL ANALYSIS (PER SERVING)							
Energy	Protein	Carbohydrate	Fat	Fiber	Calcium	Iron	Sodium
270 kcal	23 g	6 g	18 g	1 g	23 mg	3 mg	300 mg

*Here's an easy Asian-style
dish that's ready in under
30 minutes.*

Variation

Replace the chicken stock
with beef stock and replace
the chicken with 1 lb (500 g)
boneless beef sirloin or
striploin steak, thinly sliced.
If desired, replace the
peas with 1 cup (250 mL)
chopped broccoli.

Asian Vegetable Chicken Bowl

2 cups	reduced-sodium chicken stock	500 mL
1 tsp	sesame oil	5 mL
1 tsp	hoisin sauce	5 mL
1	carrot, thinly sliced	1
4	boneless skinless chicken breasts, thinly sliced	4
1 cup	frozen peas	250 mL
¾ cup	couscous	175 mL
2	green onions, sliced	2

1. In a medium saucepan, bring stock, sesame oil and hoisin sauce to a boil over high heat. Add carrot and chicken; reduce heat and simmer for 10 minutes or until carrot is tender and chicken is no longer pink inside.
2. Stir in peas and couscous. Remove from heat, cover and let stand for 5 minutes or until liquid is absorbed. Serve sprinkled with green onions.

NUTRITIONAL ANALYSIS (PER SERVING)							
Energy	Protein	Carbohydrate	Fat	Fiber	Calcium	Iron	Sodium
275 kcal	33 g	25 g	5 g	5 g	31 mg	2 mg	155 mg

Warm Chicken Salad with Peanut Dressing

| 2 | boneless skinless chicken breasts | 2 |

Peanut Dressing

¼ cup	peanut butter (smooth or chunky)	60 mL
2 tbsp	lime or lemon juice	30 mL
1 tbsp	hot water	15 mL
2 tsp	reduced-sodium soy sauce	10 mL
1	clove garlic, minced	1

Salad

1	small apple, chopped	1
1	stalk celery, thinly sliced	1
½ cup	drained canned sliced water chestnuts	125 mL
½ cup	grated carrot	125 mL
½ cup	bean sprouts	125 mL

1. In a large skillet, bring 1 inch (2.5 cm) water to a boil. Add chicken, reduce heat to medium-low, cover and simmer for about 12 minutes or until chicken is no longer pink inside. Transfer to a plate and let cool for 10 minutes.

2. *Peanut Dressing:* In a small bowl, whisk together peanut butter, lime juice, hot water, soy sauce and garlic, adding more hot water, if necessary, to thin.

3. *Salad:* Cut chicken into 1-inch (2.5 cm) pieces. Place in a large bowl and add apple, celery, water chestnuts and carrot. Add peanut dressing and stir to coat. Garnish with bean sprouts.

NUTRITIONAL ANALYSIS (PER SERVING)

Energy	Protein	Carbohydrate	Fat	Fiber	Calcium	Iron	Sodium
226 kcal	19 g	17 g	10 g	4 g	34 mg	1 mg	398 mg

Mix and Match Stir-Fry

Kitchen Tips

For the vegetables, try any combination of sliced carrots, celery, bell peppers or zucchini, broccoli or cauliflower florets, or trimmed snow peas or green or yellow beans.

If you're using pork, cook it in step 2 until just a hint of pink remains inside. If you're using chicken, cook it until no longer pink inside.

½ cup	orange juice	125 mL
2 tbsp	hoisin sauce	30 mL
1 tbsp	rice vinegar	15 mL
1 tbsp	reduced-sodium soy sauce	15 mL
1 tbsp	cornstarch	15 mL
1	clove garlic, minced	1
1 tbsp	vegetable oil	15 mL
12 oz	thinly sliced boneless beef top sirloin, pork tenderloin or boneless skinless chicken breasts or cubed firm tofu	375 g
4 cups	mixed vegetables (see tip, at left)	1 L

1. In a bowl, whisk together orange juice, hoisin sauce, vinegar, soy sauce, 1 tbsp (15 mL) water, cornstarch and garlic. Set aside.
2. In a wok or large nonstick skillet, heat oil over medium-high heat. Stir-fry meat for 3 to 5 minutes or until browned and cooked through (see tip, at left). Transfer to a plate.
3. Add vegetables to wok and stir-fry for 3 minutes. Add 2 tbsp (30 mL) water, cover and steam for 2 minutes or until vegetables are tender-crisp.
4. Return meat and any juices to wok. Add sauce and bring to a boil, stirring. Cook, stirring, for 1 minute or until sauce is thickened.

NUTRITIONAL ANALYSIS (PER SERVING)

Energy	Protein	Carbohydrate	Fat	Fiber	Calcium	Iron	Sodium
321 kcal	32 g	26 g	9 g	3 g	51 mg	2 mg	484 mg

Pork Tenderloin Stir-Fry

This Asian-inspired stir-fry is sure to be a hit, and it makes an easy workday meal.

Tip

Hoisin sauce contains a lot of sodium, so save meals made with it for special occasions.

2 tbsp	vegetable oil	30 mL
1 lb	pork tenderloin, cut crosswise into ¼-inch (0.5 cm) slices	500 g
1	red bell pepper, cut into 1-inch (2.5 cm) pieces	1
1	green bell pepper, cut into 1-inch (2.5 cm) pieces	1
½	red onion, chopped	1/2
2 cups	mushrooms, quartered	500 mL
¼ cup	hoisin sauce	60 mL
¼ cup	plum sauce	60 mL
1 tsp	minced garlic	5 mL
2 cups	hot cooked rice	500 mL

1. In a wok or a large skillet, heat oil over medium-high heat. Stir-fry pork for 5 minutes or until just a hint of pink remains inside. Using a slotted spoon, transfer pork to a plate.

2. Add red pepper, green pepper, onion and mushrooms to wok and stir-fry for about 10 minutes, or until vegetables are tender and most of the water has been cooked out of the mushrooms.

3. Return pork and accumulated juices to wok. Stir in hoisin sauce, plum sauce and garlic; cook, stirring, until sauce is bubbling. Serve over rice.

NUTRITIONAL ANALYSIS (PER SERVING)							
Energy	Protein	Carbohydrate	Fat	Fiber	Calcium	Iron	Sodium
401 kcal	28 g	50 g	10 g	3 g	18 mg	3.2 mg	707 mg

Asian Tenderloin

A few simple ingredients really perk up ordinary pork tenderloin in this dish. It's just a little spicy — not too much for young palates.

Kitchen Tips

Hoisin sauce is a traditional Asian ingredient that is widely available at most large grocery stores or Asian specialty food shops. It is very high in sodium, though, so serve dishes with hoisin sauce only on special occasions.

For a little more heat, adults may want to increase the amount of hot pepper sauce.

¼ cup	plum sauce	60 mL
¼ cup	hoisin sauce	60 mL
2	cloves garlic, minced	2
⅛ tsp	hot pepper sauce	0.5 mL
½ tsp	salt	2 mL
¼ tsp	freshly ground black pepper	1 mL
1 lb	pork tenderloin	500 g

1. In a shallow dish, stir together plum sauce, hoisin sauce, garlic, hot pepper sauce, salt and pepper. Add tenderloin and turn to coat well. Cover and marinate for about 1 hour.

2. Preheat barbecue or grill. Remove tenderloin from marinade and set aside. Transfer marinade to a small saucepan and bring to a boil; cook for 5 minutes.

3. Place tenderloin on barbecue and grill over high heat for about 3 minutes per side. Reduce heat to medium and cook for about 15 minutes or until juices run clear when pierced with a fork. Baste frequently with marinade throughout cooking.

NUTRITIONAL ANALYSIS (PER SERVING)

Energy	Protein	Carbohydrate	Fat	Fiber	Calcium	Iron	Sodium
204 kcal	26 g	18 g	3 g	0 g	12 mg	2 mg	1000 mg

If you have leftovers, warm them and serve in a pita with lettuce and sliced cucumber for lunch.

Kitchen Tip

You can use jarred roasted red bell pepper or roast your own. To roast a red bell pepper, place it directly on the oven rack and broil for 15 to 20 minutes, turning every 5 minutes, until skin is charred. Place in a paper or plastic bag and let cool, then peel, seed and chop.

Ham and Roasted Red Pepper Frittata

- *Preheat oven to 350°F (180°C)*
- *9-inch (23 cm) pie plate, greased*

6	eggs	6
½ cup	2% milk	125 mL
1 tsp	Dijon mustard	5 mL
¼ tsp	freshly ground black pepper	1 mL
½ cup	diced ham or smoked turkey	125 mL
¼ cup	chopped roasted red bell pepper (see tip, at left)	60 mL
1	green onion, sliced	1
⅓ cup	shredded Cheddar cheese	75 mL

1. In a large bowl, whisk together eggs, milk, mustard and pepper. Stir in ham, roasted pepper and green onion. Pour into prepared pie plate and sprinkle with cheese.

2. Bake in preheated oven for about 30 minutes or until puffed and set. Let cool on a rack for 5 minutes. Cut into wedges.

NUTRITIONAL ANALYSIS (PER SERVING)							
Energy	Protein	Carbohydrate	Fat	Fiber	Calcium	Iron	Sodium
196 kcal	17 g	3 g	13 g	0 g	145 mg	2 mg	191 mg

Pot roast makes a hearty traditional family meal — and it's an easy way to satisfy hungry appetites.

Kitchen Tip

Cheaper cuts of meat may be tougher, but are often more flavorful. In this recipe, just about any cut of meat becomes fork tender after cooking slowly in liquid. Blade, chuck, rump or cross-rib are all good choices.

Family Beef Pot Roast with Vegetables

1	4-lb (2 kg) beef pot roast (see tip, at left)	1
⅓ cup	all-purpose flour	75 mL
¼ tsp	salt	1 mL
¼ tsp	freshly ground black pepper	1 mL
¼ tsp	garlic powder	1 mL
2 tbsp	vegetable oil	30 mL
1 cup	reduced-sodium beef or vegetable stock (or tomato juice), divided	250 mL
6	small potatoes, peeled	6
3	onions, quartered	3
6	small carrots, thickly sliced	6
¼ cup	water	60 mL

1. Wipe beef dry with paper towels. In a large plastic bag, combine flour, salt, pepper and garlic powder. Place roast in bag and shake to coat. Remove from bag; reserve extra flour.

2. In a large heavy-bottomed saucepan with a lid, heat oil over medium-high. Add roast and brown well on all sides. Reduce heat. Add ½ cup (125 mL) of the stock; cover and simmer for 1½ hours. (Or bake in a preheated 325°F/160°C oven.) Add vegetables and remaining stock. Continue cooking for another 1 hour or until tender. Add extra liquid, if necessary, during cooking time.

3. Transfer beef and vegetables to a serving plate. In a bowl, whisk together reserved flour and water until smooth. Whisk mixture into juices remaining in pan; cook, stirring constantly, until smooth.

NUTRITIONAL ANALYSIS (PER SERVING)							
Energy	Protein	Carbohydrate	Fat	Fiber	Calcium	Iron	Sodium
898 kcal	110 g	40 g	31 g	5 g	88 mg	10 mg	322 mg

Beef Satays

Don't be discouraged by the long list of ingredients in this recipe — it's really fast and easy to make. Serve as an appetizer or a main meal.

Kitchen Tips

For a lower-fat version, replace beef with boneless skinless chicken breasts. (You'll also get less iron, however.)

Hot pepper sauce can replace the Chinese chili sauce.

This recipe is peanut-free, but if you'd like a traditional peanut flavor in the sauce, add 2 tsp (10 mL) peanut butter.

• *Baking sheet, lined with foil*

Satay Sauce

2 tsp	lime juice, divided	10 mL
1	green onion, minced	1
⅓ cup	unsweetened coconut milk	75 mL
1 tsp	granulated sugar	5 mL
½ tsp	soy sauce	2 mL
¼ tsp	ground cumin	1 mL
¼ tsp	ground coriander	1 mL
¼ tsp	Chinese chili sauce	1 mL
Pinch	ground turmeric	Pinch

Marinade

¼ cup	hoisin sauce	60 mL
¼ cup	plum sauce	60 mL
2 tbsp	white vinegar	30 mL
1 tbsp	honey	15 mL
½ tsp	Chinese chili sauce	2 mL
1	green onion, minced	1
1 tbsp	minced cilantro	15 mL
1 lb	top sirloin or beef fillet, cut into 4- by ½- by ⅛-inch (10 cm by 1 cm by 2 mm) strips	500 g

1. *Sauce:* In a small saucepan, combine 1 tsp (5 mL) of the lime juice with the green onion, coconut milk, sugar, soy sauce, cumin, coriander, chili sauce and turmeric. Bring to a slow boil and cook for about 1 minute. Remove from heat and allow to cool to room temperature. Stir in remaining lime juice. (Sauce can be made up to a day ahead and refrigerated.)

2. *Marinade:* In a bowl, combine hoisin sauce, plum sauce, vinegar, honey, chili sauce, green onion and cilantro. Add beef strips and toss to coat. Cover and refrigerate for at least 1 hour.

Kitchen Tip

You may want to use less chili sauce, and a smaller amount of cilantro, if your kids are encountering these ingredients for the first time.

3. Remove beef from marinade and transfer to prepared baking sheet. Preheat broiler. Place sheet as close to heat as possible and broil for about 5 minutes or until beef is cooked.

NUTRITIONAL ANALYSIS (PER SERVING)							
Energy	Protein	Carbohydrate	Fat	Fiber	Calcium	Iron	Sodium
140 kcal	14 g	12 g	4 g	0 g	20 mg	1 mg	389 mg

Makes 4 servings

This easy meal is perfect for busy weeknight suppers — it's ready in about 20 minutes.

Kitchen Tip

For speediest cooking, use instant-type rice.

Speedy Beef Stroganoff

1 lb	lean ground beef	500 g
1 cup	sliced mushrooms	250 mL
1	onion, sliced	1
1½ cups	beef stock	375 mL
2 tbsp	ketchup	30 mL
1½ cups	fast-cooking rice (see tip, at left)	375 mL
½ cup	sour cream	125 mL

1. In a skillet over medium-high heat, cook ground beef, breaking up meat with a spoon, until browned and crumbly. Drain fat. Add mushrooms and onion; cook for 5 minutes. Stir in stock and ketchup. Bring to a boil. Add rice and sour cream. Remove from heat, cover and let stand for 5 minutes.

NUTRITIONAL ANALYSIS (PER SERVING)							
Energy	Protein	Carbohydrate	Fat	Fiber	Calcium	Iron	Sodium
347 kcal	32 g	35 g	8 g	1 g	72 mg	3 mg	208 mg

Beef and Vegetable Stew

1½ tbsp	vegetable oil	22 mL
1 lb	stewing beef, cubed	500 g
4 cups	beef stock	1 L
½ tsp	dried parsley	2 mL
1	bay leaf	1
½ tsp	dried thyme	2 mL
¼ tsp	freshly ground black pepper	1 mL
1	can (28 oz/796 mL) diced tomatoes, drained	1
2	potatoes, peeled and cut into 1-inch (2.5 cm) cubes	2
3	carrots, peeled and sliced	3
4	stalks celery, sliced into 1-inch (2.5 cm) pieces	4
2 cups	mushrooms, quartered	500 mL
1	medium onion, chopped	1
¼ cup	cornstarch	60 mL
¼ cup	cold water	60 mL

1. In a large stock pot, heat oil over medium-high heat. Add beef and sauté until meat is browned. Stir in beef stock. Add parsley, bay leaf, thyme and pepper. Reduce heat and simmer for 1 hour.

2. Stir in tomatoes, potatoes, carrots, celery, mushrooms and onion. In a small bowl, whisk together cornstarch and water until dissolved; whisk into tomato mixture. Cover and simmer for another 1 hour and 15 minutes.

NUTRITIONAL ANALYSIS (PER SERVING)							
Energy	Protein	Carbohydrate	Fat	Fiber	Calcium	Iron	Sodium
248 kcal	15 g	23 g	11 g	3 g	53 mg	3 mg	347 mg

We've adapted the Mexican dish chiles rellenos *(stuffed chile peppers) to make it more child-friendly. Instead of stuffing chile peppers, we sprinkle diced canned chiles, which are much milder, over the meat.*

Kitchen Tip

Instead of using the large baking pan, you can divide the ingredients among two 8-inch (2 L) square pans. Bake for 20 minutes in step 2. Serve one pan for dinner and let the other one cool, then cover securely with foil and freeze for up to 3 months. Thaw in the refrigerator, then reheat in a 350°F (180°C) oven for 15 minutes.

Mexican Beef, Chile 'n' Cheese Bake

- *Preheat oven to 350°F (180°C)*
- *13- by 9-inch (3 L) baking pan, greased*

1 lb	lean ground beef	500 g
1	small onion, chopped	1
1	can (4 oz/127 mL) diced mild green chile peppers, drained	1
4	eggs, lightly beaten	4
1½ cups	shredded Cheddar cheese, divided	375 mL
1 cup	cottage cheese	250 mL
1 cup	tomato sauce	250 mL
½ tsp	ground cumin	2 mL
½ tsp	chili powder	2 mL
	Light sour cream (optional)	

1. In a nonstick skillet, cook beef and onion over medium heat, breaking up beef with a spoon, until beef is lightly browned and crumbly. Drain off fat. Spread beef mixture evenly in prepared pan. Sprinkle chiles over beef.

2. In a bowl, whisk together eggs, ½ cup (125 mL) of the Cheddar cheese and cottage cheese. Spoon over beef. Bake in preheated oven for 30 minutes.

3. Meanwhile, in a small bowl, combine tomato sauce, cumin and chili powder. Spoon evenly over egg mixture; sprinkle with remaining Cheddar cheese. Bake for 10 minutes or until sauce is bubbling and cheese is melted. Top each serving with a spoonful of sour cream (if using).

NUTRITIONAL ANALYSIS (PER SERVING)							
Energy	Protein	Carbohydrate	Fat	Fiber	Calcium	Iron	Sodium
219 kcal	23 g	4 g	12 g	1 g	198 mg	2 mg	480 mg

Basic Beef Mixture

Ground beef forms the basis of many dishes that kids love — including sloppy joes, pizza, shepherd's pie, chili, or just as a topping for baked or mashed potatoes. Make a big batch of this recipe and freeze in smaller amounts. The recipe originated from The Beef Information Centre.

2 lbs	lean or medium ground beef	1 kg
4	cloves garlic, minced	4
2	medium onions, finely chopped	2
2 cups	tomato sauce or pasta sauce	500 mL
2 tsp	dried basil	10 mL
2 tsp	dried oregano	10 mL
½ tsp	salt	2 mL
¼ tsp	freshly ground black pepper	1 mL

1. In a large skillet over medium-high heat, cook beef, garlic and onion, using a spoon to break up the meat, for 10 minutes or until beef is no longer pink. Drain fat.

2. Add tomato sauce, basil, oregano, salt and pepper. Bring to a boil; reduce heat and simmer for 5 minutes. Divide beef mixture into 1-cup (250 mL) portions. Refrigerate for up to 2 days or freeze for up to 3 months.

NUTRITIONAL ANALYSIS (PER ½ CUP/125 ML)

Energy	Protein	Carbohydrate	Fat	Fiber	Calcium	Iron	Sodium
106 kcal	15 g	4 g	3 g	1 g	14 mg	2 mg	355 mg

Uses

Sloppy Joes: In a saucepan, combine 1 cup (250 mL) Basic Beef Mixture, 2 tbsp (25 mL) finely chopped green pepper and 2 tbsp (25 mL) finely chopped celery. Heat thoroughly and serve over cooked rice, toasted bun or bread. Makes 1¼ cups (300 mL).

Pizza: Spread 1 cup (250 mL) Basic Beef Mixture over a 12-inch (30 cm) prebaked pizza shell or flatbread crust. Top with ½ cup (125 mL) shredded Cheddar and ½ cup (125 mL) mozzarella cheese. Place pizza on a baking sheet; broil until cheese is melted. Makes one 12-inch (30 cm) pizza.

Baked Potato Topping: Bake or microwave 1 potato. Cut a cross in top of potato; squeeze to open. Top with ¼ cup (60 mL) heated Basic Beef Mixture and serve. Makes 1 serving.

Shepherd's Pie: In a shallow ovenproof casserole, combine 1 cup (250 mL) Basic Beef Mixture, ½ cup (125 mL) frozen mixed vegetables and ½ cup (125 mL) sliced canned mushrooms. Top with 2 cups (500 mL) cooked mashed potatoes. Bake in 350°F (180°C) oven for 15 minutes. Makes 3 to 4 servings.

Last-Minute Chili: In a small saucepan, combine 1 cup (250 mL) Basic Beef Mixture, ½ cup (125 mL) tomato sauce, ½ cup (125 mL) drained kidney beans and 1 tsp (5 mL) chili powder. Makes 2 cups (500 mL).

The great thing about the basic meat mixture in this recipe is that it's easy to change it up to suit your family's tastes or your mood on a particular night. Teriyaki, Mexican-style, BBQ or Italian-style — it's your choice!

Kitchen Tip

To lower the amount of sodium in this recipe, use reduced-sodium teriyaki sauce.

Variations

Mexican Meatloaf Muffins: Replace the teriyaki sauce with salsa and replace the gingerroot with an equal amount of chili powder.

BBQ Meatloaf Muffins: Replace the teriyaki sauce with barbecue sauce and omit the gingerroot.

Italian Meatloaf Muffins: Replace the teriyaki sauce with tomato pasta sauce and replace the gingerroot with an equal amount of dried basil or oregano.

Teriyaki Meatloaf Muffins

- *Preheat oven to 400°F (200°C)*
- *12-cup muffin pan, 8 cups greased*
- *Rimmed baking sheet*

1	egg, beaten	1
2	cloves garlic, minced	2
½	onion, grated	½
½ cup	finely grated carrot	125 mL
¼ cup	dry bread crumbs	60 mL
6 tbsp	thick teriyaki sauce, divided	90 mL
1 tsp	minced gingerroot (or pinch ground ginger)	5 mL
½ tsp	hot pepper sauce	2 mL
¼ tsp	salt	1 mL
¼ tsp	freshly ground black pepper	1 mL
1 lb	lean ground beef, pork or turkey	500 g

1. In a large bowl, combine egg, garlic, onion, carrot, bread crumbs, 2 tbsp (30 mL) of the teriyaki sauce, ginger, hot pepper sauce, salt and pepper. Add beef and mix thoroughly.

2. Divide mixture among prepared muffin cups, flattening tops slightly. Spread remaining teriyaki sauce over muffins. Place muffin pan on rimmed baking sheet.

3. Bake in preheated oven for about 20 minutes or until meat thermometer inserted in center of a muffin registers at least 165°F (74°C). Let cool for 5 minutes.

NUTRITIONAL ANALYSIS (PER MUFFIN)							
Energy	Protein	Carbohydrate	Fat	Fiber	Calcium	Iron	Sodium
105 kcal	13 g	6 g	3 g	1 g	15 mg	1 mg	608 mg

Great on their own or enjoy with spaghetti or other thin pasta. Serve with a sprinkling of freshly grated Parmesan.

Kitchen Tip

This is a good opportunity for older children to help with preparing the dish.

Meatball Medley

1½ lbs	lean ground beef	750 g
3 tbsp	water	45 mL
1	small onion, diced	1
1	egg	1
2 tbsp	grated Parmesan cheese	30 mL
1 tsp	dried basil	5 mL
½ tsp	salt	2 mL
¼ tsp	freshly ground black pepper	1 mL
¼ tsp	dried sage	1 mL
4 tsp	vegetable oil	20 mL

Sauce

1	large onion, chopped	1
4	cloves garlic, minced	4
2¼ cups	sliced mushrooms	550 mL
2 tsp	dried basil	10 mL
¾ tsp	dried sage	4 mL
¼ tsp	hot pepper flakes	1 mL
4 tsp	all-purpose flour	20 mL
3 cups	beef stock	750 mL
3 tbsp	tomato paste	45 mL
1 tbsp	red wine vinegar	15 mL
1	bay leaf	1
3	carrots, sliced	3
½ tsp	salt	2 mL
1	red bell pepper, chopped	1
1	yellow bell pepper, chopped	1
1	medium zucchini, chopped	1
1 cup	frozen peas	250 mL

1. *Meatballs:* In a large bowl, combine beef, water, onion, egg, cheese, basil, salt, pepper and sage. Mix well. With moistened hands, shape meat mixture into about 24 meatballs.

Kitchen Tip

To freeze, prepare recipe up to the end of step 4. Freeze, then thaw when ready to use. Warm meatball mixture over low heat, then proceed with step 5.

2. In a large skillet, heat oil over medium heat. In batches, if necessary, cook meatballs, turning often, for about 10 minutes. Transfer cooked meatballs to a plate and set aside.

3. *Sauce:* In the same skillet, combine onion, garlic, mushrooms, basil, sage and hot pepper flakes. Cook, stirring, for about 3 minutes or until the onions are tender. Sprinkle with flour and cook, continuing to stir frequently, for another 3 minutes.

4. Increase heat to high and gradually pour in the stock. Bring to a boil, scraping up any brown bits from the bottom and sides of the skillet. Stir in tomato paste, vinegar, bay leaf, carrots and salt. Reduce heat to low. Add reserved meatballs and simmer for 30 minutes or until the carrots are tender.

5. Stir in red and yellow peppers; cook for 3 minutes. Add zucchini and peas; simmer for about 8 minutes or until heated throughout. Remove and discard bay leaf before serving.

NUTRITIONAL ANALYSIS (PER SERVING)

Energy	Protein	Carbohydrate	Fat	Fiber	Calcium	Iron	Sodium
144 kcal	16 g	9 g	5 g	2 g	32 mg	2 mg	281 mg

*Ask kids to name their
favorite foods and
chances are that pizza and
hamburgers will rank near
the top of the list. Here's a
dish that combines the best
of both.*

Kitchen Tip

Regular ground beef is
less expensive than the
lean or extra-lean variety,
and actually makes juicier
burgers. Broiling or grilling
allows some of the fat to drip
away.

Pizza-Style Hamburgers

* *Preheat barbecue or broiler*

1 lb	ground beef (see tip, at left)	500 g
1	egg, beaten	1
¼ cup	finely chopped green pepper	60 mL
2 tbsp	finely chopped onion	30 mL
¼ cup	dry bread crumbs or small-flake rolled oats	60 mL
½ cup	pizza sauce or tomato sauce	125 mL
½ tsp	dried basil	2 mL
½ tsp	dried oregano	2 mL
6	slices mozzarella cheese	6
6	hamburger buns, split and warmed	6

1. In a bowl, combine beef, egg, green pepper, onion,
bread crumbs, pizza sauce, basil and oregano. Do
not overmix. With moistened hands, shape mixture
into 6 evenly shaped flat patties. (For younger
children, you may wish to make a larger number
of smaller burgers.)

2. Grill on preheated barbecue or under the broiler for
about 5 minutes per side or until well done and center
is no longer pink. During last few minutes of cooking
time, top each burger with cheese; cook until cheese
starts to melt. Serve on warm buns.

NUTRITIONAL ANALYSIS (PER BURGER)							
Energy	Protein	Carbohydrate	Fat	Fiber	Calcium	Iron	Sodium
321 kcal	28 g	28 g	11 g	2 g	224 mg	3 mg	528 mg

Food Safety Tip

Unlike beef burgers, which should be completely cooked through to destroy any harmful bacteria, lamb burgers can be served with some pink remaining at the center.

Lamb Burgers

• *Preheat barbecue or broiler*

2 lbs	lean ground lamb (see tip, at left)	1 kg
8 oz	goat cheese	250 g
2 to 4	cloves garlic, mashed	2 to 4
¼ cup	chopped fresh parsley or mint	60 mL
½ tsp	ground cumin	2 mL
½ tsp	hot pepper flakes	2 mL
½ tsp	salt	2 mL
½ tsp	freshly ground black pepper	2 mL

1. In a large bowl, combine lamb, cheese, garlic, parsley and seasonings. With moistened hands, shape meat into 8 patties. (For younger children, you may wish to make a larger number of smaller burgers.) Place patties on a plate, cover and chill until ready to cook.

2. Grill on preheated barbecue or under the broiler. Cook until meat is brown on the outside but still slightly pink at the center.

NUTRITIONAL ANALYSIS (PER BURGER)							
Energy	Protein	Carbohydrate	Fat	Fiber	Calcium	Iron	Sodium
409 kcal	34 g	1 g	29 g	0 g	76 mg	3 mg	354 mg

Braised Lamb

Winter comfort food doesn't get much better than this! Use lamb or beef — either will make a great family dinner.

Kitchen Tip

If you use beef instead of lamb, cooking time may vary, depending on the cut of beef. Check frequently for tenderness. Beef will also create a slightly thinner sauce — although it's still delicious to sop up with pieces of crusty bread.

3 tbsp	olive oil	45 mL
2 lbs	lean lamb or beef, cut into cubes (see tip, at left)	1 kg
3	medium onions, chopped	3
1	large clove garlic, minced	1
3 tbsp	all-purpose flour	45 mL
1½ cups	apple juice	375 mL
1 cup	chicken stock or beef stock	250 mL
3 tbsp	tomato paste	45 mL
½ tsp	salt	2 mL
¼ tsp	freshly ground black pepper	1 mL

1. In a large saucepan, heat oil on medium-high heat. Add lamb in small batches; cook for 5 minutes or until browned on all sides, removing pieces as they brown. Reduce heat to medium. Add onions and garlic; cook, stirring, for 3 minutes or until softened (but not browned). Add flour and cook, stirring, for 1 minute. Stir in apple juice, stock and tomato paste.

2. Return lamb to saucepan. Bring to a boil; reduce heat, cover and cook for 1½ hours or until meat is tender. Season with salt and pepper to taste.

NUTRITIONAL ANALYSIS (PER SERVING)							
Energy	Protein	Carbohydrate	Fat	Fiber	Calcium	Iron	Sodium
526 kcal	51 g	21 g	26 g	2 g	47 mg	4 mg	404 mg

Makes 4 servings

This easy vegetarian dish, simmered in a sweet, mildly seasoned sauce, makes a terrific midweek family dinner.

Spanish Rice with Tofu

1 tbsp	canola oil	15 mL
1	small onion, finely chopped	1
¼ cup	finely chopped green bell pepper	60 mL
2 cups	chopped tomatoes	500 mL
⅔ cup	long-grain white rice	150 mL
½ cup	ketchup	125 mL
Pinch	freshly ground black pepper	Pinch
1 cup	diced firm tofu	250 mL
½ cup	shredded Cheddar cheese	125 mL

1. In a large saucepan, heat oil over medium heat. Sauté onion and green pepper for 5 minutes or until softened.

2. Stir in tomatoes, rice, ketchup and pepper. Add 1 cup (250 mL) water and bring to a boil. Reduce heat to low, cover and simmer for 20 minutes.

3. Gently stir in tofu. Sprinkle with cheese, cover and simmer for 10 minutes or until cheese is melted and bubbly.

NUTRITIONAL ANALYSIS (PER SERVING)							
Energy	Protein	Carbohydrate	Fat	Fiber	Calcium	Iron	Sodium
312 kcal	13 g	39 g	13 g	3 g	250 mg	2 mg	431 mg

Egg Foo Yong

The bean sprouts add crunch to the softer texture of the eggs in this tasty Asian-style dish.

Variation

Use a different leftover cooked meat, such as chicken or beef.

4	eggs, lightly beaten	4
1	green onion, finely chopped	1
1 cup	bean sprouts	250 mL
½ cup	diced cooked pork	125 mL
2 tsp	reduced-sodium soy sauce	10 mL
1 tbsp	canola oil	15 mL

1. In a small bowl, combine eggs, green onion, bean sprouts, pork and soy sauce.

2. In a skillet, heat oil over medium heat. Pour in egg mixture and cook, stirring, for 5 minutes or until egg is set. Serve warm.

NUTRITIONAL ANALYSIS (PER SERVING)

Energy	Protein	Carbohydrate	Fat	Fiber	Calcium	Iron	Sodium
219 kcal	17 g	3 g	16 g	0 g	54 mg	2 mg	186 mg

When you're short on time, we suggest serving these beans with carrot sticks, celery sticks and buttered whole wheat rolls or toast.

Variation

If your family likes mustard, add 1 to 2 tsp (5 to 10 mL) with the salsa.

Easy Fiesta Beans

* *Preheat broiler*
* *8-cup (2 L) casserole dish, greased*

1	can (14 oz/398 mL) nonfat refried beans	1
1	can (14 oz/398 mL) baked beans	1
½ cup	salsa	125 mL
¾ cup	shredded Cheddar cheese, divided	175 mL
2	green onions, finely chopped (optional)	2

1. In a medium saucepan, combine refried beans, baked beans and salsa. Heat over medium heat, stirring frequently, for about 5 minutes or until heated through. Stir in ¼ cup (60 mL) of the cheese until melted.

2. Spoon bean mixture into prepared casserole dish and sprinkle with remaining cheese and green onions (if using). Broil for about 2 minutes or until cheese is melted and lightly browned.

NUTRITIONAL ANALYSIS (PER SERVING)

Energy	Protein	Carbohydrate	Fat	Fiber	Calcium	Iron	Sodium
217 kcal	11 g	29 g	6 g	7 g	162 mg	2 mg	704 mg

This curry has a mild flavor; if your family likes it stronger, increase the curry paste to 1 to 1½ tbsp (15 to 22 mL). Serve over brown rice, with plain yogurt spooned on top of the curry.

Kitchen Tip

Indian curry paste is available in jars in the spice aisle of most supermarkets. When stored in the refrigerator after opening, it stays fresh longer than curry powder. If you prefer, you can substitute an equal amount of curry powder.

Chickpea and Potato Curry with Spinach

1 tbsp	vegetable oil	15 mL
1	onion, chopped	1
2	cloves garlic, minced	2
2 tsp	mild Indian curry paste	10 mL
2 tsp	minced gingerroot (or ½ tsp/2 mL ground ginger)	10 mL
¼ tsp	freshly ground black pepper	1 mL
Pinch	salt	Pinch
1	can (28 oz/796 mL) diced tomatoes	1
½ cup	reduced-sodium vegetable stock or water	125 mL
2 tbsp	tomato paste	30 mL
1 lb	mini potatoes, quartered	500 g
2 cups	canned chickpeas, rinsed and drained	500 mL
4 cups	lightly packed baby spinach leaves	1 L

1. In a large nonstick skillet, heat oil over medium heat. Sauté onion and garlic for 3 minutes. Stir in curry paste, ginger, pepper and salt; sauté for 2 minutes or until onion is softened.

2. Add tomatoes, stock and tomato paste; bring to a boil. Stir in potatoes and chickpeas. Reduce heat to low, cover and simmer for about 40 minutes or until potatoes are tender. Stir in spinach, cover and simmer for 5 minutes.

NUTRITIONAL ANALYSIS (PER SERVING)

Energy	Protein	Carbohydrate	Fat	Fiber	Calcium	Iron	Sodium
183 kcal	8 g	32 g	4 g	6 g	70 mg	3 mg	612 mg

Quinoa is an ancient grain that was a staple for the Incans and is still a big part of the diet of their descendants. It has a mild, nutty flavor and is a rich source of protein and iron. This dish can be a meal in itself or a side dish.

Kitchen Tip

For variety, try adding leftover cooked vegetables (broccoli, green beans) or protein (cooked chicken, tofu) to this dish.

Parmesan Quinoa

1 tbsp	olive oil or vegetable oil	15 mL
½	red onion, finely chopped	½
1	clove garlic, minced	1
1 cup	quinoa, rinsed	250 mL
2¼ cups	reduced-sodium vegetable stock	550 mL
1	carrot, grated	1
¼ cup	grated Parmesan cheese	60 mL
Pinch	salt	Pinch
¼ tsp	freshly ground black pepper	1 mL

1. In a large saucepan, heat oil over medium heat. Sauté onion for 3 minutes. Add garlic and quinoa; sauté for 2 to 3 minutes.
2. Add stock and bring to a boil. Reduce heat to low, cover and simmer for about 15 minutes or until liquid is absorbed and quinoa is tender. Fluff with a fork, then stir in cheese, salt and pepper.

NUTRITIONAL ANALYSIS (PER SERVING)

Energy	Protein	Carbohydrate	Fat	Fiber	Calcium	Iron	Sodium
133 kcal	5 g	19 g	5 g	3 g	56 mg	2 mg	138 mg

Quinoa, a staple in both ancient and modern South American cuisine, takes on the flavors of whatever it is cooked with. It is the only grain that has all nine essential amino acids, making it a complete protein.

Quinoa with Tomatoes, Herbs and Cheese

1 tbsp	canola oil	15 mL
½ cup	finely chopped onion	125 mL
3	cloves garlic, minced	3
Pinch	freshly ground black pepper	Pinch
2 cups	reduced-sodium chicken or vegetable stock	500 mL
1 cup	quinoa, rinsed	250 mL
4	tomatoes, chopped	4
⅓ cup	grated Parmesan cheese	75 mL
¼ cup	chopped fresh basil (or 1 tbsp/15 mL dried)	60 mL

1. In a large saucepan, heat oil over medium heat. Sauté onion for 3 minutes. Add garlic and pepper; sauté for 1 minute.
2. Add stock and quinoa; bring to a boil. Reduce heat to medium-low, cover and simmer for 15 minutes or until liquid is absorbed and quinoa is tender.
3. Remove from heat and stir in tomatoes. Cover and let stand for 5 minutes. Fluff with a fork, then sprinkle with cheese and basil.

NUTRITIONAL ANALYSIS (PER SERVING)

Energy	Protein	Carbohydrate	Fat	Fiber	Calcium	Iron	Sodium
180 kcal	7 g	25 g	6 g	3 g	85 mg	2 mg	97 mg

Salads
and Sides

Strawberry Salad

Just the name of this salad is appealing to kids. They'll love it even more when they taste it!

Variation

Try replacing the strawberries with mandarin segments and add ¼ cup (50 mL) mushrooms.

1	bunch fresh spinach (about 6 oz/150 g), washed and torn into bite-sized pieces	1
2 cups	lettuce, washed and torn into bite-sized pieces	500 mL
2 cups	sliced fresh strawberries	500 mL
2 tbsp	sesame seeds	30 mL

Dressing

2 tbsp	olive oil	30 mL
2 tbsp	vinegar	30 mL
1 tbsp	granulated sugar	15 mL
Pinch	paprika	Pinch

1. In a salad bowl, toss spinach and lettuce until combined. Add strawberries. Sprinkle with sesame seeds.

2. *Dressing:* In a small bowl, whisk together oil, vinegar, sugar and paprika. Just before serving, pour dressing over salad and toss lightly.

NUTRITIONAL ANALYSIS (PER SERVING)							
Energy	Protein	Carbohydrate	Fat	Fiber	Calcium	Iron	Sodium
69 kcal	1 g	7 g	5 g	2 g	31 mg	1 mg	35 mg

This crunchy salad makes a nice change from plain iceberg lettuce. It's terrific in the summer with burgers and corn on the cob.

Deluxe Coleslaw

1 cup	mayonnaise	250 mL
2 tbsp	2% milk	30 mL
2 tbsp	vinegar or lemon juice	30 mL
1 tsp	brown sugar	5 mL
½ tsp	salt	2 mL
¼ tsp	freshly ground black pepper	1 mL
¼ tsp	paprika	1 mL
1	medium head cabbage, shredded	1
1	large stalk celery, thinly sliced	1
1	large carrot, shredded	1
2 tbsp	minced onion	30 mL

1. In a small bowl, mix together mayonnaise, milk, vinegar, brown sugar, salt, pepper and paprika.
2. In a large bowl, toss together the cabbage, celery, carrot, onion. Add mayonnaise mixture and combine well. Cover and refrigerate for at least 1 hour before serving.

NUTRITIONAL ANALYSIS (PER ½ CUP/125 ML)							
Energy	Protein	Carbohydrate	Fat	Fiber	Calcium	Iron	Sodium
100 kcal	0.7 g	4 g	9 g	1 g	23 mg	0.3 mg	149 mg

*Take your salad apart
and arrange each item
separately, serving the
dressing as a dip.*

Tomato, Cucumber and Romaine with Buttermilk Ranch Dip

¼ cup	light mayonnaise	60 mL
¼ cup	light sour cream or plain yogurt	60 mL
¼ cup	buttermilk	60 mL
1	small clove garlic, minced	1
1 tbsp	finely chopped fresh parsley	15 mL
½ tsp	dried dillweed	2 mL
½ tsp	Dijon mustard	2 mL
Pinch	salt	Pinch
Pinch	freshly ground black pepper	Pinch
1	4-inch (10 cm) piece English cucumber	1
8	small inner leaves romaine lettuce	8
1 cup	cherry or grape tomatoes	250 mL

1. In a small bowl, whisk together mayonnaise, sour cream, buttermilk, garlic, parsley, dill, mustard, salt and pepper.

2. Cut cucumber piece in half lengthwise, then cut into sticks.

3. Arrange cucumber sticks, romaine and tomatoes on a large plate, with the dip in the center.

NUTRITIONAL ANALYSIS (PER SERVING)							
Energy	Protein	Carbohydrate	Fat	Fiber	Calcium	Iron	Sodium
69 kcal	2 g	5 g	4 g	1 g	53 mg	0.5 mg	142 mg

Chopped Salad

*This salad is perfect when
you don't have enough
lettuce to make a tossed
salad. Add a handful of
croutons for extra crunch.*

2 cups	chopped romaine lettuce	500 mL
1	carrot, diced	1
1	stalk celery, diced	1
⅓ cup	chopped mushrooms	75 mL
⅓ cup	chopped English cucumber	75 mL
⅓ cup	chopped broccoli florets	75 mL
⅓ cup	chopped bell peppers	75 mL
⅓ cup	chopped tomatoes	75 mL
2 tbsp	olive oil	30 mL
2 tbsp	balsamic vinegar	30 mL
1 tsp	Dijon mustard	5 mL
¼ tsp	granulated sugar	1 mL
Pinch	salt	Pinch
Pinch	freshly ground black pepper	Pinch

1. In a large bowl, combine lettuce, carrot, celery, mushrooms, cucumber, broccoli, bell peppers and tomatoes.

2. In a small bowl, whisk together oil, vinegar, mustard, sugar, salt and pepper. Pour over salad and toss to coat.

NUTRITIONAL ANALYSIS (PER SERVING)							
Energy	Protein	Carbohydrate	Fat	Fiber	Calcium	Iron	Sodium
62 kcal	0.7 g	8 g	4 g	1 g	14 mg	0.3 mg	60 mg

A can of mixed beans is the perfect base for this crunchy salad. You can also serve it in a lettuce-lined whole-grain pita.

Kitchen Tip

A 19-oz (540 mL) can of beans will yield about 2 cups (500 mL), rinsed and drained.

Mixed Bean and Vegetable Salad

2 cups	canned mixed beans, rinsed and drained	500 mL
1	stalk celery, thinly sliced	1
½	yellow or green bell pepper, chopped	½
1 cup	halved or quartered cherry tomatoes	250 mL
2 tbsp	chopped fresh parsley	30 mL
1 tbsp	olive oil	15 mL
1 tbsp	red wine vinegar	15 mL
½ tsp	Dijon mustard	2 mL
1	clove garlic, minced	1
Pinch	salt	Pinch
Pinch	freshly ground black pepper	Pinch

1. In a large bowl, combine beans, celery, yellow pepper, tomatoes and parsley.

2. In a small bowl, whisk together oil, vinegar, mustard, garlic, salt and pepper. Pour over bean mixture and toss to coat.

NUTRITIONAL ANALYSIS (PER SERVING)							
Energy	Protein	Carbohydrate	Fat	Fiber	Calcium	Iron	Sodium
97 kcal	5 g	15 g	2 g	4 g	30 mg	1 mg	294 mg

Kids will enjoy this colorful,
tasty bean salad at lunch,
and it's full of protein and
fiber for long-lasting energy.
Serve with fresh whole-grain
bread or alongside chicken
or fish.

Edamame and Bean Salad

2 cups	green beans, trimmed and cut into 1-inch (2.5 cm) pieces	500 mL
2 cups	yellow wax beans, trimmed and cut into 1-inch (2.5 cm) pieces	500 mL
2 cups	shelled edamame	500 mL
1 cup	chopped tomatoes (about 2 medium)	250 mL
2 tsp	dried basil	10 mL
1 tbsp	rice vinegar	15 mL
2 tsp	fresh lime juice	10 mL
1 tsp	liquid honey	5 mL
1 tsp	Dijon mustard	5 mL
1 tbsp	olive oil	15 mL
¼ tsp	salt	1 mL
¼ tsp	freshly ground black pepper	1 mL

1. In a large pot, bring ¾ cup (175 mL) water to a boil over high heat. Add green beans, yellow beans and edamame; cover and steam for 5 to 7 minutes or until tender-crisp. Drain and rinse under cold water. Transfer to a large bowl and stir in tomatoes.

2. In a small bowl or a measuring cup, combine basil, vinegar, lime juice, honey and mustard. Whisk in olive oil and season with salt and pepper. Pour over bean mixture and toss to coat.

NUTRITIONAL ANALYSIS (PER SERVING)							
Energy	Protein	Carbohydrate	Fat	Fiber	Calcium	Iron	Sodium
97 kcal	5 g	9 g	4 g	4 g	51 mg	1 mg	111 mg

You can increase the chili powder and hot pepper sauce if your family likes things spicy. If you are packing it for a lunch the next day, add a lime wedge to squeeze over it.

Black Bean and Rice Salad

⅔ cup	long-grain brown rice	150 mL
2 cups	canned black beans, rinsed and drained	500 mL
1 cup	frozen corn kernels, thawed	250 mL
1	red bell pepper, chopped	1
1	green onion, sliced	1
2 tbsp	vegetable oil	30 mL
2 tbsp	fresh lime juice	30 mL
½ tsp	chili powder	2 mL
Dash	hot pepper sauce	Dash
Pinch	ground cumin	Pinch
Pinch	salt	Pinch

1. In a saucepan, bring 1⅓ cups (325 mL) salted water to a boil. Add rice, reduce heat to low, cover and simmer for about 40 minutes or until rice is tender and water is absorbed. Transfer to a large bowl.
2. Add beans, corn, red pepper and green onion to the rice.
3. In a small bowl, whisk together oil, lime juice, chili powder, hot pepper sauce, cumin and salt. Pour over rice mixture and toss to combine. Serve warm or cover and refrigerate for 2 hours, until chilled, or for up to 1 day.

NUTRITIONAL ANALYSIS (PER SERVING)

Energy	Protein	Carbohydrate	Fat	Fiber	Calcium	Iron	Sodium
111 kcal	4 g	18 g	3 g	3 g	20 mg	0.9 mg	238 mg

Quinoa is an ancient grain native to South America. It is a complete protein, and has a nutty taste and a chewy texture.

Broccoli and Quinoa Salad

½ cup	quinoa, rinsed	125 mL
2 cups	chopped broccoli florets	500 mL
⅓ cup	dried cranberries or raisins	75 mL
¼ cup	unsalted roasted sunflower seeds	60 mL
¼ cup	light mayonnaise	60 mL
¼ cup	plain yogurt	60 mL
1 tsp	grated lemon zest	5 mL
1 tbsp	fresh lemon juice	15 mL
1 tsp	liquid honey	5 mL
Pinch	salt	Pinch
Pinch	freshly ground black pepper	Pinch

1. In a saucepan, bring quinoa and 1⅓ cups (325 mL) water to boil. Reduce heat to low, cover and simmer for about 15 minutes or until quinoa is tender and water is absorbed. Transfer to a large bowl and let cool.

2. Add broccoli, cranberries and sunflower seeds to the quinoa.

3. In a small bowl, whisk together mayonnaise, yogurt, lemon zest, lemon juice, honey, salt and pepper. Pour over quinoa mixture and toss to coat.

NUTRITIONAL ANALYSIS (PER SERVING)							
Energy	Protein	Carbohydrate	Fat	Fiber	Calcium	Iron	Sodium
155 kcal	3 g	25 g	5 g	2 g	30 mg	0.8 mg	107 mg

Greek Pasta Salad

2 cups	penne pasta	500 mL
2	plum (Roma) tomatoes, chopped	2
1	green bell pepper, chopped	1
2 cups	shredded romaine lettuce	500 mL
1 cup	chopped English cucumber	250 mL
1/4 cup	thinly sliced red onion	60 mL
2 tbsp	olive oil	30 mL
2 tbsp	red wine vinegar	30 mL
1	clove garlic, minced	1
1/4 tsp	dried oregano	1 mL
1/4 tsp	freshly ground black pepper	1 mL
1/4 cup	crumbled feta cheese	60 mL

1. In a large saucepan, cook penne in boiling water according to package instructions until tender but firm. Drain and rinse under running water to cool. Drain well.
2. In a large bowl, combine penne, tomatoes, green pepper, romaine, cucumber and red onion.
3. In a small bowl, whisk together oil, vinegar, garlic, oregano and pepper. Pour over salad and toss to coat. Sprinkle with feta cheese.

NUTRITIONAL ANALYSIS (PER SERVING)

Energy	Protein	Carbohydrate	Fat	Fiber	Calcium	Iron	Sodium
107 kcal	3 g	15 g	3 g	1 g	24 mg	0.5 mg	37 mg

*This recipe is wonderful
served as a warm entrée or
as a cold pasta salad.*

Variations

If desired, replace snow
peas with frozen peas.

Add or substitute your
favorite vegetables for those
called for in the recipe.

Try this dish topped with
slivers of grilled chicken
breast.

Creamy Pasta and Vegetable Salad

¼ cup	fresh parsley sprigs	60 mL
¼ cup	fresh basil leaves (or 1 tbsp/15 mL dried)	60 mL
1	green onion, cut into chunks	1
½ cup	2% milk	125 mL
¼ cup	mayonnaise	60 mL
1 tbsp	lemon juice	15 mL
½ tsp	dry mustard	2 mL
½ tsp	granulated sugar	2 mL
Pinch	salt	Pinch
Pinch	freshly ground black pepper	Pinch
2 cups	rotini	500 mL
1 cup	slivered carrot strips	250 mL
1 cup	diagonally sliced snow peas	250 mL
¼ cup	finely chopped green or red bell pepper (optional)	60 mL

1. In a food processor or by hand, finely chop parsley, basil and green onion.
2. In a bowl, whisk together milk, mayonnaise and lemon juice until smooth. Stir in herb-onion mixture. Add mustard, sugar, salt and pepper; stir to blend.
3. In a large pot of boiling water, cook pasta for 10 minutes. Add carrots and snow peas; cook for 2 minutes or until pasta is tender but firm and vegetables are tender-crisp. Drain well.
4. If serving warm, immediately add mayonnaise mixture to pasta while still hot and toss to coat.
5. If serving cold, rinse pasta and vegetables under running water until cool. Drain and toss with mayonnaise mixture. Serve at once or cover and refrigerate for several hours until needed.

NUTRITIONAL ANALYSIS (PER SERVING)

Energy	Protein	Carbohydrate	Fat	Fiber	Calcium	Iron	Sodium
82 kcal	2 g	10 g	4 g	1 g	24 mg	0.5 mg	68 mg

This side dish makes a great accompaniment to meat, especially ham, pork or chicken. Apples add sweetness without extra sugar.

Baked Carrot and Apple Casserole

- *Preheat oven to 350°F (180°C)*
- *4-cup (1 L) casserole dish, greased*

3 cups	sliced carrots	750 mL
2 cups	sliced apples (unpeeled)	500 mL
2 tbsp	butter or margarine	30 mL
1 tbsp	liquid honey	15 mL
¼ tsp	ground nutmeg	1 mL

1. In a large saucepan of boiling water, cook carrots for 10 minutes or until just tender; drain.

2. In prepared casserole dish, combine carrots, apples, butter and honey.

3 Cover and bake in preheated oven for 35 minutes or until apples are tender. Sprinkle with nutmeg.

NUTRITIONAL ANALYSIS (PER SERVING)							
Energy	Protein	Carbohydrate	Fat	Fiber	Calcium	Iron	Sodium
91 kcal	0.7 g	14 g	4 g	3 g	25 mg	0.2 mg	72 mg

Glazed Carrots

3 tbsp	butter or margarine, divided	45 mL
¼ cup	water	60 mL
Pinch	salt	Pinch
1 lb	carrots, thinly sliced	500 g
1 tsp	granulated sugar	5 mL
2 tbsp	minced fresh basil	30 mL

1. In a large skillet, heat 1 tbsp (15 mL) of the butter over medium-low heat, along with water and salt. Once butter has melted, stir in carrots. Cook, covered, for 8 to 10 minutes or until tender. Drain carrots and set aside.

2. Using the same skillet, melt remaining butter. When butter begins to sizzle, add sugar. Shake pan a few times, then add carrots and basil; cook, tossing carrots gently, for 3 to 5 minutes or until glazed.

NUTRITIONAL ANALYSIS (PER SERVING)							
Energy	Protein	Carbohydrate	Fat	Fiber	Calcium	Iron	Sodium
126 kcal	1 g	12 g	9 g	3 g	43 mg	0.4 mg	213 mg

Kitchen Tip

A lot of dirt can hide between the layers of a leek, so be sure to trim and wash well before boiling.

Parmesan Leeks

- *Preheat broiler*
- *6-cup (1.5 L) casserole, greased*

3	leeks, trimmed, well washed and cut into bite-size pieces	3
1 tbsp	butter or margarine	15 mL
1 tbsp	all-purpose flour	15 mL
¼ cup	2% milk	60 mL
¼ tsp	salt	1 mL
Pinch	freshly ground black pepper	Pinch
2 tbsp	grated Parmesan cheese	30 mL

1. In a large saucepan of boiling water, cook leeks for 5 to 10 minutes or until tender. Drain all but ¼ cup (60 mL) cooking liquid; set aside. Transfer leeks to prepared casserole.

2. In a small saucepan, melt butter over medium heat. Whisk in flour, milk and reserved leek cooking liquid. Reduce heat to simmer; whisk until smooth. Add salt and pepper. Pour sauce mixture over the leeks. Sprinkle with Parmesan cheese. Broil until golden brown.

NUTRITIONAL ANALYSIS (PER SERVING)							
Energy	Protein	Carbohydrate	Fat	Fiber	Calcium	Iron	Sodium
92 kcal	3 g	12 g	4 g	1 g	86 mg	2 mg	224 mg

Zucchini is a quick and delicious side for any dinner or lunch. This recipe is simple but very tasty — great on its own as a snack, or served with meat, fish, chicken or tofu.

Kitchen Tip

When it's in season, substitute yellow summer squash for half the zucchini, for a slightly different flavor.

Simple Parmesan Zucchini

1 tbsp	vegetable oil	15 mL
2	zucchini, cut into thin slices	2
3 tbsp	freshly grated Parmesan cheese	45 mL

1. In a nonstick skillet, heat oil over medium-high heat. Sauté zucchini for 4 to 5 minutes or until lightly browned. Remove from heat and add cheese, stirring for 10 to 15 seconds. Serve immediately.

NUTRITIONAL ANALYSIS (PER SERVING)

Energy	Protein	Carbohydrate	Fat	Fiber	Calcium	Iron	Sodium
62 kcal	3 g	3 g	5 g	1 g	56 mg	0.4 mg	67 mg

Baby bok choy is delicious, cooks quickly and is a perfect complement to any dinner, but especially chicken or fish.

Quick and Easy Bok Choy Stir-Fry

2 tbsp	vegetable oil	30 mL
4 to 6	baby bok choy, ends trimmed, leaves separated	4 to 6
1 tsp	chopped gingerroot (or ¼ tsp/1 mL dried ginger)	5 mL
1 tsp	chopped garlic (or ¼ tsp/1 mL garlic powder)	5 mL
¼ cup	reduced-sodium vegetable stock	60 mL
½ tsp	reduced-sodium soy sauce	2 mL

1. In a medium saucepan, heat oil over medium heat. Sauté bok choy, ginger and garlic for 2 minutes or until bok choy is slightly wilted. Add stock, cover and simmer for about 3 minutes or until bok choy is tender. Stir in soy sauce.

NUTRITIONAL ANALYSIS (PER SERVING)

Energy	Protein	Carbohydrate	Fat	Fiber	Calcium	Iron	Sodium
82 kcal	2 g	3 g	7 g	1 g	134 mg	1 mg	113 mg

Chinese Veggies

Kitchen Tips

Adjust cooking time to prepare vegetables to desired softness.

If you don't have any homemade chicken stock, use ready-to-use chicken broth, preferably a reduced-sodium variety.

1 tbsp	vegetable oil	15 mL
1 lb	broccoli florets, chopped	500 g
1	onion, thinly sliced	1
1 tbsp	minced gingerroot	15 mL
3	baby bok choy	3
4 oz	snow peas	125 g
3	celery stalks, thinly sliced	3
5	green onions, thinly sliced	5
¾ cup	reduced-sodium chicken stock	175 mL

1. In a wok or a large skillet, heat oil over high heat. Add broccoli, onions and ginger; stir-fry for 1 minute. Add bok choy, snow peas, celery and green onions. Pour in stock. Toss vegetables until well coated. Bring to a boil, cover and cook for 2 to 3 minutes or until the vegetables are tender-crisp.

NUTRITIONAL ANALYSIS (PER SERVING)							
Energy	Protein	Carbohydrate	Fat	Fiber	Calcium	Iron	Sodium
70 kcal	4 g	10 g	3 g	4 g	72 mg	2 mg	60 mg

Braised winter vegetables are a marvelous accompaniment to roasts of chicken, beef or pork.

Braised Winter Vegetables

- *Preheat oven to 400°F (200°C)*
- *Large roasting pan*

3	carrots, peeled and cut into chunks	3
3	small white turnips, peeled and cut into chunks	3
½	rutabaga, peeled and cut into chunks	½
1	large sweet potato, peeled and cut into chunks	1
3 tbsp	olive oil	45 mL
½ tsp	salt	2 mL
¼ tsp	freshly ground black pepper	1 mL
	Chopped fresh parsley	

1. Place carrots, turnips, rutabaga and sweet potato in roasting pan. Sprinkle with oil, salt and pepper. Cover pan and roast in preheated oven for 35 minutes or until vegetables are tender. Serve garnished with chopped parsley.

NUTRITIONAL ANALYSIS (PER SERVING)							
Energy	Protein	Carbohydrate	Fat	Fiber	Calcium	Iron	Sodium
111 kcal	1 g	12 g	7 g	3 g	41 mg	0.5 mg	254 mg

Makes 4 servings

Children really seem to like the flavor of sweet potatoes — as you'll discover with this recipe.

Kitchen Tip

These potatoes can be baked at the same time that you cook a roast.

Stuffed Baked Sweet Potatoes

- *Preheat oven to 350°F (180°C)*
- *Small baking pan*

2	sweet potatoes (medium size)	2
¼ cup	orange juice	60 mL
2 tbsp	butter or margarine	30 mL
¼ tsp	grated orange zest	1 mL
¼ tsp	ground nutmeg	1 mL
¼ tsp	salt	1 mL
Pinch	freshly ground black pepper	Pinch

1. Wash potatoes and pierce with a fork in several places. Place on oven rack in preheated oven. Bake for 1 hour or until potatoes are tender.

2. When cool enough to handle, cut each potato in half. With a spoon, carefully remove pulp to a bowl, being sure not to damage shell. Mash pulp with orange juice, butter, orange zest, nutmeg, salt and pepper. Stuff shells with mixture and transfer to baking pan.

3. Bake stuffed shells for 10 minutes or until heated through. (Before serving to small children, test the stuffing to make sure it is not too hot inside. You may wish to remove filling from shell.)

NUTRITIONAL ANALYSIS (PER SERVING)							
Energy	Protein	Carbohydrate	Fat	Fiber	Calcium	Iron	Sodium
109 kcal	1 g	13 g	6 g	2 g	14 mg	0.4 mg	221 mg

Here's a simply wonderful, easily made casserole that's great for a crowd!

Kitchen Tip

Double the recipe and freeze one portion to have on hand for surprise guests. It's easy to reheat.

Swedish Potatoes

* Preheat oven to 350°F (180°C)
* 8-cup (2 L) casserole, greased

6	large potatoes, peeled and cut into chunks	6
¾ cup	sour cream	175 mL
½	package (8 oz/250 g) cream cheese, softened	½
2 tbsp	finely chopped onion	30 mL
½ tsp	salt	2 mL
¼ tsp	freshly ground black pepper	1 mL
¾ cup	fine dry bread crumbs	175 mL

1. In a large saucepan, cook potatoes in boiling water until tender. Drain and mash.
2. In a small bowl, beat together sour cream, cream cheese, onion, salt and pepper. Add mixture to mashed potatoes and stir until smooth.
3. Spoon potato mixture into prepared casserole. Top with bread crumbs. Bake in preheated oven for 30 minutes or until hot and golden brown.

NUTRITIONAL ANALYSIS (PER SERVING)							
Energy	Protein	Carbohydrate	Fat	Fiber	Calcium	Iron	Sodium
319 kcal	8 g	55 g	8 g	4 g	94 mg	1 mg	304 mg

These are absolutely the very best roasted crispy potatoes you will ever eat. They're our all-time favorite!

Garlic Roasted Potatoes

- *Preheat oven to 400°F (200°C)*
- *Shallow baking pan, greased*

4	Yukon Gold potatoes, cut into chunks	4
2 tbsp	olive oil	30 mL
1 or 2	cloves garlic, sliced	1 or 2
	Salt and freshly ground pepper	

1. Place potato chunks in a plastic bag. Add oil and garlic. Seal bag and toss until potatoes are coated. Transfer to prepared baking pan. Sprinkle with salt and pepper. Bake in preheated oven for 35 minutes or until potatoes are tender and golden brown.

NUTRITIONAL ANALYSIS (PER SERVING)							
Energy	Protein	Carbohydrate	Fat	Fiber	Calcium	Iron	Sodium
171 kcal	4 g	24 g	7 g	3 g	3 mg	2 mg	5 mg

Kids will rave about these, so be sure to make extra! Serve warm or cold, alone or with sour cream, as a side dish or a snack. They'll keep in the fridge for up to 2 days.

Tasty Potato Pancakes

3	potatoes, peeled and shredded	3
2	eggs, lightly beaten	2
½	onion, finely chopped	½
Pinch	salt	Pinch
2 to 3 tbsp	vegetable oil (approx.), divided	30 to 45 mL

1. In a medium bowl, combine potatoes, eggs, onion and salt. Form into 2-inch (5 cm) diameter patties.

2. In a skillet, heat 2 tbsp (30 mL) of the oil over medium-high heat. Cook patties, in batches, for 2 to 3 minutes per side or until lightly browned on both sides, adding oil to the skillet and adjusting heat between batches as necessary. Transfer to a plate lined with paper towels.

NUTRITIONAL ANALYSIS (PER PANCAKE)							
Energy	Protein	Carbohydrate	Fat	Fiber	Calcium	Iron	Sodium
156 kcal	3 g	18 g	9 g	2 g	17 mg	0.6 mg	74 mg

Arborio is an Italian short-grain rice that can absorb great quantities of flavorful stock to create creamy risotto, a true comfort food. Dress it up by adding some vegetables.

Italian Vegetable Risotto

1 tbsp	olive oil, divided	15 mL
½ cup	finely chopped onion	125 mL
1 cup	Arborio rice	250 mL
3 cups	reduced-sodium chicken stock, heated to boiling and kept hot	750 mL
1	small zucchini, diced	1
½ cup	frozen peas, thawed	125 mL
½ cup	shredded mozzarella cheese	125 mL
¼ cup	grated Parmesan cheese	60 mL
¼ tsp	ground nutmeg	1 mL

1. In a medium saucepan, heat 2 tsp (10 mL) of the oil over medium heat. Sauté onion for 5 minutes or until softened. Stir in rice until coated with oil.

2. Add ½ cup (125 mL) stock, reduce heat and simmer, stirring constantly, until liquid is absorbed. Continue adding stock, ½ cup (125 mL) at a time, stirring frequently, until each addition is absorbed before stirring in the next, until all the stock has been added and absorbed and rice is tender and creamy, about 20 minutes. After all the stock has been absorbed, if rice is not yet tender and creamy, you may need to add some hot water.

3. Meanwhile, in a nonstick skillet, heat remaining oil over medium-high heat. Sauté zucchini for 5 minutes or until tender. Add peas and sauté for 1 minute.

4. Stir mozzarella and Parmesan into rice until cheese is melted. Stir in zucchini and peas. Sprinkle with nutmeg and serve immediately.

NUTRITIONAL ANALYSIS (PER SERVING)

Energy	Protein	Carbohydrate	Fat	Fiber	Calcium	Iron	Sodium
183 kcal	8 g	30 g	4 g	2 g	106 mg	0.6 mg	192 mg

Assemble this vegetable casserole ahead, refrigerate and then bake just before serving. Everyone who's tried this recipe loves it!

Kitchen Tip

Instead of fresh broccoli, use an equal quantity of frozen chopped broccoli. It should be thawed before combining with the rice, but need not be blanched.

Rice and Broccoli Casserole

- *Preheat oven to 350°F (180°C)*
- *Shallow 8-cup (2 L) casserole, greased*

2 cups	broccoli florets (see tip, at left)	500 mL
2 cups	cooked rice	500 mL
1	small onion, finely chopped	1
2	eggs	2
1½ cups	2% milk	375 mL
½ tsp	salt	2 mL
¼ tsp	freshly ground black pepper	1 mL
¼ tsp	ground nutmeg	1 mL
¼ cup	grated Parmesan cheese	60 mL

1. In a colander, blanch broccoli over boiling water for 2 minutes. Transfer to a bowl and combine with rice and onion. Transfer to prepared casserole.
2. In a small bowl, whisk together eggs, milk, salt, pepper and nutmeg. Pour over rice mixture. Sprinkle with cheese. Cover and refrigerate until ready to bake.
3. Bake in preheated oven for 35 minutes or until mixture is bubbling and set in the center.

NUTRITIONAL ANALYSIS (PER SERVING)							
Energy	Protein	Carbohydrate	Fat	Fiber	Calcium	Iron	Sodium
159 kcal	7 g	23 g	4 g	2 g	132 mg	1 mg	297 mg

*Couscous is quick to prepare
and very versatile. Use
your family's favorite frozen
vegetables to liven it up.*

Couscous Pilaf

1 tbsp	vegetable oil	15 mL
1	small onion, chopped	1
1	clove garlic, minced	1
½ tsp	dried basil	2 mL
¼ tsp	salt	1 mL
¼ tsp	freshly ground black pepper	1 mL
1½ cups	reduced-sodium chicken stock or water	375 mL
1 cup	frozen vegetables	250 mL
1 cup	whole wheat couscous	250 mL

1. In a large saucepan, heat oil over medium heat. Sauté onion, garlic, basil, salt and pepper for about 5 minutes or until onion is softened.

2. Add stock and frozen vegetables; bring to a boil. Stir in couscous. Remove from heat, cover and let stand for 5 minutes or until liquid is absorbed.

NUTRITIONAL ANALYSIS (PER SERVING)

Energy	Protein	Carbohydrate	Fat	Fiber	Calcium	Iron	Sodium
86 kcal	3 g	15 g	2 g	2 g	14 mg	0.6 mg	189 mg

Creamy Cheddar Sauce

This sauce is perfect with so many vegetables and is bound to make your little ones ask for more. Try it on cooked cauliflower, broccoli, carrots, green beans or anything else you think they will like.

⅓ cup	2% milk	75 mL
⅓ cup	mayonnaise	75 mL
1 cup	shredded Cheddar cheese	250 mL
Pinch	freshly ground black pepper	Pinch
Pinch	freshly grated nutmeg	Pinch
	Cooked vegetables	

1. In a small saucepan over medium heat, whisk together milk and mayonnaise until smooth. Add cheese, pepper and nutmeg. Cook until cheese has melted. (Be sure the sauce does not boil.) Pour over vegetables. Toss and serve.

NUTRITIONAL ANALYSIS (PER 1 TBSP/15 ML)

Energy	Protein	Carbohydrate	Fat	Fiber	Calcium	Iron	Sodium
86 kcal	3 g	0.5 g	8 g	0 g	76 mg	0.1 mg	101 mg

Snacks

*This easy dip is a treat for
the whole family when
served with vegetables or
nachos.*

Mild Salsa Cheese Dip

½ cup	mild salsa	125 mL
1 cup	shredded Cheddar cheese	250 mL
½	package (8 oz/250 g) cream cheese	½
1 to 2 tbsp	ketchup	15 to 30 mL
	Assorted raw vegetables or corn nacho chips	

1. In a small saucepan over medium heat, combine salsa, Cheddar cheese and cream cheese. Cook, stirring, until cheeses are melted. Stir in ketchup until mixture is smooth. Serve with vegetables or nachos.

NUTRITIONAL ANALYSIS (PER ¼ CUP/60 ML)

Energy	Protein	Carbohydrate	Fat	Fiber	Calcium	Iron	Sodium
238 kcal	9 g	6 g	20 g	0 g	236 mg	0.4 mg	474 mg

*This dip is a perennial
favorite with snackers young
and old. Serve with torn pita
pieces or raw vegetables.*

Creamy Spinach Dip

1	package (10 oz/284 g) frozen chopped spinach, thawed, excess liquid squeezed out	1
½ cup	plain yogurt	125 mL
½	package (8 oz/250 g) cream cheese	½
2 tbsp	finely chopped onion	30 mL
½ tsp	Worcestershire sauce	2 mL
Pinch	salt	Pinch
Pinch	freshly ground black pepper	Pinch

1. In a food processor, combine spinach, yogurt, cream cheese and onion; process with on/off turns until smooth. Add Worcestershire sauce, salt and pepper; process to blend. Transfer dip to a bowl; cover and refrigerate for several hours or overnight to allow flavors to develop.

NUTRITIONAL ANALYSIS (PER ¼ CUP/60 ML)

Energy	Protein	Carbohydrate	Fat	Fiber	Calcium	Iron	Sodium
73 kcal	3 g	3 g	6 g	1 g	77 mg	0.5 mg	156 mg

Want to make a big plate of veggies disappear? Just serve this dip — kids find it irresistible!

Ranch Dip for Kids

⅔ cup	sour cream	150 mL
⅓ cup	light mayonnaise	75 mL
1 tbsp	cider vinegar	15 mL
1 tsp	dried dillweed	5 mL
1 tsp	Dijon mustard	5 mL
Pinch	salt	Pinch
Pinch	freshly ground black pepper	Pinch

1. In a small bowl, whisk together sour cream, mayonnaise and vinegar until smooth. Add dill, mustard, salt and pepper. Whisk to blend. Cover and refrigerate for up to 1 week.

NUTRITIONAL ANALYSIS (PER ¼ CUP/60 ML)

Energy	Protein	Carbohydrate	Fat	Fiber	Calcium	Iron	Sodium
148 kcal	2 g	3 g	13 g	0 g	33 mg	0.2 mg	262 mg

You can buy commercially prepared cheese spreads — but when this tasty homemade version is so quick and easy to prepare, why bother?

Kitchen Tip

Vary the strength of flavor by using mild, medium or old Cheddar cheese — or, for a completely different taste, use mozzarella or Swiss.

Cheddar Cheese Spread

1 cup	shredded Cheddar cheese	250 mL
¼ cup	cream cheese	60 mL
¼ cup	mayonnaise	60 mL
Pinch	dry mustard	Pinch
Pinch	Worcestershire sauce	Pinch

1. In a food processor — or in a bowl, with an electric mixer — combine Cheddar, cream cheese, mayonnaise, mustard and Worcestershire sauce; process until very smooth. Cover and refrigerate for up to 2 weeks or freeze for longer storage.

NUTRITIONAL ANALYSIS (PER 1 TBSP/15 ML)

Energy	Protein	Carbohydrate	Fat	Fiber	Calcium	Iron	Sodium
66 kcal	2 g	0.3 g	6 g	0 g	55 mg	0.1 mg	78 mg

Serve this spread on crackers, toast or apple slices. It's a perfect snack (or breakfast) for enticing finicky young appetites.

Kitchen Tip

If your child is able to eat apple skin, then leave apples unpeeled to provide added fiber.

To prepare apple slices, core and peel (if desired; see above) as many apples as are needed for the meal. Cut into thin slices. Dip each slice in a mixture of lemon juice and water to prevent browning.

Store unused spread in refrigerator.

Apple 'n' Cheese Spread

½	package (8 oz/250 g) cream cheese, at room temperature	½
½ cup	shredded mild Cheddar cheese	125 mL
2 tsp	lemon juice	10 mL
½ tsp	dry mustard	2 mL
1	apple, peeled and grated (see tip, at left)	1
	Crackers, toast or apple slices (see tip, at left)	

1. In a bowl, with an electric mixer, or in a food processor, blend cream cheese until smooth. Add Cheddar cheese, lemon juice and mustard; blend until creamy. Stir in grated apple; cover and refrigerate for 2 hours to allow flavors to blend. Before serving, bring dip to room temperature (for best spreading consistency).

NUTRITIONAL ANALYSIS (PER ¼ CUP/60 ML)

Energy	Protein	Carbohydrate	Fat	Fiber	Calcium	Iron	Sodium
177 kcal	5 g	7 g	15 g	1 g	33 mg	0.2 mg	185 mg

Makes 48 crisps

Everyone loves these crisp crackers. They're easy and economical to make — and taste great, whether on their own or with a dip. Vary the seasonings to suit your family's preferences.

Pita Crisps

- *Preheat oven to 350°F (180°C)*
- *Baking sheet, ungreased*

3 tbsp	olive oil	45 mL
1	clove garlic, minced	1
½ tsp	dried basil	2 mL
½ tsp	dried oregano	2 mL
Pinch	salt	Pinch
Pinch	freshly ground black pepper	Pinch
3	5-inch (12.5 cm) whole wheat pitas, each cut into 8 wedges, then separated to make 16 triangles	3

1. In a small bowl, combine oil, garlic, basil, oregano, salt and pepper. Brush mixture lightly over "inside" surface of each triangle and place, brushed side up, on baking sheet. Bake in preheated oven for 12 minutes or until crisp and golden brown.

2. Remove from oven to a wire rack. Allow to cool before storing in an airtight container.

NUTRITIONAL ANALYSIS (PER 6 CRISPS)							
Energy	Protein	Carbohydrate	Fat	Fiber	Calcium	Iron	Sodium
108 kcal	2 g	11 g	6 g	1 g	24 mg	0.8 mg	39 mg

Makes 12 wedges

Tired of plain old cheese and crackers? Try this quick and easy treat.

Kitchen Tip

For a little more zest, add layers of sour cream and salsa to cheese layer. Or reduce quantity of cheese to ¼ cup (60 mL) and add a combination of ¼ cup (60 mL) diced cooked chicken and ¼ cup (60 mL) diced cooked vegetables.

Cheese Quesadillas

2 tsp	vegetable oil, divided	10 mL
4	medium (8-inch/20 cm) flour tortillas	4
1 cup	shredded Cheddar cheese, divided	250 mL

1. In a nonstick skillet, heat half of the oil over medium-high heat. Place tortilla in skillet and sprinkle half of the cheese evenly over tortilla. Cover with second tortilla shell and press down firmly. Heat for about 1½ minutes, then flip tortilla over and cook for another minute or until light brown and cheese has melted. Transfer to a rack and let cool slightly (so little hands are not burned) before cutting into 6 wedges. Repeat procedure with remaining ingredients.

NUTRITIONAL ANALYSIS (PER WEDGE)

Energy	Protein	Carbohydrate	Fat	Fiber	Calcium	Iron	Sodium
93 kcal	4 g	8 g	5 g	1 g	88 mg	0.6 mg	156 mg

Makes 2½ cups (625 mL)

Here's a great alternative to commercially prepared cereal-based snacks. It's quick to make and provides more food energy than the cereal alone. Young children love to feed themselves the small, easily handled bits and pieces.

Stovetop Cereal Snack

1 tbsp	butter or margarine	15 mL
1 tsp	Worcestershire sauce	5 mL
1½ cups	o-shaped oat cereal	375 mL
½ cup	shredded wheat squares	125 mL
½ cup	stick pretzels, broken	125 mL

1. In a large nonstick skillet, melt butter over medium-low heat. Stir in Worcestershire sauce, cereal and squares; cook, stirring constantly, for 5 minutes or until brown. Remove from heat and allow to cool before adding pretzel sticks. Toss lightly and transfer to an airtight container.

NUTRITIONAL ANALYSIS (PER ½ CUP/125 ML)

Energy	Protein	Carbohydrate	Fat	Fiber	Calcium	Iron	Sodium
96 kcal	2 g	16 g	3 g	2 g	44 mg	2 mg	170 mg

Oatmeal Cereal Cookies

Variation

Replace 1/3 cup (75 mL) of the dried fruit with semisweet chocolate chips.

- *Preheat oven to 350°F (180°C)*
- *Baking sheets, lined with parchment paper or greased*

1 cup	quick-cooking rolled oats	250 mL
1 cup	all-purpose flour	250 mL
1/2 tsp	baking powder	2 mL
1/2 tsp	baking soda	2 mL
1/2 tsp	ground cinnamon	2 mL
1/4 tsp	salt	1 mL
2/3 cup	butter, softened	150 mL
2/3 cup	packed brown sugar	150 mL
1	egg	1
1 tsp	vanilla extract	5 mL
1 cup	dried fruit, such as blueberries, cranberries, raisins, chopped apricots	250 mL
1 cup	crisp rice cereal	250 mL
1 cup	bran flakes cereal	250 mL

1. In a medium bowl, whisk together oats, flour, baking powder, baking soda, cinnamon and salt. Set aside.

2. In a large bowl, cream butter and brown sugar until fluffy. Beat in egg and vanilla. Stir in oats mixture until blended. Stir in dried fruit, rice cereal and bran cereal.

3. Drop by heaping tablespoonfuls (15 mL) onto prepared baking sheets, at least 2 inches (5 cm) apart. Bake in preheated oven for about 12 minutes or until golden with crispy edges. Transfer to wire racks to cool.

NUTRITIONAL ANALYSIS (PER COOKIE)							
Energy	Protein	Carbohydrate	Fat	Fiber	Calcium	Iron	Sodium
74 kcal	0.9 g	10 g	3 g	1 g	10 mg	0.7 mg	65 mg

Makes 6 dozen cookies

These banana-bread bites are the perfect size for little mouths!

Kitchen Tip

Try replacing raisins with other dried fruit, such as chopped dried apricots. Or, for those with a serious sweet tooth, try using chocolate chips!

Soft Banana and Oatmeal Cookies

- *Preheat oven to 350°F (180°C)*
- *Large baking sheet, ungreased*

1 cup	packed brown sugar	250 mL
1 cup	granulated sugar	250 mL
1 cup	shortening	250 mL
1 cup	mashed ripe bananas	250 mL
3	eggs, lightly beaten	3
1 tsp	vanilla extract	5 mL
2 cups	all-purpose flour	500 mL
1 tsp	baking soda	5 mL
½ tsp	salt	2 mL
2 cups	quick-cooking rolled oats	500 mL
1 cup	raisins, rinsed and patted dry	250 mL

1. In a large bowl, with an electric mixer, cream together brown sugar, granulated sugar and shortening; beat until light and fluffy. Beat in bananas, eggs and vanilla.

2. In another bowl, combine flour, baking soda and salt. Gradually stir into banana butter mixture; blend well. Stir in rolled oats and raisins.

3. Drop spoonfuls of batter onto baking sheet. Bake in preheated oven for 15 minutes or until golden brown.

NUTRITIONAL ANALYSIS (PER COOKIE)							
Energy	Protein	Carbohydrate	Fat	Fiber	Calcium	Iron	Sodium
78 kcal	1 g	12 g	3 g	1 g	7 mg	0.4 mg	38 mg

Makes 6 dozen cookies

Baking cookies is a fun way to get kids interested in food preparation, and this recipe is a great one to start with, as it's a healthy choice.

Oatmeal Raisin Cookies

- *Preheat oven to 375°F (190°C)*
- *Large baking sheet, ungreased*

1 cup	butter or margarine	250 mL
1 cup	lightly packed brown sugar	250 mL
2 cups	all-purpose flour	500 mL
2 cups	quick-cooking rolled oats	500 mL
½ cup	hot water	125 mL
1 tsp	baking soda	5 mL
1 tsp	baking powder	5 mL
1 tsp	vanilla extract	5 mL
½ tsp	salt	2 mL
1 cup	raisins or currants	250 mL

1. In a large bowl, with an electric mixer, cream together butter and brown sugar. Add flour, oats, water, baking soda, baking powder, vanilla and salt; mix well. Fold in raisins.

2. Form dough into balls and place on cookie sheet. Flatten each ball with a fork and bake for 10 minutes or until golden brown.

NUTRITIONAL ANALYSIS (PER COOKIE)							
Energy	Protein	Carbohydrate	Fat	Fiber	Calcium	Iron	Sodium
62 kcal	0.8 g	9 g	3 g	1 g	4 mg	0.4 mg	53 mg

Raisin Spice Cookies

- *Preheat oven to 375°F (190°C)*
- *Large baking sheet, lightly greased*

½ cup	shortening	125 mL
¼ cup	butter, softened	60 mL
1 cup	packed brown sugar	250 mL
1	egg	1
⅓ cup	molasses	75 mL
2¼ cups	all-purpose flour	550 mL
1 tsp	baking soda	5 mL
½ tsp	salt	2 mL
½ tsp	ground cinnamon	2 mL
¼ tsp	ground ginger	1 mL
Pinch	ground allspice	Pinch
1½ cups	raisins	375 mL
	Granulated sugar for coating	

1. In a bowl, with an electric mixer, cream together shortening and butter; beat until fluffy. Blend in brown sugar, egg and molasses.

2. In another bowl, sift together flour, baking soda, salt, cinnamon, ginger and allspice. Gradually stir into butter mixture. Add raisins and mix well. Cover and refrigerate for about 30 minutes or until dough is firm enough to handle.

3. With your hands, roll 1 to 2 tsp (5 to 10 mL) dough into balls. Roll in sugar to coat and place on prepared baking sheet. Bake for 10 minutes or until browned.

NUTRITIONAL ANALYSIS (PER COOKIE)							
Energy	Protein	Carbohydrate	Fat	Fiber	Calcium	Iron	Sodium
72 kcal	0.7 g	12 g	3 g	0 g	10 mg	0.5 mg	50 mg

Rindy's Ginger Chews

These easy cookies, created by Daina's good friend Rindy, will be a welcome addition to your cookie repertoire. They are especially delicious with a tall glass of cold milk.

Kitchen Tips

You can use corn syrup in place of molasses, but you'll miss out on the added iron and calcium molasses provides!

These cookies should be moist when you take them out of the oven, and will remain nice and chewy once they're cooled.

- *Preheat oven to 350°F (180°C)*
- *Large baking sheets, greased*

2½ cups	all-purpose flour	625 mL
1½ tsp	baking soda	7 mL
1 tsp	ground cinnamon	5 mL
1 tsp	ground ginger	5 mL
½ tsp	ground cloves	2 mL
¼ tsp	salt	1 mL
1 cup	packed dark brown sugar	250 mL
6 tbsp	granulated sugar, divided	90 mL
2	eggs	2
½ cup	butter, melted	125 mL
½ cup	light (fancy) molasses	125 mL

1. In a bowl, combine flour, baking soda, cinnamon, ginger, cloves and salt. Set aside.
2. In a large bowl, whisk together brown sugar, ¼ cup (60 mL) of the granulated sugar, eggs, butter and molasses. Stir in flour mixture.
3. Pour remaining sugar onto a plate. Dust your hands with flour and roll about 1 tsp (5 mL) dough into a ball. Roll lightly in sugar and place on baking sheet. Repeat until all dough is used, spacing balls 1 inch (2.5 cm) apart.
4. Bake in preheated oven for about 15 minutes or until tops are starting to crack. Let cool on pan on a wire rack for 10 minutes.

NUTRITIONAL ANALYSIS (PER COOKIE)							
Energy	Protein	Carbohydrate	Fat	Fiber	Calcium	Iron	Sodium
72 kcal	0.9 g	13 g	2 g	0 g	10 mg	0.5 mg	57 mg

Crispy Poppy Seed Cookies

- *Preheat oven to 375°F (190°C)*
- *Baking sheets, greased*

3½ cups	all-purpose flour	875 mL
1 tsp	baking powder	5 mL
⅛ tsp	salt	0.5 mL
⅔ cup	granulated sugar	150 mL
⅓ cup	poppy seeds	75 mL
3	eggs	3
½ cup	vegetable oil	125 mL
⅓ cup	fresh orange juice	75 mL

1. In a bowl, combine flour, baking powder and salt.
2. In a large bowl, whisk together sugar, poppy seeds, eggs, oil and orange juice. Stir in flour mixture until blended (dough should be quite stiff).
3. Dust your hands with flour and roll about 1 tsp (5 mL) dough into a ball. Place on baking sheet, then flatten with a fork. Repeat until all dough is used, spacing balls 1 inch (2.5 cm) apart and dipping fork in water between cookies.
4. Bake in preheated oven for about 10 minutes or until light brown. Let cool on pan on a wire rack for 5 minutes.

NUTRITIONAL ANALYSIS (PER 4 COOKIES)							
Energy	Protein	Carbohydrate	Fat	Fiber	Calcium	Iron	Sodium
189 kcal	4 g	25 g	9 g	1 g	53 mg	2 mg	57 mg

*Here's a great way to get
more fruit into your child's
diet. Applesauce makes
them extra good. In fact,
healthy ingredients aside,
this is one of the best
chocolate chip cookies
we've ever tasted!*

Soft Chocolate Chip Cookies

- *Preheat oven to 375°F (190°C)*
- *Baking sheet, greased*

1 cup	loosely packed brown sugar	250 mL
½ cup	unsweetened applesauce	125 mL
¼ cup	butter or margarine, softened	60 mL
1	egg	1
1 tbsp	vanilla extract	15 mL
1⅓ cups	all-purpose flour	325 mL
1½ tsp	baking powder	7 mL
½ tsp	salt	2 mL
1 cup	miniature chocolate chips	250 mL

1. In a bowl, with an electric mixer, cream together brown sugar, applesauce, butter, egg and vanilla; beat until light and fluffy.

2. In another bowl, combine flour, baking powder and salt. Gradually stir into applesauce mixture; blend well. Fold in chocolate chips.

3. Drop spoonfuls of batter onto prepared baking sheet 2 inches (5 cm) apart. Bake in preheated oven for 10 minutes or until golden brown. Place sheet on a wire rack and allow to cool for 3 minutes before removing.

NUTRITIONAL ANALYSIS (PER COOKIE)							
Energy	Protein	Carbohydrate	Fat	Fiber	Calcium	Iron	Sodium
101 kcal	1 g	15 g	4 g	0 g	11 mg	0.3 mg	81 mg

Peanut Butter Cookies

These cookies are huge
favorites with kids (except
in cases of peanut allergy,
of course).

Kitchen Tip

Using reduced-sodium
peanut butter will lower
the sodium content of
this recipe.

- Preheat oven to 375°F (190°C)
- Baking sheet, greased

1 cup	creamy peanut butter	250 mL
½ cup	butter or margarine	125 mL
¾ cup	packed brown sugar	175 mL
½ cup	granulated sugar	125 mL
1	egg	1
1 tsp	vanilla extract	5 mL
1 cup	all-purpose flour	250 mL
1 tsp	baking soda	5 mL
¼ tsp	salt	1 mL

1. In a bowl, with an electric mixer, cream together peanut butter, butter, brown sugar and granulated sugar; beat until light and fluffy. Beat in egg and vanilla.
2. In another bowl, combine flour, baking soda and salt. Gradually stir into peanut butter mixture; blend well.
3. Drop spoonfuls of batter 2 inches (5 cm) apart on prepared baking sheet. Press down with fork. (Dip fork in water, if necessary, to prevent dough from sticking.) Bake in preheated oven for 10 minutes or until golden brown.

NUTRITIONAL ANALYSIS (PER COOKIE)

Energy	Protein	Carbohydrate	Fat	Fiber	Calcium	Iron	Sodium
103 kcal	2 g	11 g	6 g	1 g	9 mg	0.4 mg	105 mg

*These soft cookies are
as delicious as they are
unusual. Kids love them.*

Kitchen Tip

If you have the time, try
making your own pumpkin
purée instead of using the
canned variety for this
recipe. With a sharp knife,
cut a sugar pumpkin in half
and scoop out the seeds. Cut
pumpkin into 1-inch (2 cm)
squares (flesh and rind) and
transfer to a large pot of
boiling water. Cook for about
20 minutes or until tender.
Drain and cool. Remove flesh
from rind and transfer to a
food processor; purée until
smooth. Freeze in batches
for use in recipes throughout
the year.

Soft Pumpkin Cookies

- Preheat oven to 350°F (180°C)
- Baking sheets, ungreased

1½ cups	raisins	375 mL
½ cup	butter or margarine, softened	125 mL
1¼ cups	packed brown sugar	300 mL
1 cup	canned pumpkin purée (not pie filling)	250 mL
2 tbsp	applesauce	30 mL
1	egg	1
1 tsp	vanilla extract	5 mL
½ tsp	ground ginger	2 mL
½ tsp	ground cinnamon	2 mL
2¼ cups	all-purpose flour	550 mL
1 tsp	baking soda	5 mL
1 tsp	baking powder	5 mL

1. In a small bowl, soak raisins in hot water for 5 minutes, then rinse and pat dry with a paper towel. Set aside.
2. In a large bowl, cream together butter and brown sugar until fluffy. Add pumpkin purée, applesauce, egg, vanilla, ginger and cinnamon; beat until well mixed.
3. In another bowl, sift together flour, baking soda and baking powder. Gradually add to pumpkin mixture, stirring until just combined. Stir in raisins.
4. Drop spoonfuls of batter onto baking sheet. Bake in preheated oven for 12 minutes or until golden brown.

NUTRITIONAL ANALYSIS (PER COOKIE)							
Energy	Protein	Carbohydrate	Fat	Fiber	Calcium	Iron	Sodium
64 kcal	0.8 g	12 g	2 g	1 g	10 mg	0.4 mg	45 mg

Makes 25 squares

Easy and quick to make (no more than 10 minutes), these squares combine the great flavors of oatmeal and chocolate.

Kitchen Tip

For a change, try using butterscotch chips instead of chocolate.

Chocolate Oatmeal Squares

- *Preheat oven to 375°F (190°C)*
- *8-inch (2 L) square baking pan, greased*

1¼ cups	all-purpose flour	300 mL
1 cup	large-flake rolled oats	250 mL
½ cup	packed brown sugar	125 mL
½ tsp	ground cinnamon	2 mL
⅔ cup	butter or margarine	150 mL
1 cup	chocolate chips	250 mL

1. In a food processor, combine flour, oats, brown sugar and cinnamon. Add butter and process with on/off turns until mixture resembles coarse crumbs. Set aside ½ cup (125 mL) of mixture; press remainder into bottom of prepared pan.
2. Bake in preheated oven for 10 minutes or until golden brown. Remove from oven and sprinkle chips over surface. Sprinkle with reserved crumbs. Return to oven and bake for 25 minutes or until chocolate has melted and surface is golden brown. Cut into squares while still warm.

NUTRITIONAL ANALYSIS (PER SQUARE)

Energy	Protein	Carbohydrate	Fat	Fiber	Calcium	Iron	Sodium
148 kcal	2 g	18 g	8 g	1 g	9 mg	0.6 mg	36 mg

Raspberry Granola Bars

This snack is also good for breakfast, combining cereal and jam in one bite.

Kitchen Tip
Try making this recipe with other types of jam — strawberry, cherry, blueberry or your favorite.

- *Preheat oven to 375°F (190°C)*
- *8-inch (2 L) square baking pan, greased*

¾ cup	Homemade Microwave Granola (see recipe, page 154)	175 mL
½ cup	graham wafer crumbs	125 mL
¼ cup	butter or margarine, melted	60 mL
1	egg white	1
1½ cups	raspberry jam	375 mL

1. In a bowl, combine granola, graham wafer crumbs, melted butter and egg white; stir until well mixed. Reserve ¼ cup (50 mL) of mixture; press remainder into bottom of prepared pan. Bake in preheated oven for 7 minutes.
2. Spread jam evenly over baked crust. Top with reserved crumbs, return to oven and bake for 30 minutes or until bubbly. Remove from oven and run a sharp knife around edge of pan. Allow to cool completely before cutting into bars.

NUTRITIONAL ANALYSIS (PER BAR)							
Energy	Protein	Carbohydrate	Fat	Fiber	Calcium	Iron	Sodium
126 kcal	1 g	23 g	4 g	1 g	4 mg	0.3 mg	40 mg

Adding dried fruit to classic rice crisp squares gives them extra fiber and nutrients. The cranberries also give them a nice festive look.

Kitchen Tip

To prevent marshmallow mixture from sticking to your hands when pressing into pan, lightly coat your fingers with margarine.

If your kids are accustomed to regular rice crisp treats, they may view any change with suspicion. Try making this recipe with fruit added to only half of the bars, and let the children became used to it gradually.

Fruit Rice Crisp Bars

- *13- by 9-inch (3 L) baking dish, greased*

¼ cup	butter or margarine	60 mL
½	package (8 oz/250 g) marshmallows	½
1 tsp	vanilla extract	5 mL
5 cups	crisp rice cereal	1.25 L
½ cup	dried cranberries or raisins	125 mL

1. In a large saucepan, melt butter over low heat. Stir in marshmallows and vanilla; blend until smooth. Remove from heat. Add rice cereal and dried fruit; stir until well combined. Press into prepared baking dish. Allow to cool completely before cutting into bars.

NUTRITIONAL ANALYSIS (PER BAR)

Energy	Protein	Carbohydrate	Fat	Fiber	Calcium	Iron	Sodium
50 kcal	0.4 g	9 g	2 g	0 g	0.8 mg	2 mg	50 mg

Try this nutritious alternative to sugary frozen treats.

Kitchen Tip

Use a variety of puréed fruits to create different flavors.

Frozen Yogurt Pops

1 cup	plain yogurt	250 mL
¾ cup	frozen fruit juice concentrate, thawed, or puréed fruit	175 mL
¾ cup	2% milk	175 mL

1. In a bowl, combine yogurt, fruit juice concentrate and milk; stir to mix well. Pour into 8 small paper cups; freeze until partially frozen. Insert a wooden stick into center of each; freeze until firm. To serve, peel away paper cups. (Alternatively, pour mixture into an 8-compartment plastic popsicle mold; place handles on top and freeze.)

NUTRITIONAL ANALYSIS (PER POP)

Energy	Protein	Carbohydrate	Fat	Fiber	Calcium	Iron	Sodium
62 kcal	2 g	10 g	0.8 g	0 g	85 mg	0.1 mg	37 mg

Makes 16 slices

Millet is a cereal grain that makes a crunchy addition to this banana bread.

Banana Bread

- *Preheat oven to 350°F (180°C)*
- *9- by 5-inch (2 L) loaf pan, lined with parchment paper or greased*

1 cup	whole wheat or multigrain flour	250 mL
1 cup	all-purpose flour	250 mL
¼ cup	millet	60 mL
1 tsp	baking powder	5 mL
1 tsp	baking soda	5 mL
¼ tsp	salt	1 mL
2	ripe bananas	2
½ cup	packed brown sugar	125 mL
2	eggs	2
½ cup	buttermilk	125 mL
2 tbsp	vegetable oil	30 mL
1 tsp	vanilla extract	5 mL

1. In a large bowl, whisk together whole wheat flour, all-purpose flour, millet, baking powder, baking soda and salt. Set aside.

2. In another bowl, mash bananas. Whisk in sugar, eggs, buttermilk, oil and vanilla. Stir into flour mixture until just combined.

3. Pour into prepared loaf pan. Bake in preheated oven for 45 to 50 minutes or until cake tester inserted in center comes out clean. Let cool in pan on a wire rack for 15 minutes. Remove from pan and let cool on rack.

NUTRITIONAL ANALYSIS (PER SLICE)

Energy	Protein	Carbohydrate	Fat	Fiber	Calcium	Iron	Sodium
132 kcal	3 g	24 g	3 g	2 g	28 mg	0.9 mg	160 mg

Gingerbread is one of the ultimate comfort foods, appealing to young and old alike. The addition of apple gives this gingerbread extra moisture and a fresh flavor. It's the molasses that gives this recipe its boost of iron. Serve as a snack or a dessert.

Kitchen Tip

Serve this gingerbread with applesauce or sweetened whipped cream.

Apple Gingerbread

- *Preheat oven to 350°F (180°C)*
- *13- by 9-inch (3 L) baking pan, greased*

2 cups	all-purpose flour	500 mL
¼ cup	granulated sugar	60 mL
2 tsp	baking powder	10 mL
1 tsp	baking soda	5 mL
1 tsp	ground ginger	5 mL
½ tsp	ground cinnamon	2 mL
½ tsp	ground nutmeg	2 mL
½ tsp	salt	2 mL
½ cup	butter or margarine	125 mL
2	eggs	2
½ cup	molasses	125 mL
⅓ cup	2% milk	75 mL
1	medium apple, peeled and grated	1

1. In a bowl, combine flour, sugar, baking powder, baking soda, spices, and salt. Set aside.

2. In a large bowl, with an electric mixer, cream together butter, eggs and molasses. Stir in dry ingredients, a little at a time, alternating with small additions of milk. Fold in apples. Pour into prepared baking pan.

3. Bake in preheated oven for 35 minutes or until cake tester inserted in center comes out clean. Cool on a wire rack before cutting into 15 pieces.

NUTRITIONAL ANALYSIS (PER PIECE)							
Energy	Protein	Carbohydrate	Fat	Fiber	Calcium	Iron	Sodium
172 kcal	3 g	25 g	7 g	1 g	50 mg	1 mg	293 mg

Applesauce and grated zucchini keep this loaf moist.

Chocolate Zucchini Bread

- *Preheat oven to 350°F (180°C)*
- *9- by 5-inch (2 L) loaf pan, lined with parchment paper or greased*

1 cup	all-purpose flour	250 mL
½ cup	whole wheat flour	125 mL
½ cup	unsweetened cocoa powder	125 mL
1 tsp	baking soda	5 mL
¼ tsp	baking powder	1 mL
¼ tsp	salt	1 mL
⅔ cup	packed brown sugar	150 mL
2	eggs	2
¾ cup	unsweetened applesauce	175 mL
⅓ cup	vegetable oil	75 mL
1 tsp	grated orange zest	5 mL
1 tsp	vanilla extract	5 mL
1 cup	grated zucchini	250 mL

1. In a large bowl, whisk together all-purpose flour, whole wheat flour, cocoa powder, baking soda, baking powder and salt. Set aside.

2. In another bowl, whisk together brown sugar, eggs, applesauce, oil, orange zest and vanilla. Pour over flour mixture and sprinkle with zucchini; stir until just combined.

3. Pour into prepared loaf pan. Bake in preheated oven for 50 to 60 minutes or until cake tester inserted in center comes out clean. Let cool in pan on a wire rack for 15 minutes. Remove from pan and let cool on rack.

NUTRITIONAL ANALYSIS (PER SLICE)							
Energy	Protein	Carbohydrate	Fat	Fiber	Calcium	Iron	Sodium
135 kcal	3 g	20 g	6 g	2 g	19 mg	1 mg	136 mg

Makes 18 slices

This is a wonderfully moist snacking cake. And because it's egg-free, it is also a terrific choice for children with an egg allergy.

Variation

This cake also tastes great with added raisins. Just combine 2 cups (500 mL) raisins with ½ cup (125 mL) of the flour called for in the recipe; toss until well coated (this keeps raisins from sinking to the bottom of the cake); set aside. Proceed with recipe and stir coated raisins into batter just before pouring into the pan.

Applesauce Cake

- *Preheat oven to 350°F (180°C)*
- *9-inch (2.5 L) tube pan, greased and floured*

2 cups	lightly packed brown sugar	500 mL
1 cup	butter or margarine, softened	250 mL
2½ cups	applesauce	625 mL
4 cups	all-purpose flour	1 L
1 tsp	ground cloves	5 mL
1 tsp	ground cinnamon	5 mL
1 tbsp	baking soda	15 mL

1. In a large bowl, with an electric mixer, cream together brown sugar and butter. Stir in applesauce.

2. In another bowl, sift together flour, cloves, cinnamon and baking soda. Add sifted ingredients a little at a time to applesauce mixture, beating after each addition until just combined. Pour into prepared tube pan. Bake in preheated oven for 1 hour or until toothpick inserted in cake comes out clean.

NUTRITIONAL ANALYSIS (PER SLICE)							
Energy	Protein	Carbohydrate	Fat	Fiber	Calcium	Iron	Sodium
287 kcal	3 g	47 g	11 g	1 g	11 mg	1 mg	284 mg

This simple lemon pound cake makes an easy summer dessert, served simply with fresh berries. A slice also makes a fun treat in a lunch box. Pound cake freezes very well.

Lemon Pound Cake

- *Preheat oven to 300°F (150°C)*
- *8-inch (2 L) square baking pan*

3	egg whites	3
1½ cups	granulated sugar, divided	375 mL
½ cup	sour cream	125 mL
½ tsp	baking soda	2 mL
½ cup	butter or margarine, softened	125 mL
3	egg yolks	3
	Juice of 1 lemon	
2 cups	all-purpose flour	500 mL
¾ tsp	baking powder	4 mL

1. In a bowl, with an electric mixer, beat egg whites until soft peaks form. Gradually beat in ¾ cup (175 mL) of the sugar. Set aside.

2. In a measuring cup, stir together sour cream and baking soda. Set aside.

3. In a large bowl, with an electric mixer, cream together butter and remaining sugar. Blend in egg yolks and lemon juice. Add flour and baking powder a little at a time, alternating with additions of sour cream mixture, beating after each addition until just combined.

4. Gently fold in beaten egg whites. Pour batter into prepared pan and bake for 50 minutes or until a toothpick inserted in the cake comes out clean. Allow to cool before serving.

NUTRITIONAL ANALYSIS (PER SLICE)							
Energy	Protein	Carbohydrate	Fat	Fiber	Calcium	Iron	Sodium
176 kcal	3 g	26 g	7 g	0 g	28 mg	0.9 mg	123 mg

Here's the great flavor of cake in the handy shape of a muffin — a real treat for younger children.

Apple Snacking Cupcakes

- Preheat oven to 400°F (200°C)
- 12-cup muffin pan, greased or paper-lined

½ cup	butter or margarine	125 mL
1 cup	granulated sugar	250 mL
2	eggs	2
1 tsp	vanilla extract	5 mL
1 cup	all-purpose flour	250 mL
1 cup	whole wheat flour	250 mL
1 tbsp	baking powder	15 mL
1 tsp	baking soda	5 mL
½ tsp	ground cinnamon	2 mL
½ tsp	ground nutmeg	2 mL
2 cups	unsweetened applesauce	500 mL

1. In a large bowl, with an electric mixer, cream butter and sugar. Blend in eggs and vanilla; beat until light and fluffy.

2. In another bowl, combine all-purpose flour, whole wheat flour, baking powder, baking soda, cinnamon and nutmeg. Add to butter mixture, a little at a time, alternating with applesauce; mix well after each addition.

3. Spoon batter into prepared muffin cups. Bake in preheated oven for 20 minutes or until muffins are firm to the touch. Allow to cool for 10 minutes before removing from pan to wire rack.

NUTRITIONAL ANALYSIS (PER CUPCAKE)							
Energy	Protein	Carbohydrate	Fat	Fiber	Calcium	Iron	Sodium
178 kcal	2 g	25 g	9 g	1 g	35 mg	0.7 mg	308 mg

Desserts

Makes 8 servings

Here's the perfect fruit to serve with vanilla ice cream or yogurt.

Kitchen Tip

For this recipe, pears should be a bit on the firm side. Leave them unpeeled; the skins will turn an attractive deep amber color when roasted.

Honey Roasted Pears

- Preheat oven to 400°F (200°C)
- 13- by 9-inch (3 L) baking dish, greased

8	firm Bosc pears, cut into quarters	8
3 tbsp	butter or margarine	45 mL
¾ cup	apple cider	175 mL
⅓ cup	liquid honey	75 mL
1 tbsp	lemon juice	15 mL
2 tsp	vanilla extract	10 mL

1. Place pears in prepared baking dish. Dot with butter.

2. In a small saucepan, combine cider, honey, lemon juice and vanilla. Bring to a boil. Pour over pears. Cover and bake in preheated oven for 20 minutes. Uncover and bake for another 30 minutes or until pears are tender. Let stand for 10 minutes before serving.

NUTRITIONAL ANALYSIS (PER SERVING)							
Energy	Protein	Carbohydrate	Fat	Fiber	Calcium	Iron	Sodium
201 kcal	0.7 g	42 g	5 g	6 g	18 mg	0.3 mg	33 mg

A combination of popular flavors creates a winning effect in this dessert.

Kitchen Tip

To add an extra-special touch, serve with whipped cream or ice cream.

Apple 'n' Maple Dessert

- *Preheat oven to 375°F (190°C)*
- *8-inch (2 L) square baking pan, greased*

4	large apples, peeled and thinly sliced	4
½ cup	dried cranberries	125 mL
½ cup	maple syrup, divided	125 mL
2	eggs	2
2 tbsp	melted butter or margarine	30 mL
¼ cup	2% milk	60 mL
2 tsp	vanilla extract	10 mL
½ cup	all-purpose flour	125 mL
2 tsp	baking powder	10 mL
	Ground cinnamon	

1. In a bowl, toss together apple slices and cranberries. Transfer to prepared pan and drizzle with ¼ cup (50 mL) of the maple syrup.

2. In a bowl, with an electric mixer, beat eggs until fluffy. Beat in butter, milk, vanilla and remaining maple syrup.

3. In another bowl, stir together flour and baking powder. Add to egg mixture and blend until smooth.

4. Spoon batter evenly over fruit. Sprinkle batter with cinnamon. Bake in preheated oven for 40 minutes or until apples are tender and batter is golden brown.

NUTRITIONAL ANALYSIS (PER SERVING)

Energy	Protein	Carbohydrate	Fat	Fiber	Calcium	Iron	Sodium
275 kcal	4 g	54 g	6 g	3 g	80 mg	1 mg	238 mg

Light and simply delicious, this dessert suits any occasion — and kids love it!

Zesty Lemon Yogurt Mousse

1	package (¼ oz/7 g) unflavored gelatin powder	1
¼ cup	cold water	60 mL
¾ cup	granulated sugar, divided	175 mL
	Grated zest of 1 lemon	
½ cup	fresh lemon juice	125 mL
1 cup	plain yogurt	250 mL
⅔ cup	half-and-half (10%) cream	150 mL

1. In a small saucepan, sprinkle gelatin over cold water; let stand for 1 minute to soften. Stir over low heat until gelatin is dissolved. Remove from heat and stir in half the sugar and the lemon zest and lemon juice. Stir in yogurt.

2. In a bowl, whisk together remaining sugar and cream until sugar is dissolved; fold into lemon mixture.

3. Spoon into 6 serving dishes. Cover and refrigerate for at least 2 hours, until chilled, or for up to 1 day.

NUTRITIONAL ANALYSIS (PER SERVING)							
Energy	Protein	Carbohydrate	Fat	Fiber	Calcium	Iron	Sodium
96 kcal	3 g	18 g	2 g	0 g	79 mg	0.1 mg	36 mg

Chocolate Banana Pudding

2¹⁄₃ cups	2% milk, divided	575 mL
¹⁄₂ cup	granulated sugar	125 mL
1	egg	1
¹⁄₃ cup	unsweetened cocoa powder	75 mL
3 tbsp	cornstarch	45 mL
1	banana, sliced	1
1 tsp	vanilla extract	5 mL

1. In a large saucepan, combine 2 cups (500 mL) of the milk and the sugar. Heat over medium heat, stirring to dissolve sugar, until bubbles form around edge of pan.
2. Meanwhile, in a large bowl, whisk together remaining milk, egg, cocoa powder and cornstarch until smooth. While whisking briskly, gradually add hot milk mixture. Pour back into saucepan and cook, stirring constantly, for 8 to 10 minutes or until thickened (do not let boil). Remove from heat.
3. Stir in banana and vanilla. Serve warm or pour into a bowl, place plastic wrap directly on surface of pudding and refrigerate for about 2 hours, until chilled.

NUTRITIONAL ANALYSIS (PER SERVING)							
Energy	Protein	Carbohydrate	Fat	Fiber	Calcium	Iron	Sodium
154 kcal	6 g	28 g	4 g	2 g	147 mg	0.9 mg	59 mg

As easy to make as it is delicious, this old-fashioned dessert will please all members of the family. The soft custard (often called crème Anglaise) can be served hot or cold over cake or fruit, or, as here, with meringues floating in it.

Kitchen Tip

If you have a vanilla bean, add it to the milk while it is warming. Remove from milk before poaching meringues.

Floating Islands

2 cups	2% milk	500 mL
4	eggs, separated, at room temperature	4
½ cup	granulated sugar, divided	125 mL
1 tsp	vanilla extract (see tip, at left)	5 mL
	Assorted fresh fruit	

1. In a large skillet, bring milk to a simmer over medium heat, stirring occasionally (do not let boil).

2. Meanwhile, in a medium bowl, beat egg whites until soft peaks form. Gradually beat in ¼ cup (60 mL) of the sugar; beat until whites are stiff but not dry. Scoop up small spoonfuls and drop into the simmering milk; poach 4 spoonfuls at a time, turning once, for about 3 minutes per side. Using a slotted spoon, transfer meringues to a dessert plate. Repeat until all whites have been used, dividing meringues evenly among 4 plates.

3. In a large bowl, whisk together egg yolks and remaining sugar until light and slightly thickened. While whisking briskly, gradually ladle hot poaching milk into egg yolk mixture. Pour back into skillet. Reduce heat to low and cook, stirring constantly, until mixture thickens enough to coat the back of a metal spoon (do not let boil). Strain, if necessary. Stir in vanilla.

4. Ladle custard around meringues. Serve with fruit.

NUTRITIONAL ANALYSIS (PER SERVING)

Energy	Protein	Carbohydrate	Fat	Fiber	Calcium	Iron	Sodium
187 kcal	10 g	24 g	7 g	0 g	166 mg	0.8 mg	112 mg

Speedy Rice Pudding with Golden Raisins

- *8-cup (2 L) microwave-safe casserole with lid*

3½ cups	2% milk	875 mL
¼ cup	long-grain white rice	60 mL
¼ cup	long-grain brown rice	60 mL
½ cup	granulated sugar	125 mL
1	cinnamon stick	1
1	egg	1
⅓ cup	golden raisins	75 mL
1 tsp	vanilla extract	5 mL

1. In casserole, combine milk, white rice, brown rice, sugar and cinnamon stick. Cook, uncovered, on High for 7 minutes or until boiling. Cook, stirring every 5 minutes, on Medium-High for another 20 minutes or until rice is tender.

2. In a small bowl, whisk together egg with ¼ cup (50 mL) of the hot rice mixture. Return egg mixture to casserole and stir well

3. Stir in raisins and cook on Medium for 3 minutes or until slightly thickened. Remove and discard cinnamon stick; stir in vanilla. Let pudding stand for 5 minutes before serving. Serve warm or cover and refrigerate.

NUTRITIONAL ANALYSIS (PER SERVING)

Energy	Protein	Carbohydrate	Fat	Fiber	Calcium	Iron	Sodium
206 kcal	7 g	38 g	4 g	1 g	177 mg	0.8 mg	71 mg

Arroz con leche *is Spanish for "rice with milk," and this recipe makes a wonderful creamy rice pudding, cooked in milk. It also has a touch of cinnamon, along with vanilla and raisins. It's a hit with all ages, especially when served warm.*

Arroz con Leche

2 cups	2% milk	500 mL
2/3 cup	short- or medium-grain rice	150 mL
1	cinnamon stick (about 3 inches/7.5 cm)	1
1	can (14 oz or 300 mL) sweetened condensed milk	1
1/2 cup	golden raisins	125 mL
1 tsp	vanilla extract	5 mL

1. In a saucepan, combine 2% milk, $3/4$ cup (175 mL) water, rice and cinnamon stick; bring to a boil over medium heat. Reduce heat to low and simmer, stirring frequently, for 15 minutes or until rice is softened. Discard cinnamon stick.

2. Stir in condensed milk, raisins and vanilla. Simmer, stirring occasionally, for 15 minutes or until most of the liquid is absorbed, raisins are plump and rice has a pudding-like consistency. Serve warm.

NUTRITIONAL ANALYSIS (PER SERVING)							
Energy	Protein	Carbohydrate	Fat	Fiber	Calcium	Iron	Sodium
369 kcal	10 g	65 g	8 g	2 g	293 mg	0.9 mg	120 mg

Here's a sensational variation on apple crisp — one of our all-time favorites. The "Scotch" in the title refers to the oatmeal crisp topping.

Kitchen Tip

Use apples or pears — or a combination. For added color, try adding a few cranberries.

Scotch Custard Apple Pudding

- *Preheat oven to 350°F (180°C)*
- *8-inch (2 L) square shallow baking pan, greased*

4 cups	sliced peeled apples or pears (about 4 medium)	1 L
¾ cup	packed brown sugar	175 mL
½ cup	rolled oats	125 mL
½ cup	all-purpose flour	125 mL
⅓ cup	butter or margarine	75 mL
⅔ cup	2% milk	150 mL
1	egg	1
1 tsp	vanilla extract	5 mL
	Ground cinnamon	

1. Arrange fruit in prepared pan.

2. In a food processor or blender, combine brown sugar, oats, flour and butter. Process with on/off turns until mixture resembles coarse crumbs. Sprinkle over fruit.

3. In a small bowl, whisk together milk, egg and vanilla. Pour over crumb mixture. Sprinkle lightly with cinnamon. Bake in a preheated oven for 45 minutes or until bubbly and top is golden brown. Serve warm or at room temperature.

NUTRITIONAL ANALYSIS (PER SERVING)							
Energy	Protein	Carbohydrate	Fat	Fiber	Calcium	Iron	Sodium
322 kcal	4 g	51 g	12 g	2 g	72 mg	1 mg	102 mg

This old-fashioned dessert is a natural candidate for adding to your "all-time favorites" recipe file.

Kitchen Tip

Choose from a wide variety of fruits, including peaches, apples, berries, rhubarb and pitted sour cherries. See chart (below, right) for preparation instructions.

Fruit Crisp

- *Preheat oven to 350°F (180°C)*
- *7- by 11-inch (2 L) baking pan*

5 cups	prepared fruit (see tip, at left)	1.25 L
1 cup	packed brown sugar	250 mL
1 cup	all-purpose flour	250 mL
¾ cup	quick-cooking rolled oats	175 mL
1 tsp	ground cinnamon	5 mL
½ tsp	ground nutmeg	2 mL
½ cup	butter or margarine	125 mL

1. Arrange prepared fruit in baking pan.

2. In a bowl, combine brown sugar, flour, rolled oats, cinnamon and nutmeg. Cut in butter until crumbly. Sprinkle mixture over fruit. Bake in preheated oven for 40 minutes or until fruit is cooked and topping is golden brown.

NUTRITIONAL ANALYSIS (PER SERVING)							
Energy	Protein	Carbohydrate	Fat	Fiber	Calcium	Iron	Sodium
442 kcal	5 g	72 g	17 g	3 g	57 mg	2 mg	120 mg

Preparing Fruit for Crisps and Cobblers

FRUIT	PREPARATION
Apples and peaches	Peel, core and cut into slices.
Blueberries	Pick over. Remove and discard stems. Wash.
Rhubarb	Cut into small pieces and toss with ⅔ cup (150 mL) granulated sugar.
Sour cherries	Wash, pit and toss with ¾ cup (175 mL) granulated sugar.
Strawberry-rhubarb combination	Hull and slice strawberries. Cut rhubarb into small pieces and toss with ¾ cup (175 mL) granulated sugar.

Pumpkin is not just for Thanksgiving, and fruit crisps are not just for fall. This crisp is cut into squares, which will keep for several days in the refrigerator.

Crustless Pumpkin Crisp

- *Preheat oven to 350°F (180°C)*
- *11- by 7-inch (2 L) glass baking dish, greased*

½ cup	lightly packed brown sugar	125 mL
2	eggs	2
1	can (14 oz/398 mL) pumpkin purée (not pie filling)	1
1 cup	low-fat evaporated milk	250 mL
1 tsp	ground cinnamon	5 mL
½ tsp	ground nutmeg	2 mL
½ tsp	ground ginger	2 mL
1 tsp	vanilla extract	5 mL

Crisp Topping

1 cup	large-flake (old-fashioned) rolled oats	250 mL
½ cup	lightly packed brown sugar	125 mL
2 tbsp	all-purpose flour	30 mL
½ tsp	ground cinnamon	2 mL
½ tsp	ground nutmeg	2 mL
⅓ cup	butter or margarine	75 mL

1. In a medium bowl, whisk together brown sugar, eggs, pumpkin, milk, cinnamon, nutmeg, ginger and vanilla. Pour into prepared baking dish.

2. *Crisp Topping:* In another bowl, combine rolled oats, brown sugar, flour, cinnamon and nutmeg. Cut in butter with two knives. Sprinkle over pumpkin mixture.

3. Bake in preheated oven for 40 minutes or until firm in center. Let cool completely in pan on a wire rack. Cover and refrigerate until set, then cut into squares.

NUTRITIONAL ANALYSIS (PER SQUARE)							
Energy	Protein	Carbohydrate	Fat	Fiber	Calcium	Iron	Sodium
257 kcal	6 g	40 g	9 g	2 g	115 mg	0.8 mg	159 mg

This versatile cobbler recipe combines your favorite fruit with a thick biscuit crust. Delicious served hot or cold!

Kitchen Tip

This recipe works well with sliced apples or peaches, pears, blueberries, pitted cherries or plums. See page 326 for preparation instructions.

For a special treat, serve with a scoop of ice cream or frozen vanilla yogurt.

Fruit Cobbler

* *Preheat oven to 350°F (180°C)*
* *13- by 9-inch (3 L) baking pan, greased*

6 cups	prepared fruit (see tip, at left)	1.5 L
3/4 cup	granulated sugar	175 mL
1 tbsp	tapioca	15 mL
2 tsp	grated lemon zest	10 mL

Batter

1 1/4 cups	all-purpose flour	300 mL
1/3 cup	cornmeal	75 mL
1/3 cup	granulated sugar	75 mL
2 1/2 tsp	baking powder	12 mL
1/4 tsp	baking soda	1 mL
1/4 tsp	salt	1 mL
1/3 cup	butter or margarine	75 mL
1 1/3 cups	buttermilk	325 mL
1 tbsp	granulated sugar	15 mL
1 tsp	ground cinnamon	5 mL

1. In a bowl, combine fruit, sugar, tapioca and zest. Transfer to prepared pan. Allow to stand for 15 minutes.

2. Meanwhile, in a food processor or blender, combine flour, cornmeal, sugar, baking powder, baking soda and salt; process until mixed. Add butter and process with on/off turns until mixture resembles coarse crumbs.

3. In a large bowl, combine flour-butter mixture and buttermilk; stir just until moistened. Spoon batter over fruit. Sprinkle with sugar and cinnamon. Bake in preheated oven for 30 minutes or until topping is golden and fruit bubbles around sides. Serve warm or cold.

NUTRITIONAL ANALYSIS (PER SERVING)							
Energy	Protein	Carbohydrate	Fat	Fiber	Calcium	Iron	Sodium
236 kcal	4 g	44 g	7 g	2 g	88 mg	1 mg	328 mg

Instead of a birthday cake, why not try a birthday cookie? This one is always a favorite at kids' birthday parties.

Chocolate Chip Pizza Cookie

* *Preheat oven to 350°F (180°C)*
* *Baking sheet, greased*

⅓ cup	butter or margarine	75 mL
½ cup	packed brown sugar (preferably golden brown)	125 mL
¼ cup	granulated sugar	60 mL
1	egg	1
1 tsp	vanilla extract	5 mL
1½ cups	all-purpose flour	375 mL
½ tsp	baking soda	2 mL
¼ tsp	salt	1 mL
1½ cups	chocolate chips	375 mL

1. In a bowl, with an electric mixer, cream together butter, brown sugar, granulated sugar, egg and vanilla. Blend in flour, baking soda and salt. Stir in chocolate chips.

2. Place dough on baking sheet and roll or pat into large round circle (like a pizza). Bake in preheated oven for 8 minutes or until golden brown. Cut into 16 pizza wedges and serve.

NUTRITIONAL ANALYSIS (PER WEDGE)							
Energy	Protein	Carbohydrate	Fat	Fiber	Calcium	Iron	Sodium
233 kcal	3 g	33 g	10 g	0 g	10 mg	0.6 mg	108 mg

No fuss, no muss — these scrumptious treats require only one bowl for mixing.

Kitchen Tips

To make a peanut-free version of this recipe (in cases of peanut allergy, for example), replace peanut butter with an equal amount of butter or margarine.

To prevent batter from sticking when pressing it into the baking pan, lightly coat your hands with oil.

Peanut Butter Brownies

- *Preheat oven to 350°F (180°C)*
- *8-inch (2 L) square baking pan, greased*

¾ cup	cake-and-pastry flour	175 mL
¾ cup	granulated sugar	175 mL
⅓ cup	unsweetened cocoa	75 mL
½ tsp	baking powder	2 mL
½ tsp	salt	2 mL
¼ cup	butter or margarine, softened	60 mL
¼ cup	creamy peanut butter (see tip, at left)	60 mL
1	egg	1
1 tsp	vanilla extract	5 mL

1. In a large bowl, combine flour, sugar, cocoa, baking powder and salt. Make a hole in center and stir in butter, peanut butter, egg and vanilla. Stir until fairly smooth. Press batter into prepared pan. Bake in preheated oven for 25 minutes or until cake tester inserted in center comes out clean. Cool on wire rack before cutting into 16 squares.

NUTRITIONAL ANALYSIS (PER BROWNIE)							
Energy	Protein	Carbohydrate	Fat	Fiber	Calcium	Iron	Sodium
104 kcal	2 g	14 g	5 g	1 g	7 mg	0.7 mg	133 mg

Also known as "matrimonial squares," these delicious date squares are a terrific source of iron!

Date Squares

- *Preheat oven to 350°F (180°C)*
- *8-inch (2 L) square baking dish, ungreased*

1½ cups	rolled oats	375 mL
1½ cups	all-purpose flour	375 mL
1⅓ cups	packed brown sugar, divided	325 mL
¼ tsp	salt	1 mL
½ tsp	baking soda	2 mL
¾ cup	butter, softened	175 mL
1 lb	pitted dates, chopped	500 g
1¼ cups	water	300 mL
1 tsp	lemon juice	5 mL

1. In a large bowl, combine rolled oats, flour, 1 cup (250 mL) of the brown sugar, salt and baking soda. With pastry blender or with a pair of knives, cut butter into dry ingredients until mixture resembles coarse crumbs. Set aside.

2. In a saucepan over medium heat, combine dates, water and remaining brown sugar. Bring to a boil and cook for 5 minutes or until thickened. Remove from heat and stir in lemon juice.

3. *Assembly:* Lightly press one-half of oat mixture into baking dish. Spread filling over base, then crumble remaining oat mixture on top. Bake in preheated oven for 20 minutes or until golden brown. Cool on wire rack before cutting into 16 squares.

NUTRITIONAL ANALYSIS (PER SQUARE)							
Energy	Protein	Carbohydrate	Fat	Fiber	Calcium	Iron	Sodium
307 kcal	3 g	56 g	9 g	3 g	41 mg	1 mg	143 mg

This moist and delicious cake combines apples with the wonderful aromas of cinnamon and nutmeg. Apples are a great fruit to bake with, and they are readily accesible all year round. This cake is perfect for little hands and works equally well as a dessert or as a mid-day snack!

Apple Cake

- *Preheat oven to 400°F (200°C)*
- *8-inch (2 L) square baking pan, greased*

1 cup	all-purpose flour	250 mL
1 tsp	baking soda	5 mL
1 tsp	ground cinnamon	5 mL
¾ tsp	ground nutmeg	4 mL
¼ tsp	salt	1 mL
¼ cup	butter or margarine, softened	60 mL
1 cup	granulated sugar	250 mL
1	egg	1
2 cups	sliced peeled apples	500 mL

1. In a bowl, combine flour, baking soda, cinnamon, nutmeg and salt; stir to mix well.

2. In a bowl, with an electric mixer, cream together butter and sugar. Blend in egg. Fold in apple slices. Gradually add flour mixture, stirring after each addition. Pour batter into prepared pan. Bake in preheated oven for 30 minutes or until toothpick inserted in center comes out clean. Cool on a wire rack before serving.

NUTRITIONAL ANALYSIS (PER SERVING)							
Energy	Protein	Carbohydrate	Fat	Fiber	Calcium	Iron	Sodium
95 kcal	1 g	17 g	3 g	1 g	6 mg	0.4 mg	140 mg

Makes 12 servings

What's the "surprise" in this cake? Well, how about beets? Seriously! They add great flavor and texture, as well as good nutrition (they're a good source of iron and folate). And this cake is so moist, you don't need any icing.

Kitchen Tips

For a chocolate-mint flavor, add ¾ tsp (4 mL) peppermint extract.

If making a cake with beets is just a little too "surprising" for you, replace them with 4 bananas, mashed, and ½ cup (125 mL) milk.

Chocolate Surprise Cake

- *Preheat oven to 325°F (160°C)*
- *8-inch (2 L) square baking pan, greased*

1¾ cups	all-purpose flour	425 mL
6 tbsp	cocoa powder	90 mL
1½ tsp	baking powder	7 mL
¼ tsp	salt	1 mL
1	can (19 oz/540 g) beets, drained and puréed	1
1 cup	granulated sugar	250 mL
½ cup	packed brown sugar	125 mL
¾ cup	vegetable oil	175 mL
¼ cup	butter or margarine, softened	60 mL
2	eggs	2
1 tsp	vanilla extract	5 mL

1. In a bowl, sift together flour, cocoa powder, baking powder and salt.

2. In a bowl, with an electric mixer, combine beets, granulated sugar, brown sugar, oil, butter, eggs and vanilla. Beat slowly until blended, then on high for 1 to 2 minutes or until thoroughly mixed. Gradually blend in flour-cocoa mixture.

3. Transfer batter to prepared baking pan and bake for 40 minutes or until toothpick inserted in center comes out clean. Cool on a wire rack before serving.

NUTRITIONAL ANALYSIS (PER SERVING)							
Energy	Protein	Carbohydrate	Fat	Fiber	Calcium	Iron	Sodium
332 kcal	4 g	41 g	19 g	2 g	35 mg	2 mg	250 mg

Makes 12 servings

Most kids love chocolate and bananas. No wonder this cake is so popular!

Kitchen Tip

This recipe is a great use for any overripe bananas that have been lurking in the freezer waiting to be used.

Chocolate Chip and Banana Cake

- *Preheat oven to 350°F (180°C)*
- *13- by 9-inch (3 L) baking pan, greased*

⅓ cup	butter or margarine, softened	75 mL
½ cup	granulated sugar	125 mL
½ cup	lightly packed brown sugar	125 mL
3	eggs	3
3	mashed ripe bananas	3
2 tsp	vanilla extract	10 mL
1½ cups	all-purpose flour	375 mL
½ cup	whole wheat flour	125 mL
1 tbsp	baking powder	15 mL
½ tsp	baking soda	2 mL
½ tsp	salt	2 mL
1 cup	2% milk	250 mL
1	package (12 oz/375 g) chocolate chips	1

1. In a bowl, with an electric mixer, cream together butter, granulated sugar and brown sugar; beat until light and fluffy. Beat in eggs, one at a time. Blend in bananas and vanilla.
2. In another bowl, combine all-purpose flour, whole wheat flour, baking powder, baking soda and salt. Stir into egg mixture, a little at a time, alternately with milk. Stir in chocolate chips.
3. Transfer batter to prepared pan and bake in preheated oven for about 35 minutes or until tester inserted in center comes out clean. Cool on a wire rack before slicing.

NUTRITIONAL ANALYSIS (PER SERVING)							
Energy	Protein	Carbohydrate	Fat	Fiber	Calcium	Iron	Sodium
357 kcal	6 g	55 g	13 g	2 g	61 mg	1 mg	346 mg

Orange Bundt Cake

Full of tangy citrus flavor, this is one of our favorites.

Kitchen Tip

This cake is excellent when served with your choice of seasonal fresh fruit. Try sliced strawberries, peaches, nectarines or apricots.

- *Preheat oven to 350°F (180°C)*
- *10-inch (3 L) Bundt pan, greased and floured*

½ cup	butter or margarine	125 mL
2½ cups	granulated sugar, divided	625 mL
2	eggs	2
1¼ cups	plain yogurt	300 mL
	Zest of 1 orange	
2 cups	all-purpose flour	500 mL
2 tsp	baking powder	10 mL
½ cup	fresh orange juice	125 mL

1. In a bowl, with an electric mixer, cream together butter and 2 cups (500 mL) of the sugar; beat until light and fluffy. Beat in eggs until blended.

2. In a small bowl, combine yogurt and orange zest; set aside.

3. In another bowl, combine flour and baking powder. Stir into butter mixture, a little at a time, alternating with yogurt mixture.

4. Spoon batter into prepared pan. Bake in preheated oven for 50 minutes or until tester inserted in center comes out clean. Remove from oven to rack and cool for 5 minutes. Invert cake onto a plate with a rim. Insert a toothpick, 1 inch (2.5 cm) deep, several times into surface of cake.

5. In a measuring cup, whisk together orange juice and remaining ½ cup (125 mL) sugar. Drizzle mixture over warm cake. Allow to cool before serving.

NUTRITIONAL ANALYSIS (PER SERVING)

Energy	Protein	Carbohydrate	Fat	Fiber	Calcium	Iron	Sodium
277 kcal	4 g	49 g	9 g	1 g	70 mg	1 mg	175 mg

Makes 12 servings

The mixture of chocolate and orange makes this a nice change from plain chocolate cake, and the orange juice glaze makes it extra-moist and absolutely delicious. It's a favorite with all ages!

Orange and Chocolate Marble Cake

- *Preheat oven to 350°F (180°C)*
- *8-inch (2 L) baking pan, greased*

1 cup	butter or margarine, softened	250 mL
1 cup	granulated sugar	250 mL
3	egg yolks	3
1¾ cups	all-purpose flour	425 mL
¾ tsp	baking soda	4 mL
¾ tsp	baking powder	4 mL
1 cup	plain yogurt	250 mL
	Grated zest of 1 orange	1
2 oz	unsweetened chocolate, melted (see tip, at right)	50 g
3	egg whites	3
Pinch	cream of tartar	Pinch

Glaze

½ cup	orange juice	125 mL
¼ cup	granulated sugar	60 mL

1. In a bowl, with an electric mixer, cream together butter and sugar. Beat in egg yolks, one at a time.

2. In another bowl, sift together flour, baking soda and baking powder. Add to butter mixture a little at a time, alternating with additions of yogurt. Beat after each addition until combined.

3. Divide batter between two clean bowls. Into one bowl, stir in orange zest. Stir melted chocolate into the other.

4. In another bowl, with an electric mixer, beat egg whites until foamy. Add cream of tartar; beat whites to form stiff peaks. Gently fold one-half of the whites into the orange batter and one-half of the whites into the chocolate batter.

Kitchen Tip

To melt chocolate, microwave on High for about 1 minute or until soft, then stir until completely melted and smooth.

5. Place batters alternately by spoonful into baking pan. Bake in preheated oven for 1 hour and 10 minutes or until tester inserted in center comes out clean. Let cool for 5 minutes.

6. *Glaze:* In a small bowl, whisk together orange juice and sugar. Pour glaze over cake while still in pan. Let cool completely and serve.

NUTRITIONAL ANALYSIS (PER SERVING)

Energy	Protein	Carbohydrate	Fat	Fiber	Calcium	Iron	Sodium
309 kcal	5 g	33 g	19 g	1 g	60 mg	2 mg	253 mg

Pineapple gives this cake its wonderful tropical flavor — and helps to keep it moist for several days.

Kitchen Tip

If you wish, use any leftover pineapple to make a frosting: In a bowl, with an electric mixer, cream ¼ cup (60 mL) butter or margarine until light and fluffy. Gradually beat in confectioner's (icing) sugar, ¼ cup (60 mL) at a time, adding extra crushed pineapple and juice as mixture thickens. (You will probably use about 1½ cups/375 mL sugar, depending on amount of pineapple and juice added.)

Pineapple Sour Cream Cake

- *Preheat oven to 350°F (180°C)*
- *13- by 9-inch (3 L) baking pan, greased*

2 cups	cake-and-pastry flour	500 mL
2 tsp	baking powder	10 mL
1 tsp	baking soda	5 mL
¼ cup	butter or margarine	60 mL
2	eggs	2
1 cup	granulated sugar	250 mL
1 cup	crushed canned pineapple and juice	250 mL
¾ cup	sour cream	175 mL

1. In a bowl, combine flour, baking powder and baking soda. Set aside.

2. In a bowl, with an electric mixer, beat butter and eggs until frothy. Gradually add sugar, beating until very thick. Stir in pineapple. Add flour mixture alternately with sour cream, ending with flour; stir well after each addition.

3. Spread batter in prepared pan. Bake in preheated oven for 30 minutes or until tester inserted in center comes out clean. Cool completely on wire rack before cutting into pieces.

NUTRITIONAL ANALYSIS (PER SERVING)							
Energy	Protein	Carbohydrate	Fat	Fiber	Calcium	Iron	Sodium
241 kcal	5 g	42 g	7 g	0 g	65 mg	2 mg	294 mg

Pink is a favorite color for many children — as is this rosy, warming dessert.

Cranberry Applesauce

1 cup	apple juice or sweet apple cider	250 mL
½ cup	liquid honey	125 mL
2 tbsp	brown sugar	30 mL
2 cups	fresh or frozen cranberries	500 mL
3 cups	chopped peeled apples	750 mL
½ tsp	ground cinnamon	2 mL

1. In a saucepan over medium-high heat, combine apple juice, honey and sugar. Bring to a boil. Add cranberries and apples. Reduce heat to medium and cook, uncovered, for 10 minutes or until fruit is tender and sauce has thickened.

2. Remove from heat and allow to cool. Add cinnamon and taste for seasoning. For a smoother texture (which young children may prefer), purée mixture in a food processor or blender.

NUTRITIONAL ANALYSIS (PER ½ CUP/125 ML)

Energy	Protein	Carbohydrate	Fat	Fiber	Calcium	Iron	Sodium
171 kcal	0.2 g	43 g	0.1 g	2 g	5 mg	0.1 mg	5 mg

Makes 1¼ cups
(300 mL)

Tangy Fruit Sauce

This sauce is wonderful served on pancakes (see page 144), as a topping for ice cream or with angel food cake.

¼ cup	granulated sugar	60 mL
2 tbsp	cornstarch	30 mL
½ cup	orange juice	125 mL
½ cup	water	125 mL
1 cup	sliced strawberries, raspberries, blueberries or sour cherries	250 mL
1 tsp	grated lemon zest	5 mL
1 tbsp	lemon juice	15 mL

1. In a saucepan over medium heat, combine sugar, cornstarch, orange juice and water; bring to a boil. Reduce heat and cook, stirring constantly, until sauce has thickened. Stir in fruit, zest and lemon juice. Serve warm or cover and refrigerate until needed.

NUTRITIONAL ANALYSIS (PER ¼ CUP/60 ML)

Energy	Protein	Carbohydrate	Fat	Fiber	Calcium	Iron	Sodium
49 kcal	0 g	13 g	0 g	1 g	8 mg	0.2 mg	1 mg

Do you want to raise happier, healthier children? So do we.

Join the SickKids Family Knowledge Group and be part of the SickKids vision:

Healthier Children. A Better World.™

Don't Miss This Opportunity!

SickKids is looking for volunteer reviewers and editors (no experience necessary!) to ensure that the books SickKids publishes are interesting, educational, written in plain English, and genuinely help caregivers provide the best care for children.

If this interests you, please join the SickKids Family Knowledge Group (SKFKG). Membership is FREE and signing up is QUICK and EASY.

Just visit **www.skfamilyknowledgegroup.ca** or call **416-813-7654, ext 2971**.

Members will receive invitations directly to their inbox and can choose projects at their convenience. No matter what, members will receive timely and relevant information and practical tips via email from SickKids on important child health and wellness topics.

We look forward to hearing your opinions and ideas.

The SKFKG Management Team

SickKids®

Resources for Parents

American Food Safety
www.foodsafety.gov

American Academy of Pediatrics
141 Northwest Point Boulevard
Elk Grove Village, IL 60007-1098
USA
www.aap.org

American Dietetic Association
216 W. Jackson Blvd.
Chicago, IL 60606-6995
www.eatright.org

Anaphylaxis Network of Canada
www.anaphylaxis.org

Body Image
www.bodypositive.org

Canadian Pediatric Society
2204 Walkley Road, Suite 100
Ottawa, ON Canada
K1G 4G8
www.cps.ca

Canadian Organic Advisory Board
www.coab.ca

Canadian Organic Growers
www.cog.ca

Dietitians of Canada
480 University Avenue, Suite 604
Toronto, ON Canada
M5G 1V2
www.dietitians.ca

Food Allergy Network of Canada
www.foodallergy.org

FAO — Food and Agriculture Organization
www.fao.org/organicag

Health Canada
A.L. 0900C2
Ottawa, ON Canada
K1A 0K9
www.hc-sc.gc.ca
Food labeling
www.hc-sc.gc.ca/hppb/nutrition/labels/
e_before.html
Canada's Food Guide to Healthy Eating
www.hc-sc.gc.ca/hppb/nutrition/pube/
foodguid/index.html

U.S. Food and Drug Administration
5600 Fishers Lane, Rockville, MD
20857-0001
1-888-INFO-FDA (1-888-463-6332)
www.fda.gov
The Food Pyramid
www.nal.usda.gov/fnic/Fpyr/pyramid.gif

Specialty Food Shop
The Hospital for Sick Children
555 University Ave.
Toronto, ON Canada
M5G 1X8
1-800-SFS-7976 or 416-977-4360
(Wide product selection. Purchase
wheat-free, milk-free, egg-free products.
Dietitians available to answer questions.)
www.specialtyfoodshop.com

Library and Archives Canada Cataloguing in Publication

Saab, Joanne
    Better food for kids : your essential guide to nutrition for all children from age 2 to 10 /
Joanne Saab and Daina Kalnins. — 2nd ed.

Includes bibliographical references and index.
ISBN 978-0-7788-0251-8

    1. Cookery. 2. Children—Nutrition. I. Kalnins, Daina II. Title.

TX740.S15 2010   641.5'622   C2010-903264-0

References

General

Bates H. Food or pharmacy? An introduction to functional foods and nutraceuticals. Dietitians of Canada — Current Issues. 2007 Feb.

Eriksson E. Children who often drink full-fat milk weigh less. Master's Thesis, University of Gothenburg. 2009, November 4.

Fogarty AW et al. A natural experiment on the impact of fruit supplementation on asthma symptoms in children. Eur Resp J 2009;33:481–85.

Fulkerson JA et al. Family meals: Perceptions of benefits and challenges among parents of 8- to 10-year-old children. JADA 2008;108:706–9.

Heart and Stroke Foundation Report on the Health of Ontario's Kids. Toronto, ON: Heart and Stroke Foundation; 2009.

Larson NI et al. Family meals during adolescence are associated with higher diet quality and healthful meal patterns during young adulthood. JADA 2007;107:1502–10.

Nicklas T et al. Children's food consumption patterns have changed over two decades (1973–1994): The Bogalusa heart study. JADA 2004;104:1127–40.

O'Connor TM et al. Beverage intake among preschool children and its effect on weight status. Pediatrics 2006;118:1010–18.

Wilschanski M, Branski D. Recurrent abdominal pain in children: Is constipation an issue? IMAJ 2004;6:697–98.

Young people in Canada: Their health and well-being. Chapter 7: Healthy Living. Part of WHO Healthy Behavior in School-aged Children Survey, Canadian Component, 2001–02.

Allergy

Greer FR et al. Effects of early nutritional interventions on the development of atopic disease in infants and children: The role of maternal dietary restriction, breastfeeding, timing of introduction of complementary foods, and hydrolyzed formulas. Pediatr 2008;121:183–91.

Bone Health

Clark EM et al. Association between bone density and fractures in children: A systematic review and meta-analysis. Pediatrics. 2006;117:e291–97.

Poliquin S et al. Calcium and vitamin D intakes in an adult Canadian population. Can J Diet Res 2009;70:21–27.

Vatanparast H et al. Many adult Canadians are not meeting current calcium recommendations from food and supplement intake. Appl Physiol Nutr Metabol 2009;34: 191–96.

Whiting SJ et al. Factors that affects bone mineral accrual in the adolescent growth spurt. J Nutr 2004;134:696S–700S.

Exercise

Dobbins M et al. School-based physical activity programs for promoting physical activity and fitness in children and adolescents aged 6–18. Cochrane database of systematic reviews. 2009; 1 Art No. CD007651.

Rodriguez NR et al. Position of the American Dietetic Association, Dietitians of Canada, and the American College of Sports Medicine: Nutrition and athletic performance. JADA 2009;109:509–27.

Tremblay MS et al. Fitness of Canadian children and youth: Results from the 2007–2009 Canadian health measures survey. Statistics Canada, Catalogue No. 82-003-XPE Health Reports; Mar 2009.

Nutrition in Schools and Day Cares

Position of the American Dietetic Association, Society for Nutrition Education, and American School Food Service Association — Nutrition services: An essential component of comprehensive school health programs. JADA 2003;103:505–14.

Position of the American Dietetic Association: Benchmarks for nutrition programs in child care settings. JADA 2005;105:979–86.

School Food and Beverage Policy Ontario, Policy/ Program Memorandum No. 150, 2010.

Obesity

American Academy of Pediatrics — Committee on Nutrition. Policy Statement. Prevention of pediatric overweight and obesity. Pediatr 2003;112(2):424–30.

Barr-Anderson DJ et al. Characteristics associated with older adolescents who have a television in their bedrooms. Pediatrics 2008;121(4):718–24.

Brownell KD et al. The public health and economic benefits of taxing sugar-sweetened beverages. NEJM 2009;361(16):1599–1605.

Daniels SR, Greer FR and the Committee on Nutrition. Lipid screening and cardiovascular health in childhood. Pediatrics 2008;122:198–208.

Dietz WH, Robinson TN. Overweight children and adolescents. NEJM 2005;352:2100–09.

Gillman MW et al. Family dinner and diet quality among older children and adolescents. Arch Fam Med 2000;9:235–40.

Huberty JL et al. From good ideas to actions: A model-driven community collaborative to prevent childhood obesity. Prevent Med 2010;50:S36–43.

Janssen I et al. Overweight and obesity in Canadian adolescents and their associations with dietary habits and physical activity patterns. J Adolescent Health 2004;35:360–67.

Morrison JA et al. Metabolic syndrome in childhood predicts adult cardiovascular disease 25 years later: The Princeton lipid research clinics follow-up study. Pediatr 2007;120:340–45.

Nead KG et al. Overweight children and adolescents: A risk group for iron deficiency. Pediatrics. 2004;114:104–8.

Nestle M. Food marketing and childhood obesity — a matter of policy. NEJM 2006;354(24):2527–29.

Ode KL et al. Identification and treatment of metabolic complications in pediatric obesity. Rev Endocr Metab Disord 2009;10:167–88.

Olstad DL, McCargar L. Prevention of overweight and obesity in children under the age of 6 years. Appl Physiol Nutr Metab 2009;34(4):551–70.

Tremblay MS, Willms JD. Secular trends in the body mass index of Canadian children. CMAJ 2000; 163(11):1429–33.

Veerman JL et al. By how much would limiting TV food advertising reduce childhood obesity? Euro J Pub Health 2009;19(4):365–69.

Omega-3 Fatty Acids

Gebauer SK et al. N-3 fatty acid dietary recommendations and food sources to achieve essentiality and cardiovascular benefits. Am J Clin Nutr 2006;83:1526S–35S.

Heird WC, Lapillonne A. The role of essential fatty acids in development. Ann Rev Nutr 2005;25: 549–71.

Position of the American Dietetic Association and Dietitians of Canada: Dietary fatty acids. JADA 2007 Dec;107(12):2151.

Oddy WH et al. Ratio of omega-6 to omega-3 fatty acids and childhood asthma. JU Asthma 2004;41:319–26.

Prebiotics and Probiotics

Bausserman M, Michail S. The use of lactobacillus gg in irritable bowel syndrome in children: A double-blind randomized control trial. J Pediatr 2005;147:197–201.

Kalantzopoulos G. Fermented products with probiotic qualities. Anaerob 1997;3:185–90.

Savino F et al. Lactobacillus reuteri (American Type Culture Collection Strain 55730) versus simethicone in the treatment of infantile colic: Prospective randomized study. Pediatrics 2007;119:e124–130.

Neu J. Probiotics: Protecting the intestinal ecosystem? Edit J Pediatr 2005147:143–46.

Saavedra JM. Use of probiotics in pediatrics: Rationale, mechanisms of action, and practical aspects. Nutr Clin Pract; 2007;22:351–65.

Schneeman BO. Fiber, inulin and oligofructos: Similarities and differences. Journal of Nutrition 1999:129:1424S–27S.

Shafai T. Routine supplement of prebiotics and probiotics to newborn infants is not recommended. Pediatrics 2009;123(3):e543–44.

Salt

He FJ, MacGregor GA. Importance of salt in determining blood pressure in children — meta-analysis of controlled trials. Hypertension 2006;48:1–9.

Vegetarian

Messina V et al. A new food guide for North American vegetarians. Can J Diet Prac Res 2003;64(2):82–86.

Position of the American Dietetic Association: Vegetarian diets. JADA 2009; 109:1266–82.

Position of the American Dietetic Association and Dietitians of Canada: Vegetarian diets. Can J Diet Prac Res 2003 64:62–81.

Vitamin D

Maalouf J et al. Short- and long-term safety of weekly high-dose vitamin D_3 supplementation in school children. 2008;93:2693–701.

Gordon CM et al. Prevalence of vitamin D deficiency among healthy infants and toddlers. Arch Pediatr Adolesc Med 2008;162:505–12.

Index